Hemodynamics and Hemodynamic Monitoring

Edited by Nissar Shaikh

Published in London, United Kingdom

Hemodynamics and Hemodynamic Monitoring
http://dx.doi.org/10.5772/intechopen.1008598
Edited by Nissar Shaikh

Contributors
Aanchal Kapoor, Abdelrahman Balal, Abdulmalik Jaber, Alaaeldin Ahmed, Ali Msheik, Ali Sulaiman, Arshad H. Chanda, Ashok Kandasamy, Asreena Arayilakath Pattuvathil, Azha Fatima, Bakri Alali, Bhavya Naithani Dube, Fateen Shareef, Fathimath Shajahan, Hamza Bin Saleem, Hassam Zulfiqar, Henning Bay Nielsen, Jawdat Alali, M. Abdul Wasay, Mahmoud Tabouni, Malek Abusannuga, Maliha Khalid, Mallikarjun Dube, Manal Faisal Alsharafi, Mariyam Fatima, Mohammad Hemadneh, Mohammad Mateenuddin Quadri, Mojahid Mohammed Khaled Alhussein, Moza Almohannadi, Muhammad Khalid, Neeraj Kumar, Nissar Shaikh, Omar Shihadeh, Roaa Naser Suleiman, Roshan Afsha, Salma Mehjabeen, Sana Saleem, Sara Abdulla, Seema Nahid, Shajahan Idayathulla, Umm E. Amara, Umme Nashrah, Usama Bin Saleem, Yilin Zhang, Yun Xie, Zakria Attique

First published in London, United Kingdom, 2026 by IntechOpen
IntechOpen is the global imprint of INTECHOPEN LIMITED, registered in England and Wales, registration number: 11086078, 167-169 Great Portland Street, London, W1W 5PF, United Kingdom

For EU product safety concerns: IN TECH d.o.o., Prolaz Marije Krucifikse Kozulić 3, 51000 Rijeka, Croatia, info@intechopen.com or visit our website at intechopen.com.

British Library Cataloguing-in-Publication Data
A catalogue record for this book is available from the British Library

Hemodynamics and Hemodynamic Monitoring
Edited by Nissar Shaikh
p. cm.
Print ISBN 978-1-83635-532-8
Online ISBN 978-1-83635-531-1
eBook (PDF) ISBN 978-1-83635-533-5

If disposing of this product, please recycle the paper responsibly.

Meet the editor

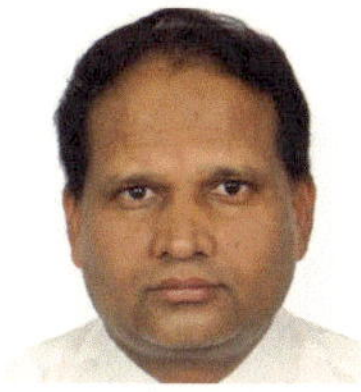

Dr. Nissar Shaikh (Shaikh Nissaruddin Maheboob), MBBS, MD, EDIC, DiD, FCCM, is a senior intensivist at Hamad Medical Corporation and is affiliated with Weill Cornell Medical College in Doha, Qatar, as well as Qatar University. He is an Associate Professor at the College of Medicine at Qatar University and an Assistant Professor at Weill Cornell Medical College in Doha, Qatar. He has published 10 medical/intensive care books, 250 peer-reviewed medical publications, and 50 book chapters. He has presented extensively at national and international conferences and has been invited to deliver lectures. He is a recipient of the Star of Excellence and other awards at Hamad Medical Corporation.

Contents

Preface **IX**

Chapter 1 **1**
Advanced Hemodynamic Monitoring: Pros, Cons, and the Future
by Malek Abusannuga, Zakria Attique, Sara Abdulla, Hassam Zulfiqar, Moza Almohannadi and Fathimath Shajahan

Chapter 2 **33**
Cerebral Hemodynamics
by Ali Msheik, Alaaeldin Ahmed, Omar Shihadeh and Ali Sulaiman

Chapter 3 **59**
Clinical Monitoring of Pediatric and Adolescent Patients Undergoing Continuous Renal Replacement Therapy (CRRT)
by Mohammad Mateenuddin Quadri, Bakri Alali and Nissar Shaikh

Chapter 4 **81**
Hemodynamic Challenges in Critically Ill Patients with Cirrhosis
by Aanchal Kapoor

Chapter 5 **97**
Maintaining Peripheral Circulation in the Surgical Patient: A Narrative Review of the Importance of Near-Infrared Spectroscopy
by Henning Bay Nielsen

Chapter 6 **121**
Methodological Issues and Safety Considerations in Enhancing Exercise Performance through Ischemic Preconditioning
by Yilin Zhang and Yun Xie

Chapter 7 **145**
Hemodynamic Stability during Spinal Anesthesia
by Maliha Khalid and Muhammad Khalid

Chapter 8 159
Minimally Invasive Cardiac Output Monitoring Devices: Principles, Applications, and Limitations
by Bhavya Naithani Dube, Mallikarjun Dube and Neeraj Kumar

Chapter 9 185
POCUS (Point of Care Ultrasound): Hemodynamic Monitoring of Future
by Arshad H. Chanda, Shajahan Idayathulla, Hassam Zulfiqar, Mariyam Fatima, Abdelrahman Balal and Mojahid Mohammed Khaled Alhussein

Chapter 10 201
Perioperative Hemodynamic Monitoring: Ensuring Stability and Improving Outcomes
by Sana Saleem, Asreena Arayilakath Pattuvathil, Hamza Bin Saleem, Usama Bin Saleem, Roaa Naser Suleiman and Manal Faisal Alsharafi

Chapter 11 213
Pulmonary Artery Catheter: The Golden Way of Advanced Hemodynamic Monitoring
by Jawdat Alali, Mahmoud Tabouni, Abdulmalik Jaber and Mohammad Hemadneh

Chapter 12 227
Non-Invasive Cardiac Output Monitoring in Perioperative Medicine
by Ashok Kandasamy

Chapter 13 245
Hemodynamic and Monitoring in Pregnancy
by Seema Nahid, Fateen Shareef, Umm E. Amara, Salma Mehjabeen, Umme Nashrah, Roshan Afsha, M. Abdul Wasay and Azha Fatima

Preface

Hemodynamics refers to the circulation of blood within the body, and hemodynamic monitoring involves assessing and continuously monitoring preload, cardiac contractility, afterload, and oxygen delivery and consumption. Since its discovery in the seventeenth century, hemodynamic monitoring has undergone exponential development. This book takes the reader from the historical foundations and gold standards of hemodynamic monitoring to both traditional methods and recent advances in hemodynamics and hemodynamic monitoring.

This book describes various aspects of hemodynamic monitoring across different patient groups, using simple, clear, and understandable language, supported by flowcharts and diagrams. It covers a wide range of topics, from the physiological hemodynamic changes of pregnancy to the pathological hemodynamic alterations seen in critically ill patients. In addition, the book explores the unique organ hemodynamics in the brain and the disturbances in hemodynamics associated with multiple organ dysfunction. Written by experts in their respective fields, the book transforms a complex subject into an engaging and accessible narrative.

I am thankful to all the authors for their hard work in writing the up-to-date chapters. The authors and I would also like to express our gratitude to Miss Maja from IntechOpen for her thorough reviews and prompt, sincere communications that led to the publication of this unique book. I am deeply in debt and thankful to my wife, Dr. Firdos, and my daughters, Dr. Amara and Dr. Jaza, for their invaluable advice and patience during the editing of this book.

Nissar Shaikh
Hamad Medical Corporation,
Weill Cornell Medical College in Doha-Qatar,
Qatar University,
Doha-Qatar

Chapter 1

Advanced Hemodynamic Monitoring: Pros, Cons, and the Future

Malek Abusannuga, Zakria Attique, Sara Abdulla, Hassam Zulfiqar, Moza Almohannadi and Fathimath Shajahan

Abstract

This chapter offers a comprehensive comparison of advanced hemodynamic monitoring methods by evaluating the well-established pulmonary artery catheter (PAC) alongside emerging semi-invasive and minimally invasive techniques. It outlines the evolution and clinical utility of PACs, emphasizing their role in managing critically ill patients with conditions such as acute myocardial infarction (MI), acute respiratory distress syndrome (ARDS), cardiogenic shock (CS), and those undergoing transplant evaluation. Although PACs provide accurate measurements of cardiac output (CO), pulmonary artery (PA) pressures, and mixed venous oxygen saturation, their diagnostic precision is counterbalanced by risks such as arrhythmias, infections, thromboembolic events, and potential data misinterpretation. Major clinical trials—including PAC-MAN, ESCAPE, VASST, and FACTT—demonstrate that despite their utility, the routine use of PACs does not consistently translate into enhanced survival outcomes across diverse patient populations. In contrast, less invasive approaches using pulse wave analysis, Doppler-based techniques, and thermodilution—employed in systems like PiCCO, VolumeView, LiDCO, FloTrac, ProAQT/PulsioFlex, Argos, and MostCare—offer benefits such as reduced procedural risks, real-time data acquisition, and easier usability, though they may encounter issues with calibration, signal dependency, and accuracy in hemodynamically unstable patients. Ultimately, while PACs remain crucial in select high-acuity scenarios, these innovative alternatives support a more individualized and safer approach to cardiovascular monitoring across a wide range of clinical settings.

Keywords: pulmonary artery catheter, invasive monitoring, minimally invasive monitoring, semi-invasive monitoring, pulse wave analysis, transpulmonary thermodilution, lithium dilution technique, Doppler-based monitoring

1. Introduction

Early anesthetic-related fatalities in the mid-nineteenth century due to chloroform administration drew attention to the necessity of precise hemodynamic monitoring, initially prioritizing respiratory observation but gradually highlighting the equal

IntechOpen

importance of cardiovascular assessment [1, 2]. While prominent figures like Dr. Joseph Lister and Dr. Edward Lawrie initially emphasized respiratory signs due to the late presentation of pulse failure, Dr. Joseph Clover's 1864 recommendation for continuous pulse evaluation represented an early recognition of how important cardiovascular monitoring is [3, 4].

Later in 1870, Adolph Fick introduced a method, now known as the Fick principle, for measuring cardiac output (CO) by comparing arterial and venous oxygen content, significantly advancing the quantification of cardiac function beyond clinical symptoms alone [5]. This concept, although not immediately implemented, set the stage for later advances. Similarly, the development of noninvasive monitoring technologies, initiated with Samuel von Basch's introduction of the sphygmograph in 1881 and expanded by Scipione Riva-Rocci's mercury sphygmomanometer in 1896, marked exponential progress in blood pressure measurement and hemodynamic monitoring [6]. Additionally, Dr. Robert Kirk's 1896 adaptation of the stethoscope for intraoperative auscultation further improved real-time assessment of cardiac performance [7]. Subsequently, influential clinicians like Dr. Charles K. Teter and Dr. Harvey Cushing advocated extensively for routine use of precordial auscultation and introduced systematic charting of intraoperative vital signs, effectively laying the foundation for contemporary methods of hemodynamic monitoring during anesthesia and critical care [1, 2, 8].

The First World War further influenced the evolution of these technologies through experiences in trauma management, particularly traumatic shock [9]. In 1929, Werner Forssmann notably performed the first human cardiac catheterization on himself, pioneering a new era of invasive cardiac monitoring despite controversy and criticism surrounding his unorthodox approach [10].

During World War II, the concept of the postoperative recovery room emerged alongside significant advancements in cardiac catheterization techniques [11]. Building upon earlier work, the 1940s saw Andre Cournand and Hilmert Ranges replicate Forssmann's catheterization method, leading to Cournand and Dickinson Richards estimating CO from venous and arterial blood oxygen content in 1942, work for which they, along with Forssmann, received the Nobel Prize in 1956 [5, 9, 12]. Alfred Blalock notably used catheterization to diagnose tetralogy of Fallot for the first time in 1944, spurring the development of pressure transducers, oxygen saturation monitoring, and dye-based intracardiac shunt assessments [5, 13].

In 1947, the Mayo Clinic established the first dedicated cardiac catheterization laboratory in the United States, facilitating the diagnosis of congenital heart defects and allowing precise measurements of cardiac pressures and oxygen levels. That same year, Lewis Dexter introduced a catheter-wedging technique into pulmonary artery branches, which Earl H. Wood used to demonstrate near-equivalence between pulmonary artery and left atrial pressures, though its time-intensive nature limited immediate clinical use [14, 15].

Subsequently, in 1949, Peterson and colleagues introduced clinically practical invasive arterial catheter placement using plastic catheters connected to capacitance manometers, permitting prolonged, comfortable monitoring and patient mobility [16]. Further refinements by Peirce and Seldinger, along with polytetrafluoroethylene's widespread adoption, improved percutaneous access and made invasive arterial pressure (AP) monitoring routine through enhanced transducer technologies and continuous flush systems, solidifying its clinical utility [2]. These advances were pivotal for perioperative and critical care, as they allowed for more precise monitoring and management of hemodynamic status in surgical patients.

In 1970, Swan and Ganz developed a balloon-tipped, flow-guided catheter method to measure pulmonary artery wedge pressure [17]. This innovation facilitated broader clinical application of the pulmonary artery catheter (PAC) in settings like operating rooms, intensive care units, and catheterization labs [18]. Over time, PAC evolved from a simple instrument providing intermittent CO readings and static pressures into an advanced monitoring device capable of continuous measurement of CO, cardiac chamber pressures, oxygen supply-demand balance, and pulmonary vascular resistance.

Given the significant advancements from intermittent measurements with the pulmonary artery catheter (PAC) to today's sophisticated continuous monitoring capabilities, it is essential to understand current methods of hemodynamic monitoring in greater depth. This chapter explores advanced hemodynamic monitoring techniques, analyzing their advantages and limitations and providing insights into future developments in the field.

2. Advanced monitoring: Pulmonary artery catheter

The pulmonary artery catheter (PAC), also known as a Swan-Ganz catheter, still plays an irreplaceable role for critically ill patients, despite its use gradually trending out. When measured with skill and interpreted by staff experienced in interpreting the data, hemodynamic monitoring reveals levels of precision unmatched as yet in anything but a few isolated clinical settings [19].

2.1 Clinical benefits and applications

2.1.1 Critical hemodynamic monitoring

Although noninvasive imaging modalities have advanced in recent years, some critical care situations still require hemodynamic assessment that only PACs can provide. These catheters enable doctors to measure blood pressure, cardiac output, and respiratory gases right at the bedside without any fluoroscopy. It is relatively easy to place a PAC, which means a patient does not have to be moved while their condition still has potential repercussions. In the long journey from an emergency room to surgery, placement time is precious. The catheter's bedside use significantly improved early management strategies for patients with acute MI or those who underwent high-risk operations. It also contributed a new means of identifying and treating mechanical complications like cardiogenic shock, papillary muscle rupture, and ventricular septal defects [20, 21].

2.2 Optimizing therapy in acute myocardial infarction

Numerous key clinical insights in myocardial infarction care were produced by bedside hemodynamic studies, especially those of the myocardial infarction research unit.

The optimal range of left heart filling pressure (pulmonary capillary wedge pressure (PCWP) 14–18 mmHg) was defined. Furosemide reduced preload pressures before diuresis.

Digitalis was shown to have potentially harmful effects in acute MI.

Vasodilator therapy with sodium nitroprusside greatly improved the outcome of patients who had acute mitral regurgitation. These findings made possible today's management of myocardial infarction (MI) [20, 21].

2.3 ARDS and fluid management

In non-cardiogenic conditions such as acute respiratory distress syndrome (ARDS), the use of pulmonary artery catheters (PACs) has been advocated to improve oxygenation through judicious volume management and inotropic support. Nonetheless, in some investigations, fluid resuscitation guided by PAC has led to untoward results, not because of the catheter itself but because of the inappropriate therapeutic strategies employed. This distinction is indicative that PACs are tools for the diagnosis and monitoring of conditions, not treatment implements of any sort; their advantages are entirely dependent on clinician skill and interpretation [20, 21].

2.3.1 Cardiogenic shock after MI

Accurate assessment of ventricular filling pressures helps tailor vasopressor and fluid therapy [20, 21].

2.3.2 Role in transplant evaluation and hemodynamic education

Heart and lung transplantation: Ascertaining transplant candidacy requires detailed hemodynamic profiling. Liver transplant: PACs help rule out porto-pulmonary hypertension. Beyond their clinical uses, PACs have also served as vital teaching tools. Their role in hemodynamic training has been foundational for generations of cardiovascular and critical care specialists [20, 21].

2.3.3 Outcomes in cardiac surgery

Clinical evidence supports the use of pulmonary artery catheters (PACs) in adult cardiac surgery, demonstrating significant benefits, including shorter hospital stays and reduced rates of cardiopulmonary complications, without increasing the risk of 30-day in-hospital mortality. These advantages suggest an overall net clinical benefit when PAC-guided management is applied appropriately in high-risk surgical populations. However, this approach is not without limitations, as it has been associated with increased infectious morbidity [20, 21].

2.3.4 PAC-guided therapy in cardiogenic shock

Recent registration data from one of the most extensive multicenter real-world patient cohorts in the acute mechanical cardiogenic shock (CS) and mechanical circulatory support (MCS) program highlight that PAC monitoring improves outcomes. Patients with complete hemodynamic data before MCS initiation had significantly better survival compared to those who had no PAC data or incomplete data. This survival advantage was particularly obvious for those most seriously ill (SCAI stages D and E). Incomplete data sets, on the other hand, did not offer any such advantage, which underscores the need for meticulous PAC use by experts when treating complex clinical conditions [20, 21].

2.3.5 PAC in abdominal aortic artery repair

The use of pulmonary artery catheters (PACs) is controversial in abdominal aortic reconstruction. A few case series have indicated better results with PAC monitoring, but the absence of control groups makes them less trustworthy. One historical retrospective showed less mortality, fewer hypotensive events, and fewer renal failures with an aggressive fluid protocol that included PAC use. Curiously, when prospectively studying two hospitals, the center with worse outcomes had higher use of PAC, leaving open questions regarding its value. In contrast, two randomized controlled trials comparing PAC with central venous catheters (CVCs) showed no significant benefit on patient outcomes [20, 21].

2.3.6 The application of PAC in neurosurgery

In the field of neurosurgery, there is a lack of evidence supporting the advantages of pulmonary artery (PA) catheterization. An uncontrolled case series, along with an observational study that included a comparison group, concentrated exclusively on the catheter's capacity to identify air embolisms, neglecting to assess clinical outcomes. Furthermore, an observational study that focused on pediatric patients with head trauma indicated that the use of PA catheters was associated with lower mortality rates compared to established norms for injuries of comparable severity. Nevertheless, the lack of internal controls and the simultaneous application of various interventions complicate the ability to directly link these outcomes to the use of PA catheterization.

2.3.7 Use of PAC in obstetric-gynecologic procedures

The evidence supporting the effectiveness of pulmonary artery (PA) catheterization in obstetric and gynecologic settings is minimal. Although it is frequently advised for severe preeclampsia and has been noted in case reports for various critical scenarios, there are no controlled outcome studies available. Some accounts emphasize its usefulness in uncommon obstetric situations, whereas others argue that it may be unnecessary, such as in cases of pregnancy-related myocardial infarction. Uncontrolled case series have investigated its application, but the absence of comparison groups hinders the ability to reach definitive conclusions [21].

2.3.8 Use of PAC in pediatric catheterization

In critically ill neonates, infants, and children, PA catheterization is utilized primarily for diagnostic purposes. However, the effect of this procedure on clinical outcomes is still uncertain, as current studies are restricted to uncontrolled case series that lack comparison groups or direct evaluation of outcomes [21].

2.4 Drawbacks and complications of the pulmonary artery catheter

Complications of central venous (CV) puncture*:* Arterial Puncture: Typically treated with external direct compression. If a dilator is inappropriately used, emergent operative or endovascular treatment is warranted. Arterial/venous hematoma, AV fistula, pseudo-aneurysm: May arise if vessels are damaged while attempting access. Thoracic duct injury: Maybe complicated by chylothorax or lymphatic fistula. Pneumothorax/hemothorax: Risk increases with repeated attempts or failure to use ultrasound. Thrombosis: From injury to the vessel and the presence of the catheter. Air embolism: Even a small amount can be fatal if it reaches systemic circulation.

2.4.1 Complications related to PAC (pulmonary artery catheter) insertion and use

Arrhythmias: Frequent during PAC placement (incidence 12.5–70%) [22–24]. Statistically most frequent: Premature ventricular contractions (PVCs) (52–68%). Non-sustained VT is also common; generally, it responds to repositioning of catheter, as previously indicated. Very rare arrhythmias may need intervention (<1%).

Mechanical complications: Rare (~0.9%) but can include valve or chordae injury, catheter knotting (especially in enlarged RV), and catheter entanglement with IVC filters, pacemakers, and other catheters. Risk reduction: Limit catheter insertion depth (<60 cm) or use fluoroscopy.

2.5 Venous embolism and thrombosis

Thrombus on PAC develops by 24 hours and becomes more pronounced by 72 hours. Inflating the balloon may result in endothelial damage. Mural thrombi in the SVC, RA, or the PA were present in >60% of PAC autopsies.

2.5.1 Infections

Infection rates: Bloodstream infections 1.3–2.3%. Risk of right-sided endocarditis (2.2–7.1%), and it is especially common in patients who have prosthetic valves.

Incorrect interpretation of pulmonary artery catheter (PAC)-derived information can cause misleading therapy and may harm the patient. Thorough understanding of PAC data acquisition and interpretation is essential to reduce any risks.

2.5.2 Equipment and data acquisition errors

Transducer leveling: Numerous technical errors of this kind. New generation pressure transducers need to be aligned at the phlebostatic axis and will calibrate automatically but require manual cross-check calibration. System responsiveness: There has to be a constant and incompressible fluid column in the pressure system. Signal dampening or loss can be due to air bubbles, debris, free connections, vessel wall impingement, or transducer failure. The following responsiveness tests are conducted: Flick test: If a flicked catheter results in a high-frequency waveform response, the catheter should be functioning at the time of placement. Flush test: Shortly after deployment, the device is flushed, which causes a steep incline and then decline and oscillation on the waveform.

2.5.3 Mistakes in the thermodilution method

Errors in timing, volume, or temperature of the injectate can affect cardiac output (CO) measurements. These problems are less frequent with newer CCO devices.

2.5.4 Catheter malposition

Catheter can become trapped in RV or injectate port in RA, especially in patients of smaller stature, leading to false hemodynamic readings.

2.5.5 Misconnection of lines

Distal PA and CVP waveforms may be interchanged if monitors are misconnected, and pressures cannot be read.

2.5.6 Factors affecting PAC data interpretation

Mixed venous oxygen saturation (SvO_2): Utility in evaluating the tissue oxygen supply and demand. Interpretation is affected by anemia, hemoglobin abnormalities, increased O_2 demand (e.g., sepsis, hypermetabolic states), and noncardiac shunts or metabolic blocks (e.g., cyanide poisoning).

2.5.7 Pulmonary capillary wedge pressure (PCWP)/PAOP

Demonstrates left arterial pressure and indirectly LV preload in the absence of mitral valve disease. Mechanical ventilation, particularly in the presence of PEEP, can elevate PCWP artificially. Best practice: Measure at end-exhalation; record the reading. If ventilation is good (e.g., HFOV), the PCWP is a less reliable measure: please follow trends or volume indices instead (EDVI, SI).

2.5.8 A right atrial pressure (CVP)

A right atrial pressure (CVP) usually estimates RV end-diastolic pressure based on healthy subjects (0–5 mmHg). Dependent on respiratory rhythm and volume (blood volume). Causes of elevated CVP: Biventricular heart failure. Regurgitation/stenosis of the tricuspid valve. Pulmonary hypertension. Pericardial constriction or tamponade. Volume overload. Pulmonary artery pressures can be elevated by high-flow states, left ventricular failure, mitral valve disease, or chronic pulmonary hypertension.

2.5.9 Infusion device effects

High-flow infusions through the PAC side port may artificially change pressure measurements. Patients′ data input errors: Using actual instead of ideal body weight in obese patients can skew indexed values like cardiac index (CI) and systemic vascular resistance index (SVRI), affecting management.

2.5.10 Pulmonary artery (PA) rupture

The most dreaded complication of PAC placement, although a rare one (incidence: 0.03–0.2%). Risk factors are age > 60 years, pulmonary hypertension, inadequate complete inflation of the balloon, or inappropriately placed catheter. Cardiopulmonary bypass. Anticoagulation therapy. PAC knotting: Rare but serious complication; occurs in ~0.03% of all PAC placements. The cause is pushing the catheter too deep into the heart, particularly the RV side. More prevalent in patients with endocardial catheter coiling. Ruptured balloon and disrupted PAC: Balloon rupture can occur with repeated inflation; early reports showed up to a 17% rupture rate. The structural failure of PACs is rare (~0.4% incidence). Causes are repeated inflations resulting in balloon cracks. Shear and intravascular retention during PAC extraction by the introducer. Size difference between PAC and introducer. Multiple PAC reinsertions that resulted in balloon damage. Nitrous oxide (N_2O) anesthesia: N_2O diffuses into the balloon, enlarges it, and can cause rupture or difficulties in manipulation. Complications: Fractured pieces of PAC can embolize in the pulmonary artery or in other locations. PAC mispositioning, migration, and entrapment: Perform reassessment on a daily basis; discontinue PAC when no longer indicated. The positions of the catheters are checked with chest

X-rays. Do not advance the PAC beyond the midline by more than 5 cm to prevent distal migration. Investigating the periphery may be associated with pulmonary infarction secondary to vascular occlusion from distal migration. Rare cases of PAC malposition: Into the brachiocephalic vein with perforation. Through septal defects (ASD, VSD) into LA, aorta, or carotids. PACs can be trapped in suture lines or by staples during cardiac surgery. Intrahepatic wedging of the PAC has been documented.

2.5.11 Venous thrombosis

The risk of thrombosis depends on the catheter site. Subclavian vein: 1.9%, internal jugular vein: 7.6%, femoral vein: 22%. Thrombus formation may develop as early as 24 hours after PAC placement. Balloon rupture and inflation may also facilitate thrombus. Autopsy studies show 61% of mural thrombi were in the SVC, RA, or PA. Eleven percent suffered pulmonary infarcts. PAC duration should be kept short in order to decrease the risk of thrombosis. The risk of life-threatening PE with PACs seems to be low.

2.5.12 Complications of heparin catheters

Introduced to reduce thrombotic events. Associated with the initiation or extension of heparin-induced thrombocytopenia (HIT), even at low doses of heparin.

2.5.13 Infusion syndromes

PACs rarely cause extravasation; introducer sheaths are more commonly involved. Causes include fibrin sheath formation, catheter defects, dislodgement, and vessel wall erosion. Risk factors: Body habitus and catheter misplacement. Consequences: Local tissue injury, therapy failure (e.g., ineffective vasopressors). High-risk medications: Chemotherapeutics, vasopressors, KCl, calcium, vancomycin, and promethazine. Compartment syndrome is possible after large-volume extravasations. Preventive measures: Radiographic confirmation of placement and ensuring free flow before infusion.

2.5.14 PAC contradistinction to other intravascular devices

PACs can get caught up in things like IVC filters, which can be surgically removed in some cases. Thus, fluoroscopy is to be employed in high-risk scenarios. Do not insert catheters deeper than 60 cm if no RV waveform is obtained to decrease the risk of knotting.

2.5.15 Other PAC-related complications

Reported issues: Retrograde coronary sinus perfusion. Cannulation of the intrathecal space. Wedging and occlusion of the hepatic vein. Hepatic vein placement occurs more frequently with femoral access.

2.6 Clinical trials and studies on pulmonary artery catheters

2.6.1 PAC in the critically ill patients: The PAC-MAN trial

The PAC-MAN trial, a large randomized controlled study conducted in the United Kingdom, sought to evaluate the clinical utility of pulmonary artery catheters (PACs) in the management of critically ill patients. In this trial, patients were randomly assigned to receive care either with the guidance of a PAC or without it. One of the primary endpoints assessed was hospital mortality. The results revealed a striking similarity in mortality rates between the two arms of the study. Specifically, mortality occurred in 68% of patients (346 out of 506) in the PAC group, compared to 66% (333 out of 507) in the control group; the difference did not reach statistical significance ($p = 0.39$). These findings indicate that the routine use of PACs does not confer a clear survival advantage in the general population of critically ill patients [25, 26].

2.6.2 PAC in cardiac surgery

The ESCAPE trial: The ESCAPE trial was randomized and had been conducted at 26 tertiary-care heart failure centers in the United States and Canada. The analysis included patients with symptomatic heart failure despite optimal standard therapies. Participants were randomly assigned to either therapy guided by clinical assessment alone (clinical assessment group) or therapy guided by both clinical assessment and PAC data (PAC group). The study shows that the use of PACs had no impact on the primary endpoint, which was defined as the number of days alive and out of the hospital. This pattern persisted in all demographic subgroups. There were no differences between groups in time to death or first hospital admission, overall mortality rates, or length of stay (LOS) in hospital. The median number of hospitalizations per patient was 2.0 for both groups [27].

2.6.3 PAC versus CVC to guide treatment of ARDS

FACTT trial: A randomized clinical trial was conducted in patients with acute lung injury to evaluate the potential risks and advantages of using a pulmonary artery catheter. The main outcome measured was mortality within 60 days following randomization or before the patient was discharged home. Main Outcomes: There was no significant difference in 60-day mortality between the PAC vs. CVC groups (27.4 vs. 26.3%, $P = 0.69$; absolute difference = 1.1%, 95% confidence interval – 4.4–6.6%). There was also no significant difference between the groups in ventilator-free days in the first 28 days. The CVC group had a modestly greater median increase in ICU-free days at 1 week. The number of days without organ failure did not differ significantly between groups. In the subgroup of patients presenting with shock at study entry, no significant differences were observed between groups regarding mortality or organ-failure-free days. Furthermore, no interaction was found between catheter type and the assigned fluid management strategy. In conclusion, CVP therapy failed to reduce mortality or organ function more than PAC-guided therapy. In addition, there was a higher incidence of complications using PAC. These results, cumulated with previous studies, do not support the routine use of PACs in acute lung injury [28].

3. Semi-invasive methods of hemodynamic monitoring

Semi-invasive hemodynamic monitoring encompasses techniques that offer continuous or advanced hemodynamic data with reduced invasiveness compared to traditional methods. These approaches typically require arterial or central venous access but avoid the need for more invasive procedures such as pulmonary artery or intracardiac catheterization [20, 21].

3.1 Classification of semi-invasive hemodynamic monitoring methods

3.1.1 Arterial pressure waveform analysis and indicator dilution techniques

These methods involve the injection of a thermal or chemical marker and detection of its dilution downstream, allowing calculation of cardiac output. Lithium dilution – LiDCO System, Transpulmonary Thermodilution – Utilized by PiCCO and VolumeView systems.

3.1.2 Doppler ultrasound-based monitoring

These technologies use Doppler ultrasound to measure blood flow velocities, from which stroke volume (SV) and cardiac output can be estimated. Esophageal Doppler Monitoring (EDM) and Transesophageal Echocardiography (TEE). Each of these techniques has specific strengths and weaknesses, which make them appropriate for particular clinical situations [20, 21].

3.1.3 Pulse wave analysis methods

A variety of commercially available hemodynamic monitoring systems utilize pulse pressure analysis to estimate cardiac output (CO) and related parameters. These systems rely on proprietary algorithms to analyze the arterial pressure (AP) waveform obtained from an arterial catheter. Depending on the design, some systems require external calibration using an indicator dilution method to establish a reference CO value, while others estimate CO without external calibration by analyzing features of the AP waveform in conjunction with biometric and demographic patient data. Based on their calibration approach, these systems can be categorized as follows [29]:

3.1.4 Externally calibrated systems

These systems require calibration with an external reference method, such as transpulmonary thermodilution or lithium dilution [29, 30]. PiCCO System – Pulsion Medical Systems, Germany. VolumeView System – Edwards Lifesciences, USA. LiDCOplus System – LiDCO Ltd., UK.

3.1.5 Internally calibrated systems

These devices use proprietary algorithms to internally adjust measurements based on patient-specific characteristics without external reference calibration [29, 30]. *FloTrac system – Edwards Lifesciences, ProAQT/PulsioFlex system – Pulsion Medical Systems, LiDCOrapid system – LiDCO Ltd., UK, Argos CO Monitor – Retia Medical, USA.*

3.1.6 Uncalibrated systems

These systems do not require any calibration and derive hemodynamic parameters solely from the arterial pressure waveform morphology [29, 30]. MostCare System – Vygon, France.

3.1.7 Minimally invasive, uncalibrated pulse wave analysis

Minimally invasive, uncalibrated pulse wave analysis techniques estimate cardiac output (CO) solely based on the morphological features of the arterial blood pressure (ABP) waveform, without the need for any external or internal calibration.

3.1.8 The MostCareUp system (Vygon, France)

The MostCareUp system (Vygon, France) is currently the only commercially available device in this category. It utilizes the Pressure Recording Analytical Method (PRAM), which continuously estimates cardiac output by analyzing both the systolic and diastolic components of the ABP waveform with a high sampling rate of 1000 Hz. Unlike other systems, PRAM does not require the input of patient-specific biometric data. Instead, it detects transient instabilities in the waveform—primarily resulting from backward-traveling reflected waves—and uses these to derive beat-to-beat estimations of arterial impedance, a key variable in calculating cardiac output. This high-resolution, real-time analysis allows the system to adapt effectively to sudden physiological changes, such as variations in heart rate, cardiac contractility, and vascular tone, thereby ensuring accurate and reliable CO estimation. Validation studies have demonstrated that cardiac output values obtained with the MostCareUp system correlate well with those derived from the gold standard pulmonary artery thermodilution technique, underscoring its clinical utility in both perioperative and critical care settings [29–31].

3.1.9 Advantages of the MostCare system

The MostCare system, based on the Pressure Recording Analytical Method (PRAM), offers a number of significant clinical and operational advantages, making it a valuable tool for advanced hemodynamic monitoring.

3.1.10 Minimally invasive approach

MostCare provides continuous cardiovascular monitoring using a standard arterial catheter, eliminating the need for more invasive procedures such as pulmonary artery catheterization. This enhances patient safety and comfort. *Real-time, beat-to-beat monitoring*: The system delivers continuous, beat-to-beat analysis of key hemodynamic parameters such as cardiac output (CO) and arterial impedance, enabling clinicians to make timely therapeutic adjustments based on dynamic cardiovascular changes. *High sensitivity to hemodynamic changes*: Utilizing a high-resolution sampling rate of 1000 Hz, the system can detect subtle fluctuations in hemodynamic status, including variations in heart rate, contractility, preload, afterload, and vascular tone. *Robust performance in unstable conditions*: The PRAM algorithm is designed to remain reliable even in rapidly changing clinical scenarios, such as during anesthesia induction, vasoactive drug administration, or acute cardiovascular events. *Dynamic electronic filter*: An exclusive patented dynamic filter automatically detects and corrects waveform artifacts, including resonance and damping abnormalities, thereby optimizing signal quality and measurement accuracy. *Device compatibility*: MostCare is compatible with any type of arterial catheter or pressure transducer commonly used in clinical practice, allowing for seamless integration into existing workflows without the need for proprietary disposables. *Exclusive parameter – Cardiac cycle efficiency (CCE)*: The system uniquely provides cardiac cycle efficiency (CCE)—a parameter that reflects the energy efficiency of the cardiovascular system. CCE offers insights into the patient's hemodynamic status and therapeutic response, making it particularly useful for tracking clinical progress. *Enhanced clinical decision-making*: The availability of continuous, precise, and dynamic hemodynamic data supports improved clinical decision-making in intensive care units, during cardiac surgery, and throughout perioperative management. *Minimal patient discomfort*: As the system utilizes existing arterial lines and requires no additional invasive devices or calibration, it minimizes patient discomfort and reduces procedural risks [29–31].

3.1.11 Limitations of the MostCare system

While the MostCare system offers several innovative features in minimally invasive hemodynamic monitoring, it is important to recognize its limitations to ensure appropriate interpretation and clinical application. *Dependence on high-quality arterial waveform*: The accuracy of the MostCare system is highly dependent on the fidelity of the arterial blood pressure (ABP) waveform. Inadequate signal quality due to underdamping, overdamping, poor catheter placement, or transducer issues can lead to erroneous cardiac output (CO) estimations. Special attention must be given to waveform validation before interpreting results [30]. *Reduced accuracy in hemodynamically unstable patients*: In clinical scenarios involving extreme arrhythmias, severe hypotension, or significant variations in vascular tone, the algorithm may not perform reliably, resulting in potential inaccuracies in CO and derived parameter estimations. *Challenges in certain patient populations*: The accuracy of pulse wave analysis may be compromised in individuals with peripheral vascular disease, obesity, or severe arterial stiffening (e.g., elderly patients), where high-fidelity arterial waveforms are difficult to obtain or interpret. *Limited validation in specific clinical settings*: Although several studies have validated MostCare's performance in perioperative and ICU settings, large-scale, multicenter trials assessing its impact on long-term outcomes and its utility across diverse clinical scenarios remain limited. *Interpretation requires clinical expertise: The system's advanced outputs,* such as beat-to-beat vascular impedance and cardiac cycle efficiency (CCE), require a strong understanding of hemodynamic physiology. Misinterpretation by inexperienced users or overreliance on numerical values without clinical context may lead to inappropriate interventions. *No external calibration*: Unlike externally calibrated systems (e.g., PiCCO or VolumeView), MostCare relies solely on waveform morphology. While this allows for ease of use, it may reduce accuracy in patients with rapidly changing cardiovascular conditions where external referencing could improve precision. *Cost and training requirements*: Initial system setup can be associated with considerable costs. Additionally, healthcare providers must undergo dedicated training to effectively operate the device and interpret its data outputs. Lack of familiarity may hinder optimal utilization. *Sensitivity to mechanical artifacts*: Movements, catheter whip, or incorrect leveling/zeroing of the pressure transducer can introduce artifacts into the waveform that affect real-time monitoring accuracy. While the dynamic filter helps mitigate these effects, complete elimination is not always guaranteed. *Limited data for pediatric and non-ICU use*: MostCare's validation and primary use have focused on adult intensive care and high-risk surgical patients. Its application in pediatric populations or outside the ICU (e.g., emergency departments or step-down units) is less well studied.

3.2 Minimally invasive, internally calibrated pulse wave analysis

This category of monitoring strikes a balance between accuracy and ease of use, making it suitable for a wide range of clinical settings, including the operating room and intensive care unit. Several commercially available systems employ this approach, including the FloTrac system (Edwards Lifesciences), the ProAQT/PulsioFlex system (Pulsion Medical Systems), the LiDCOrapid system (LiDCO Ltd., UK), and the Argos cardiac output monitor (Retia Medical, USA). These platforms offer continuous, real-time cardiac output monitoring with minimal invasiveness, enhancing clinical decision-making while reducing risks associated with more invasive methods.

3.2.1 The FloTrac system

The FloTrac system (Edwards Lifesciences, USA) is a minimally invasive, internally calibrated cardiac output monitoring platform that connects to any existing arterial line—typically radial or femoral—without requiring external calibration or additional catheterization.

3.2.2 System components

FloTrac sensor: Attaches to a standard arterial catheter. Monitoring platform: An advanced interface that displays hemodynamic parameters, including stroke volume (SV), cardiac output (CO), stroke volume variation (SVV), and systemic vascular resistance (SVR).

3.2.3 Update frequency

Hemodynamic variables, including cardiac output, are updated approximately every 20 seconds to 1 minute, providing near-continuous monitoring without the need for external calibration or bolus injections.

3.2.4 Clinical utility

The FloTrac system is particularly valuable in perioperative and critical care settings where continuous, real-time, and reliable cardiac output monitoring is required without increasing procedural invasiveness. Its ease of setup and integration with existing arterial lines make it a widely adopted tool in goal-directed therapy protocols. Advantages of the FloTrac monitoring system: *Minimally invasive approach*: Utilizes a standard arterial line (typically radial), avoiding the need for central venous or pulmonary artery catheterization. Reduces procedural complexity and patient risk associated with more invasive methods. *No external calibration required:* The FloTrac system performs internal calibration using patient demographic data and arterial waveform characteristics. Eliminates the need for external reference methods like thermodilution or lithium dilution, simplifying setup and reducing user dependency. *Continuous real-time monitoring:* Provides ongoing, beat-to-beat measurements of cardiac output (CO), stroke volume (SV), and stroke volume variation (SVV). Enhances clinical responsiveness in rapidly changing hemodynamic situations, particularly in perioperative and critical care environments. *Ease of use and integration:* Features a user-friendly interface with seamless integration into existing patient monitoring systems. Designed for quick implementation and intuitive interpretation. *Automatic vascular tone adjustment:*

The algorithm dynamically adjusts for changes in vascular compliance and resistance using real-time waveform data and patient-specific variables. Enhances measurement accuracy without the need for manual recalibration. Limitations of the FloTrac monitoring system. *Reduced accuracy in extreme hemodynamic states:* The algorithm's performance can be compromised in patients with low systemic vascular resistance, such as those with sepsis or receiving vasopressors. Significant arrhythmias (e.g., atrial fibrillation) may disrupt the reliability of stroke volume and cardiac output calculations. *Reliance on population-based models:* FloTrac utilizes demographic and biometric data (age, gender, BSA) to estimate vascular compliance. These generalized assumptions may not reflect individual patient physiology, especially in those with atypical characteristics (e.g., obesity, cachexia, or structural heart disease). *Limited validation in specific clinical contexts:* Accuracy may be reduced in certain settings, including off-pump cardiac surgery, intra-abdominal hypertension, and patients on mechanical circulatory support (e.g., ECMO, LVAD). In these cases, altered arterial waveform morphology may invalidate the system's algorithmic assumptions. *Inappropriate as sole monitor in high-risk patients:* In critically unstable or complex surgical patients, more precise, externally calibrated hemodynamic monitoring methods (e.g., thermodilution) may be necessary for safe and effective management. *Cost considerations:* The initial cost of hardware and recurring costs of disposables and licensing may limit accessibility, especially in resource-constrained settings [29–33].

3.2.5 The ProAQT/PulsioFlex system

The ProAQT system, developed by Pulsion Medical Systems, is a minimally invasive, internally calibrated pulse wave analysis system used in conjunction with the PulsioFlex monitor. It offers real-time estimation of key hemodynamic parameters, including cardiac output (CO), stroke volume (SV), and dynamic indices such as stroke volume variation (SVV) and pulse pressure variation (PPV). System components: ProAQT sensor: Connects to an existing invasive arterial line (radial or femoral). PulsioFlex monitor: Displays and analyzes hemodynamic parameters in real-time. Core algorithm and principles: The ProAQT system estimates stroke volume (SV) using pulse contour analysis of the arterial pressure waveform. It analyzes the systolic portion of the waveform (area under the curve), pulse pressure and waveform morphology, and additional variables such as waveform slope and amplitude. The core physiological equation used is $CO = SV \times HR$. Where SV (stroke volume) is derived from waveform analysis. HR (heart rate) is obtained from the monitor or patient ECG.

3.2.6 Advantages of the ProAQT/PulsioFlex monitoring system

Minimally invasive: Requires only an existing arterial catheter (e.g., radial or femoral), avoiding the need for central venous access or pulmonary artery catheterization, thereby reducing procedural risk. *Internal calibration*: Utilizes advanced internal algorithms that automatically adjust cardiac output (CO) estimations based on patient-specific demographic and biometric data, as well as arterial pressure waveform analysis—eliminating the need for external calibration methods. *Optional manual calibration*: Offers the flexibility to manually enter reference cardiac output values (e.g., from thermodilution or echocardiography) to further enhance measurement accuracy when desired. *Continuous hemodynamic monitoring:* Provides real-time, beat-to-beat monitoring of key parameters, including cardiac output (CO), stroke volume (SV), stroke volume variation (SVV), pulse pressure variation (PPV), and systemic vascular resistance (SVR). This facilitates timely and informed clinical decision-making in both perioperative and critical care settings. *Dynamic fluid responsiveness assessment*: Enables goal-directed fluid therapy by continuously evaluating preload responsiveness using dynamic indices such as SVV and PPV—especially useful in mechanically ventilated patients. *User-friendly interface and monitor integration:* The PulsioFlex monitor features an intuitive graphical interface and is compatible with standard patient monitors, supporting seamless clinical workflow and ease of use. *Clinical versatility:* Suitable for a wide range of patients, from stable to moderately unstable, and adaptable for use in various settings, including operating rooms, intensive care units, and emergency care.

3.2.7 Limitations of the ProAQT/PulsioFlex monitoring system

Reduced accuracy in extreme hemodynamic states: The reliability of the system may be compromised in patients with severe vasodilation (e.g., septic shock), low cardiac output, or significant arterial waveform distortion. In such conditions, the underlying assumptions of pulse contour analysis may not hold true. *Dependence on high-quality arterial waveform:* Accurate monitoring depends on the integrity of the arterial pressure waveform. Signal artifacts, over- or underdamping, and catheter-related issues can significantly affect the precision of derived hemodynamic variables. *Susceptibility to cardiac arrhythmias:* Significant arrhythmias (e.g., atrial fibrillation) can impair the consistency of beat-to-beat stroke volume and cardiac output measurements, limiting the system's reliability in patients with irregular heart rhythms. *Use of generalized population-based models:* Internal calibration relies on demographic and biometric data referenced against large population datasets. This may introduce inaccuracies in patients whose physiology deviates from these norms (e.g., extremes of age, body size, or unique pathologies). *Lower accuracy compared to calibrated systems:* While convenient and less invasive, ProAQT is generally considered less precise than externally calibrated methods (e.g., transpulmonary thermodilution with PiCCO) in critically ill or hemodynamically unstable patients [29–33].

3.2.8 The Argos cardiac output monitor: Core technology and principle

The Argos monitor uses multi-beat analysis (MBA)—a proprietary algorithm that estimates stroke volume (SV) by analyzing the radial arterial blood pressure waveform over multiple cardiac cycles, rather than relying solely on a single-beat analysis. This approach helps mitigate the effects of waveform artifacts, transient noise, and reflected pulse waves that often compromise the accuracy of conventional single-beat algorithms. Waveform Processing: MBA identifies the pure exponential decay of the arterial pressure waveform by excluding confounding wave reflections from peripheral vasculature. Stroke volume estimation: SV is derived using a proprietary formula that incorporates biometric inputs (e.g., age, sex, height, weight) along with the cleaned, multi-beat waveform data. Cardiac Output Calculation: As with other systems, CO is calculated using the formula $CO = SV \times HR$. This real-time analysis provides beat-to-beat estimates and enhances monitoring precision without requiring external calibration [29–33].

3.2.9 Advantages over traditional systems

The multi-beat analysis algorithm demonstrates improved performance in challenging conditions such as arrhythmias, where traditional systems like FloTrac and

ProAQT often show reduced accuracy due to variability in the waveform between beats. By averaging and analyzing across multiple beats, Argos provides more stable and reliable measurements.

3.2.10 Limitations of the Argos cardiac output monitor

Limited validation data: Clinical validation studies for the Argos system are fewer in number compared to more established cardiac output monitoring technologies, particularly in diverse or high-risk patient populations. *Dependence on arterial line quality:* The accuracy of the monitor depends on a high-quality arterial waveform. Waveform artifacts, underdamping, or overdamping can negatively affect measurement reliability, requiring careful arterial line setup and maintenance. *Less familiarity among clinicians:* As a newer technology, the system may not be widely known among clinicians. This may result in a learning curve and could limit its adoption in some institutions due to lack of user experience or training. *Potential cost constraints: Limited availability:* The device may not be readily available in all regions or healthcare settings, restricting access to centers that have adopted or partnered with the manufacturer (**Table 1**).

3.3 Externally calibrated pulse wave analysis devices

Externally calibrated pulse wave analysis systems estimate cardiac output (CO) by combining arterial pressure waveform analysis with intermittent calibration using indicator dilution techniques such as transpulmonary thermodilution or lithium dilution.

These systems require *a central venous catheter for injecting the indicator* (e.g., cold saline or lithium). A dedicated arterial catheter (typically femoral or

Feature	FloTrac	ProAQT/PulsioFlex	Argos
Calibration	Internally calibrated	Internally calibrated (optional manual input)	Internally calibrated (multi-beat analysis)
Arterial Access	Requires arterial line (radial/femoral)	Requires arterial line	Requires arterial line
Core Algorithm	Stroke volume from pulse pressure variability and demographic data	Pulse contour analysis + patient-specific data	Multi-beat waveform analysis across multiple cycles
Strengths	Widely used, easy setup, automatic adjustments	Flexible with optional manual CO input, dynamic fluid responsiveness assessment	Improved accuracy in arrhythmias, reduces pulse wave reflection error
Limitations	Less accurate in vasodilation and arrhythmias	Accuracy reduced in extreme hemodynamic states or poor waveform quality	Limited validation, newer technology, less clinical familiarity
Ideal Use	Stable patients, general OR/ICU settings	Perioperative care, fluid management	Critically ill, arrhythmias, hemodynamically unstable patients

Table 1.
The above table compares three different internally calibrated pulse wave analysis devices developed by different manufacturers, highlighting their operating principle, strengths, limitations, and clinical applications.

axillary) to detect downstream changes in the indicator's temperature or concentration. The thermodilution-derived cardiac output is used to calibrate the pulse contour analysis algorithm, enabling accurate, continuous CO measurements over time. Two primary commercially available systems using this method include the *PiCCO Plus System (Pulsion Medical Systems) and the VolumeView System (Edwards Lifesciences)* [30, 32].

3.4 PiCCO plus monitor: Pulse index continuous cardiac output monitor

System overview: The PiCCO Plus monitor integrates real-time pulse contour analysis with intermittent calibration *via* transpulmonary thermodilution. This approach is less invasive than traditional pulmonary artery catheter-based thermodilution techniques, requiring only a central venous catheter and a thermistor-tipped arterial catheter.

3.4.1 Transpulmonary thermodilution process

A cold saline bolus is injected into a central vein (typically into the superior vena cava). The bolus mixes with the circulating blood and travels through the right heart, lungs, and left heart to a thermistor in a large artery (e.g., femoral). A thermodilution curve is generated by measuring the temperature changes over time. Cardiac output is calculated using the modified Stewart-Hamilton equation: $CO = V \times (Tb - Ti) \times K / \int \Delta T(t)dt$. This provides a calibrated baseline CO value that enhances the accuracy of continuous pulse wave-derived readings.

3.4.2 Pulse wave analysis (PWA) mechanism

The PiCCO Plus system applies a three-element Windkessel model, incorporating the characteristic impedance of the aorta, arterial compliance, and systemic vascular resistance (SVR).

The arterial pressure waveform, typically recorded from the femoral artery, is analyzed to estimate the central aortic waveform by compensating for pulse wave amplification, which results from pressure changes between the central and peripheral arterial systems. Calculate stroke volume (SV) by measuring the area under the systolic portion of the arterial pressure curve and dividing it by estimated aortic compliance. Arterial compliance is calculated *via* a proprietary algorithm during each thermodilution calibration. The system also accounts for real-time SVR changes through continuous analysis. Cardiac output is then continuously reassessed by analyzing the pressure waveform morphology and the first derivative of pressure over time (dP/dt). With each new thermodilution calibration, the monitor resets the PWA-derived CO to maintain long-term accuracy and correct for any measurement drift. Hemodynamic Parameters Measured by PiCCO: Cardiac Function Parameters: cardiac output (CO), cardiac index (CI), stroke volume (SV), stroke volume index (SVI), and heart rate (HR). Preload Parameters: Global End-Diastolic Volume (GEDV): Volume of blood in all four heart chambers at end-diastole; more accurate than CVP or PAOP. Global End-Diastolic Volume Index (GEDI): GEDV adjusted for body surface area. Intrathoracic Blood Volume (ITBV): Total blood volume in heart and lungs. Intrathoracic Blood Volume Index (ITBVI): ITBV adjusted for body surface area.

3.4.3 Lung water and permeability indicators

Extravascular lung water (EVLW): Fluid in lung tissue outside of pulmonary vasculature. Extravascular lung water index (EVLWI): EVLW normalized to body weight. Pulmonary vascular permeability index (PVPI): EVLW-to-pulmonary blood volume ratio; indicates alveolar-capillary barrier integrity. Extravascular lung water (EVLW) /Extravascular lung water index (EVLWI): EVLWI represents the fluid present in the interstitial and alveolar spaces of the lungs, which is the fluid present outside of the blood vessels but inside the lung tissue. Values above 10 mL/kg may indicate pulmonary edema, and increasing values might hint toward more severe edema.

3.4.4 Clinical significance of EVLWI

Diagnosis of pulmonary edema: Aids in differentiating the cardiogenic and non-cardiogenic causes of pulmonary edema, as well as in quantifying its severity and guiding treatment. Guiding fluid management: In patients with sepsis, ARDS, etc., EVLWI can aid in making decisions regarding fluid administration or cessation of fluids to avoid overload and monitoring ARDS. Advantages of PiCCO monitoring: Minimally invasive compared to PAC. Intermittent calibration enhances accuracy. Comprehensive hemodynamic assessment. Superior preload measurement. Evaluation of lung water and capillary leak. Dynamic parameters for fluid responsiveness. Real-time monitoring. Enhanced fluid management and goal-directed therapy. Effective in mechanically ventilated patients. Rapid setup and bedside use.

Limitations of PiCCO monitoring: Requires invasive arterial and central venous access. Limited accuracy in certain cardiac conditions such as severe tricuspid regurgitation, intracardiac shunts, and irregular heart rhythms, particularly atrial fibrillation, during pulse contour analysis.

These conditions may affect thermodilution curves or pulse waveform interpretation. Requires intermittent calibration. Not suitable for all patient populations, such as patients with large intracardiac shunts and patients with open-chest procedures or extreme anatomical alterations. Dependent on high-quality arterial waveform. Potential for misinterpretation. Thermodilution requires bolus injection; the calibration process involves repeated cold saline injections, which can be cumbersome during frequent recalibration, may introduce volume overload in sensitive patients, and requires coordination and operator skill for consistent results. Cost and availability.

3.4.5 VolumeView system (EV1000 platform)

Another prominent example of an externally calibrated pulse wave analysis device is the VolumeView system, developed by Edwards Lifesciences and integrated into the EV1000 monitoring platform. Like the PiCCO Plus system, it combines transpulmonary thermodilution calibration with continuous pulse contour analysis to monitor cardiac output (CO) and other advanced hemodynamic parameters. Calibration Method – Transpulmonary Thermodilution: *The system requires* a central venous catheter (CVC) for indicator (cold saline) injection and a VolumeView arterial catheter (typically placed in the femoral artery) with an integrated thermistor for temperature measurement. Cardiac output is calculated using the modified Stewart-Hamilton formula, based on the temperature change over time following indicator injection. This calibration ensures a reliable reference for continuous pulse contour analysis. *Pulse contour analysis*: Using the three-element Windkessel model, the VolumeView system analyzes aortic impedance, arterial compliance, and systemic vascular resistance. The system evaluates the shape and slope of the arterial pressure waveform, estimates central aortic pressure, and calculates real-time stroke volume and cardiac output. Between calibrations, the algorithm continuously updates measurements using changes in vascular tone and waveform dynamics. *It gives Unique Parameter – Global Ejection Fraction (GEF):* A distinctive feature of the VolumeView system is the measurement of Global Ejection Fraction (GEF), a volumetric index of left ventricular systolic function, calculated as GEF = (4 × Stroke Volume) /Global End-Diastolic Volume (GEDV). GEF offers valuable insight into myocardial contractility, especially in shock states or heart failure. The VolumeView system has shown clinical interchangeability with the PiCCO system in cardiac output monitoring, with studies suggesting superior accuracy in GEDV estimation. Its ability to deliver comprehensive and advanced hemodynamic insights makes it a powerful tool in critical care settings [31, 32].

3.4.6 Advantages

Minimally invasive. Can generate accurate CO estimates with peripheral vascular access. Central venous or pulmonary artery catheters are not required [34, 35]. Easy to use and calibrate. Can be safely used by nursing and medical staff to provide CO measurements in less than 10 minutes. Suitable for use in both conscious and unconscious patients [36]. The lithium dose needed for calibration is very small and was shown to have negligible clinical effects [37]. Unlikely to cause arrhythmias, which are seen with cold injectate needed for thermodilution CO monitoring. Allows for continuous monitoring. A single calibration can provide accurate real-time CO estimates for up to 8 hours [38].

3.4.7 Disadvantages

Contraindicated with lithium therapy. LiDCO is contraindicated in patients on lithium therapy (for psychiatric or other conditions) due to baseline interference and potential toxicity. Use in patients on lithium therapy will overestimate CO. Interference with non-depolarizing muscle relaxants. The quaternary ammonium residues of some non-depolarizing neuromuscular blockers can interfere with the lithium sensor [39]. May require recalibration and multiple measurements to improve precision. The pulse contour analysis algorithm may need frequent recalibration, especially after major clinical changes or therapeutic interventions [40]. Relies on pulse contour analysis. This makes its measurements inaccurate in conditions that compromise pulse contour integrity, such as aortic valve regurgitation, intra-aortic balloon pumps, highly dampened arterial lines, arrhythmias, and intra- or extra-cardiac shunts [39].

3.4.8 Esophageal Doppler

Esophageal Doppler uses a flexible Doppler probe, which is placed in the mid esophagus to measure the velocity of blood flowing in the thoracic aorta. The probe is typically kept at the level of the fifth to sixth thoracic vertebrae and may be kept in place for days to weeks in sedated patients [39]. The probe emits ultrasound waves (4 MHz continuous or 5 MHz pulsed waves), which are then reflected by the circulating red blood cells in the thoracic aorta. Blood flow velocity is then determined based on the reflected waves. The aorta is assumed to be cylindrical in shape, and thus the stroke volume is calculated based on the velocity-time integral (VTI) and cross-sectional area of the aorta (CSA). The CSA is estimated using nomograms given the patient's demographic data (age, weight, and height). The VTI is measured using the reflected Doppler waves, where the integral of the velocity of Doppler flow over time (dV/dt) is used to represent the "height" of the cylinder. Advantages: Allows for rapid, real-time measurements and is minimally invasive [41]. Good agreement with other techniques, including pulmonary catheter-based CO monitors [42]. Improved outcomes when used to guide fluid management [43]. Disadvantages: Operator dependent. Changes in the position of the probe may affect readings. Assumptions made about aortic cross-sectional area can introduce errors [44]. Not suitable in patients with esophageal pathology or those with distorted aortic anatomy. Continuous monitoring is difficult in awake patients.

4. Noninvasive cardiac output monitoring

Noninvasive cardiac output monitoring has emerged as a valuable tool in modern clinical practice, offering real-time hemodynamic assessment without the risks of invasive procedures. This section explores the principles, modalities, and clinical applications of noninvasive cardiac output monitoring, highlighting its advantages and limitations. At its core, all noninvasive cardiac output (CO) monitoring techniques rely on one fundamental principle:

4.1 Various modalities can be used to infer the stroke volume, including

Echocardiography: It estimates CO using two broad approaches: Doppler-based methods (flow velocity measurement)/volumetric methods (2D/3D chamber quantification).

4.2 Advantages

Real-time, widely validated, noninvasive, cheaper, can be used for point-of-care assessment, and offers the possibility to link the CO status to its causative factor, for example, hypovolemia, cardiac dysfunction, cardiac tamponade, acute cor pulmonale, and/or vasodilator circulation.

4.3 Limitations

Angle-dependent (errors if Doppler beam is >20° off-axis). Assumes circular LVOT (elliptical shape causes errors). Difficult in mechanically ventilated patients who lack suitable TTE windows. Any measurement error in the LVOTd will be squared; therefore, there might be a large error in SV calculation. Non-echocardiographic Doppler-based cardiac output measurement [45].

4.4 Ultrasound cardiac output monitor (USCOM)

4.4.1 Principle

USCOM is a noninvasive, transthoracic continuous-wave Doppler system that measures blood flow through either the aortic or pulmonary valve. The probe is placed on the suprasternal notch or left parasternal area to obtain blood flow velocity-time integrals (VTIs), which are combined with patient biometrics to estimate stroke volume and cardiac output.

4.4.2 Advantages of USCOM: Fully noninvasive, bedside application

Rapid setup and real-time output, requires no ionizing radiation or contrast. Useful in emergency, pediatric, and critical care settings. Provides trend monitoring of CO, SVR, and inotropy index.

4.4.3 Disadvantages of USCOM

Highly operator-dependent. Difficulty obtaining windows in obese or uncooperative patients. Accuracy relies on the assumed aortic/pulmonary valve diameter. Limited validation in complex hemodynamics (e.g., valve lesions, arrhythmias).

4.4.4 Carotid Doppler ultrasonography

Principle: Carotid Doppler evaluates flow velocity in the common carotid artery using a linear ultrasound probe [46]. By measuring the velocity-time integral (VTI) and estimating vessel diameter, one can estimate stroke volume and cardiac output trends, particularly in response to interventions (e.g., passive leg raises).

4.4.5 Advantages

Noninvasive, rapid, and widely available. Useful in low-resource or emergency settings and can be repeated for dynamic assessments (e.g., fluid responsiveness).

4.4.6 Disadvantages

Not a direct measure of cardiac output; reflects central blood flow trends. Assumes stable carotid artery diameter, which may not be true in elderly or diseased vessels; operator-dependent; poor reliability for absolute CO values; may be influenced by cerebrovascular disease or carotid stenosis.

4.5 Bioimpedance

Principle: The underlying principle of thoracic electrical bioimpedance (TEB) is that blood is a good electrical conductor due to its high electrolyte content, while other thoracic tissues (e.g., fat, muscle, lung) are relatively poor conductors [47, 48]. During systole, when the left ventricle ejects blood into the aorta, the volume and velocity of blood flow in the thorax increase, which transiently decreases thoracic electrical impedance. These cyclic impedance changes are detected and mathematically analyzed to estimate stroke volume and cardiac output.

4.5.1 Advantages

Totally noninvasive. Provides real-time, continuous data. Safe for all ages, including pediatrics. Useful in ambulatory or ward-based monitoring. Quick setup and easy to use with minimal training.

4.5.2 Limitations for this technique

Highly sensitive to motion (e.g., patient movement, ventilation). Small signal changes (ΔZ) are easily masked by electrical interference (e.g., electrocautery). Unreliable in obese patients, pleural effusions, or chest wall abnormalities. Inaccurate in arrhythmias or rapid hemodynamic shifts. Dependent on assumptions about thoracic anatomy and blood resistivity. Limited validation in critically ill or surgical patients. Better for trend monitoring than absolute cardiac output values. Cannot be used in patients with a pacemaker.

4.6 Bioreactance

Bioreactance is a noninvasive cardiac output monitoring technique that evolved from the limitations of thoracic electrical bioimpedance (TEB). While both rely on changes in thoracic electrical properties during the cardiac cycle, bioreactance focuses on phase shifts in electrical currents rather than amplitude changes, aiming for better signal stability, noise resistance, and clinical accuracy (**Table 2**).

Bioreactance was introduced to address these limitations by measuring phase shifts instead of relying on subtle amplitude changes, resulting in greater accuracy and consistency, particularly in critically ill or mechanically ventilated patients.

Unlike bioimpedance, bioreactance does not measure amplitude changes, making it less susceptible to noise and more stable for continuous monitoring.

4.6.1 Advantages of bioreactance

Greater signal-to-noise ratio. Less interference from motion, respiration, or electrocautery. Better correlation with thermodilution in clinical studies. Suitable for critically ill or perioperative patients. Used in devices like the noninvasive cardiac output monitor (NICOM).

4.6.2 Limitations of bioreactance

Still affected by thoracic abnormalities (e.g., pleural effusions, chest deformities). Algorithms are proprietary and not transparent. Accuracy in very low cardiac output states is debated and requires stable ECG and signal quality.

Challenge in bioimpedance	Resulting issue
Signal highly affected by movement, respiratory artifact, and electrosurgical noise	Reduced accuracy and reliability
Amplitude-based signal changes (ΔZ) are small and easily obscured	Difficult to interpret during surgery or critical illness
Variability in thoracic anatomy, obesity, and fluid shifts interferes with measurements	Inconsistent readings
Dependent on multiple assumptions and correction factors	Limited applicability in dynamic clinical conditions

Table 2.
Challenges in bioimpedance and their resulting issues.

4.7 End-tidal CO_2 monitoring

End-tidal carbon dioxide ($EtCO_2$) is the partial pressure of carbon dioxide measured at the end of exhalation and reflects the effectiveness of ventilation, pulmonary perfusion, and metabolism. Recent innovations have extended its application to continuous cardiac output (CO) monitoring in mechanically ventilated patients using the differential Fick principle. This method estimates pulmonary blood flow by analyzing changes in CO_2 elimination and $EtCO_2$ levels during controlled, cyclic alterations in ventilation—implemented *via* integrated ventilator software. Two systems, contracting and capnodynamics, utilize these principles to provide automated, breath-by-breath CO estimates without requiring additional equipment or invasive procedures. Advantages of this approach include its noninvasiveness, real-time output, and seamless integration into existing anesthesia or ICU platforms, making it particularly useful during surgery and critical care. However, the method is limited to patients under controlled ventilation and may be less accurate in severe lung pathology or during rapid metabolic shifts. Despite these limitations, studies have demonstrated acceptable accuracy compared to thermodilution, suggesting $EtCO_2$-based monitoring is a promising tool for routine intraoperative hemodynamic assessment [49].

5. Emerging role of artificial intelligence and machine learning in hemodynamic monitoring

Artificial intelligence (AI) and machine learning (ML) are increasingly transforming science and medicine in various ways. Hemodynamic monitoring is no exception; there have been many new AI-driven methods that tackle the risks and limitations associated with the established hemodynamic measurement tools [50]. A notable advancement is the HaemoSphere monitor by Edwards Lifesciences (CA, USA), which incorporates the Hypotension Prediction Index (HPI) [50, 51]. This ML-driven system analyzes real-time hemodynamic data to anticipate hypotensive events before they occur. Using a model built on arterial waveform characteristics, the HPI can predict a drop in blood pressure up to 5 minutes in advance, with index values ranging from 0 to 100—higher scores indicating greater risk. Several studies have validated the tool's accuracy in forecasting hypotension and demonstrated its effectiveness in reducing the incidence of intraoperative hypotensive episodes (78).

Smith and Wood observed that over half of the patients who experienced cardiac arrest had exhibited at least one abnormal vital sign, such as tachycardia, hypotension, temperature abnormalities, altered mental status, or reduced urine output, within 24 hours prior to the event [52]. Building on this insight, SL Hyland and colleagues developed CircEWS and CircEWS-lite, early warning systems designed to predict circulatory failure up to 8 hours in advance [53]. Using high-resolution ICU data, these systems generate a continuously updating risk score every 5 minutes. In validation tests, the model demonstrated 90% accuracy, with 82% of cases predicted more than 2 hours before onset. To reduce alert fatigue, the system includes a silencing feature that suppresses additional alarms for 30 minutes after one is triggered, and it resets after a patient stabilizes from a circulatory failure episode.

A range of AI models has been developed to support clinical decision-making in critical care, particularly for septic shock management. Jürgen Paetz applied artificial neural networks (ANNs) to generate clinical rules for septic shock patients, while Ross et al. combined ANNs with differential equations to model inflammation and septic shock [45, 54]. Other machine learning approaches have also been applied to predict sepsis-related mortality with varying success, including diagnostic systems using radial basis function networks and supervised growing neural gas models [45]. Collectively, these innovations highlight the growing potential of AI to enhance early risk identification and timely intervention in high-stakes clinical settings.

Similarly, the application of AI in ultrasound procedures has been explored in various studies. Shaikh and colleagues investigated how inexperienced critical care trainees performed CO measurements using point-of-care ultrasonography (POCUS), comparing traditional manual methods to an AI-assisted automated approach [55]. The AI-supported method provided immediate guidance for accurately measuring aortic outflow velocity. Their findings showed that while both manual and automated techniques correlated with expert measurements, the automated system delivered greater consistency, reduced variability, and more precise measurement ranges. Although both methods resulted in overestimated readings compared to expert evaluations, the AI-assisted technique demonstrated superior accuracy. Thus, incorporating AI into ultrasound procedures has the potential to enhance measurement precision and reliability in critical care settings, facilitating better assessment of patient hemodynamic responses to treatments.

6. Future directions in hemodynamic monitoring

The future of AI in hemodynamic monitoring includes promising advancements aimed at improving patient outcomes and clinical decision-making. Medical and scientific discoveries continue to advance rapidly, profoundly influencing the future of hemodynamic monitoring, particularly in shock management [56]. A key emerging direction is personalized monitoring, wherein AI algorithms are tailored to individual patient characteristics, allowing highly precise and dynamic assessments of hemodynamic status [57]. Innovations such as small, flexible, wearable sensors capable of noninvasively and continuously monitoring various physiological parameters are already available, transmitting data wirelessly to centralized computers or healthcare workers' mobile devices [58]. These advancements facilitate real-time adaptive monitoring, enabling swift clinical interventions based on immediate patient needs.

Another significant trend is the growing adoption of automated closed-loop control systems that leverage artificial intelligence [55]. Such systems can interpret real-time data and autonomously initiate appropriate therapeutic interventions, improving compliance with treatment protocols and swiftly adapting to changing clinical conditions. Future systems may utilize predictive models based on historical data from similar patient populations to automate personalized drug titration, thus advancing precision medicine in critical care. Additionally, echocardiography probes are expected to become increasingly compact, affordable, and widely accessible, enhancing point-of-care diagnostics. However, further research is necessary to establish the optimal integration and utilization of these novel technologies in critically ill populations before they become standard practice in intensive care units.

Finally, advanced signal processing represents a significant area for future development in hemodynamic monitoring [50]. By integrating sophisticated imaging modalities and innovative sensor technologies, advanced signal processing is expected to significantly enhance the accuracy, reliability, and interpretability of hemodynamic data. These techniques can refine the detection and analysis of subtle physiological signals, potentially allowing earlier recognition of hemodynamic instability or adverse events. Such improvements would facilitate proactive clinical interventions and support more precise, patient-centered management in critical care settings.

7. Challenges in implementation

Innovations in AI and ML have considerable potential to transform hemodynamic monitoring practices, yet their implementation faces many hurdles. Some of the main concerns are ensuring high quality, diversity, and representativeness of the datasets used to train ML models [59, 60]. Furthermore, biases, inaccuracies, and a lack of diversity within these datasets can limit the generalizability and equity of ML models' predictions [59, 61]. Thus, it potentially reduces their effectiveness in diverse patient populations. Additionally, due to the inherent complexity of current ML models, such as advanced neural networks, they often lack transparency, making them difficult to interpret, rendering clinicians hesitant to trust and adopt these tools [62, 63].

Regulatory and ethical challenges further complicate the integration of AI and ML into healthcare [62, 63]. Also, some technical barriers, such as interoperability issues and seamless data exchange among healthcare systems, can slow down the utilization of this technology. Additionally, regulatory frameworks require significant enhancement to manage data privacy, security, consent, and liability. Clinicians also face a paradigm shift from traditional diagnosis-based interventions to proactive decisions based on probabilistic predictions, which raises practical and ethical dilemmas, especially when intervention risks outweigh potential benefits.

Economic factors, validation requirements, and educational needs pose additional limitations [64]. The high development and commercial costs of AI tools, exemplified by premium-priced monitoring devices, restrict widespread adoption, especially in middle-income regions. Additionally, the dynamic and rapidly changing nature of hemodynamic parameters necessitates rigorous, real-time validation of AI algorithms across varied clinical settings. Addressing these multifaceted challenges through targeted research, clear guidelines, and clinician education will be critical for effectively leveraging AI in hemodynamic monitoring.

8. Conclusion

Hemodynamic monitoring has advanced tremendously since Adolph Fick's pioneering work in 1870, as well as the subsequent advances of Forssmann and Swan-Ganz. It has become a fundamental component of perioperative and critical care. Although existing practices continue to rely on invasive techniques, there is a growing fascination with advanced noninvasive methods such as echocardiography and bioimpedance devices. These technologies have been strengthened by recent breakthroughs in AI and ML, allowing for predictive capabilities such as the HPI and proactive therapeutic interventions. Despite technical advancements, some challenges persist, including alert fatigue, limited interpretability, high prices, data quality concerns, and the need for rigorous validation.

Looking forward, bridging present methodologies with future innovations demands overcoming significant but surmountable challenges. Advanced signal processing methods, wearable sensor integration, AI-driven tailored monitoring, closed-loop control systems, and improved echocardiography are all potential new developments that could revolutionize patient-centered care, real-time adaptive therapies, and patient-centered care. To achieve these advantages, though, problems with data diversity, interoperability, clinical education, ethical difficulties, and financial accessibility must be resolved. The successful integration of future developments ultimately hinges on the cooperation of technologists, physicians, and legislators, with a focus on uniform training, transparent AI systems, meticulous validation, and suitable regulatory control. The discipline of hemodynamic monitoring is well-positioned to move beyond reactive care to a future defined by proactive, individualized, and technologically empowered clinical practice by carefully managing these complications.

Author details

Malek Abusannuga[1*], Zakria Attique[1], Sara Abdulla[1,2], Hassam Zulfiqar[1], Moza Almohannadi[1] and Fathimath Shajahan[1]

1 Department of Anesthesia/ICU and perioperative Medicine, Hamad Medical Corporation, Qatar

2 Department of Global Health and Social Medicine, Harvard Medical School, USA

*Address all correspondence to: mabusannuga@hamad.qa

References

[1] Reich DL. The history of anesthesia and perioperative monitoring. In: Reich DL, Kahn RA, Mittnacht AJC, Leibowitz AB, Stone ME, Eisenkraft JB, editors. Monitoring in Anesthesia and Perioperative Care [Internet]. Cambridge: Cambridge University Press; 2011. pp. 1-8. Available from: https://www.cambridge.org/core/product/52275504F00BA99B986CB537319B3CB0

[2] Shiraboina M, Garre S, Chandrasekaran AC, Ayya SS, Gajagouni N, Shashikanth T, et al. Evolution of perioperative hemodynamic monitoring from the hand Oon pulse to hypotension prediction index. Anaesthesia and Critical Care Medicine Journal [Internet]. 2025;**10**(1). Available from: https://medwinpublishers.com/ACCMJ/evolution-of-perioperative-hemodynamic-monitoring-from-the-hand-oon-pulse-to-hypotension-prediction-index.pdf

[3] Pierce EC. MOnitoring instruments have significantly reduced anesthetic mishaps. Journal of Clinical Monitoring. 1988;**4**(2)

[4] Clover JT. On an apparatus for administering nitrous oxide gas and ether, singly or combined. British Medical Journal. 1876;**2**(811)

[5] Thakkar AB, Desai SP. Swan, Ganz, and their catheter: Its evolution over the past half century. Annals of Internal Medicine. 2018;**169**(9)

[6] Bouchez S, De Backer D, Fraipont V, Momeni M, Rex S, De Hert S. Perioperative hemodynamic monitoring techniques: A narrative review. Acta Anaesthesiologica Belgica [Internet]. 2024;**75**(2):125-138. Available from: http://www.actaanaesthesiologica.be/archive/volume-75/issue-2/reviews/perioperative-hemodynamic-monitoring-techniques-a-narrative-review/

[7] Kirk R. On auscultation of the heart during chloroform narcosis. British Medical Journal [Internet]. 1896;**2**(12-Dec-1876):1704-1706. Available from: https://www.ncbi.nlm.nih.gov/pmc/articles/PMC2511184/

[8] Sundararaman LV, Desai SP. The anesthesia Records of Harvey Cushing and Ernest Codman. Anesthesia & Analgesia [Internet]. 2018;**126**(1):322-329. Available from: http://www.ncbi.nlm.nih.gov/pubmed/29099433

[9] Bourassa MG. The history of cardiac catheterization. The Canadian Journal of Cardiology. 2005;**21**(12):1011-1014

[10] Wieling W, Jardine DL, De Lange FJ, Brignole M, Nielsen HB, Stewart J, et al. Cardiac output and vasodilation in the vasovagal response: An analysis of the classic papers. Heart Rhythm. 2016;**13**(3)

[11] Sousa CS. Contexto histórico da recuperação anestésica. Revista de Enfermagem UFPE on line [Internet]. 2018;**12**(4):1117-1121. Available from: https://periodicos.ufpe.br/revistas/index.php/revistaenfermagem/article/view/234869

[12] Cournand A, Ranges HA. Catheterization of the right auricle in man. Proceedings of the Society for Experimental Biology and Medicine. 1941;**46**(3)

[13] Nishimura RA, Carabello BA. Hemodynamics in the cardiac catheterization laboratory of the 21st century. Circulation [Internet]. 2012;**125**(17):2138-2150. Available

from: https://www.ahajournals.org/doi/10.1161/circulationaha.111.060319

[14] Dexter L, Haynes FW, Burwell CS, Eppinger EC, Sagerson RP, Evans JM. Studies of congenital heart disease. Ii. The pressure and oxygen content of blood in the right auricle, right ventricle, and pulmonary artery in control patients, with observations on the oxygen saturation and source of pulmonary "capillary" blood 1. Journal of Clinical Investigation [Internet]. 1947;**26**(3):554-560. Available from: http://www.jci.org/articles/view/101840

[15] Hellems HK, Haynes FW, Dexter L. Pulmonary capillary pressure in man. Journal of Applied Physiology. 1949;**2**(1):24-29. Available from: https://journals.physiology.org/doi/abs/10.1152/jappl.1949.2.1.24

[16] Peterson LH, Dripps RD, Risman GC. A method for recording the arterial pressure pulse and blood pressure in man. American Heart Journal [Internet]. 1949;**37**(5):771-782. Available from: https://www.sciencedirect.com/science/article/pii/0002870349901751

[17] Swan HJC, Ganz W, Forrester J, Marcus H, Diamond G, Chonette D. Catheterization of the heart in man with use of a flow-directed balloon-tipped catheter. New England Journal of Medicine [Internet]. 1970;**283**(9):447-451. Available from: https://www.nejm.org/doi/full/10.1056/NEJM197008272830902

[18] Monnet X, Teboul JL. Transpulmonary thermodilution: Advantages and limits. Critical Care. 2017;**21**

[19] De Backer D, Vincent JL. The pulmonary artery catheter: Is it still alive? Current Opinion in Critical Care. 2018;**24**

[20] Chatterjee K. The Swan-Ganz catheters: Past, present, and future. A viewpoint. Circulation. 2009;**119**(1). [Erratum appears in Circulation. 2009 Jun 2;119(21):e548]

[21] Roizen MF, Berger DL, Gabel RA, Gerson J, Mark JB, Parks RI, et al. Practice guidelines for pulmonary artery catheterization: An updated report by the American Society of Anesthesiologists Task Force on pulmonary artery catheterization. Anesthesiology. 2003;**99**

[22] Evans DC, Doraiswamy VA, Prosciak MP, Silviera M, Seamon MJ, Rodriguez Funes V, et al. Complications associated with pulmonary artery catheters: A comprehensive clinical review. Scandinavian Journal of Surgery. 2009;**98**

[23] Iberti TJ, Fischer EP, Leibowitz AB, Panacek EA, Silverstein JH, Albertson TE. A multicenter study of physicians' knowledge of the pulmonary artery catheter. JAMA: The Journal of the American Medical Association. 1990;**264**(22)

[24] Stawicki S, Prosciak M. The pulmonary artery catheter in 2008 - a (finally) maturing modality? International Journal of Critical Illness and Injury Science. 2017;**7**

[25] Harvey S, Harrison DA, Singer M, Ashcroft J, Jones CM, Elbourne D, et al. Assessment of the clinical effectiveness of pulmonary artery catheters in management of patients in intensive care (PAC-man): A randomised controlled trial. Lancet. 2005;**366**(9484)

[26] Schmitt M, Teodorescu HN, Jain A, Jain A, Jain S. Computational intelligence processing in medical diagnosis [internet]. Physica. 2013. 513 p. Available from: https://books.google.co.uk/books?id=cWrsCAAAQBAJ

[27] Shah MR, O'Connor CM, Sopko G, Hasselblad V, Califf RM, Stevenson LW. Evaluation study of congestive heart failure and pulmonary artery catheterization effectiveness (ESCAPE): Design and rationale. American Heart Journal. 2001;**141**(4)

[28] Wheeler AP et al. Pulmonary-artery versus central venous catheter to guide treatment of acute lung injury. New England Journal of Medicine. 2006;**354**(21):2213-2224

[29] Greiwe G, Peters V, Hapfelmeier A, Romagnoli S, Kubik M, Saugel B. Cardiac output estimation by multi-beat analysis of the radial arterial blood pressure waveform versus intermittent pulmonary artery thermodilution: A method comparison study in patients treated in the intensive care unit after off-pump coronary artery bypass surgery. Journal of Clinical Monitoring and Computing. 2020;**34**(4)

[30] Greiwe G, Luehsen K, Hapfelmeier A, Rogge D, Kubik M, Schulte-Uentrop L, et al. Cardiac output estimation by pulse wave analysis using the pressure recording analytical method and intermittent pulmonary artery thermodilution: A method comparison study after off-pump coronary artery bypass surgery. European Journal of Anaesthesiology. 2020;**37**(10)

[31] Saugel B, Kouz K, Scheeren TWL, Greiwe G, Hoppe P, Romagnoli S, et al. Cardiac output estimation using pulse wave analysis—Physiology, algorithms, and technologies: A narrative review. British Journal of Anaesthesia. 2021;**126**

[32] Chamos C, Vele L, Hamilton M, Cecconi M. Less invasive methods of advanced hemodynamic monitoring: Principles, devices, and their role in the perioperative hemodynamic optimization. Perioperative Medicine. 2013;**2**(1)

[33] Kouz K, Scheeren TWL, De Backer D, Saugel B. Pulse wave analysis to estimate cardiac output. Anesthesiology. 2021;**134**

[34] Jonas MM, Kelly FE, Linton RAF, Band DM, O'Brien TK, Linton NWF. A comparison of lithium dilution cardiac output measurements made using central and antecubital venous injejction of lithium chloride. Journal of Clinical Monitoring and Computing. 1999;**15**:7-8

[35] Cecconi M, Dawson D, Grounds RM, Rhodes A. Lithium dilution cardiac output measurement in the critically ill patient: Determination of precision of the technique. Intensive Care Medicine. 2009;**35**(3)

[36] Pearse RM, Ikram K, Barry J. Equipment review: An appraisal of the LiDCO™ plus method of measuring cardiac output. Critical Care. 2004;**8**

[37] Jonas MM, Linton RAF. The pharmacokinetics of intravenous lithium chloride in patients and normal volunteers. Journal of trace and microprobe. Techniques. 2001;**19**(2)

[38] Hamilton TT, Huber LM, Jessen ME. PulseCO: A less-invasive method to monitor cardiac output from arterial pressure after cardiac surgery. Annals of Thoracic Surgery. 2002

[39] Lee AJ, Cohn JH, Ranasinghe JS. Cardiac output assessed by invasive and minimally invasive techniques. Anesthesiology Research and Practice. 2011;**2011**

[40] Garcia-Rodriguez C, Pittman J, Cassell CH, Sum-Ping J, El-Moalem H, Young C, et al. Lithium dilution cardiac output measurement: A clinical assessment of central venous and peripheral venous indicator injection. Critical Care Medicine. 2002;**30**(10)

[41] Funk DJ, Moretti EW, Gan TJ. Minimally invasive cardiac output monitoring in the perioperative setting. Anesthesia and Analgesia. 2009;**108**(3)

[42] Dicorte CJ, Latham P, Greilich PE, Cooley MV, Grayburn PA, Jessen ME. Esophageal doppler monitor determinations of cardiac output and preload during cardiac operations. Annals of Thoracic Surgery. 2000;**69**(6)

[43] Sinclair S, James S, Singer M. Intraoperative intravascular volume optimisation and length of hospital stay after repair of proximal femoral fracture: Randomised controlled trial. British Medical Journal. 1997;**315**(7113)

[44] Monnet X, Chemla D, Osman D, Anguel N, Richard C, Pinsky MR, et al. Measuring aortic diameter improves accuracy of esophageal Doppler in assessing fluid responsiveness. Critical Care Medicine. 2007;**35**(2)

[45] Ross JJ, Mason DG, Paterson IG, Linkens DA, Edwards ND. Development of a Knowledge-Based Simulator for Haemodynamic Support of Septic Shock. IEE Colloquium Simulation in Medicine (Ref No1998/526) [Internet]; 1998. pp. 3/1-3/4. Available from: https://digital-library.theiet.org/doi/abs/10.1049/ic%3A19981093

[46] Suriani I, van Houte J, de Boer EC, van Knippenberg L, Manzari S, Mischi M, et al. Carotid Doppler ultrasound for noninvasive haemodynamic monitoring: A narrative review. Physiological Measurement. 2022;**43**

[47] Drummond KE, Murphy E. Minimally invasive cardiac output monitors. Continuing Education in Anaesthesia, Critical Care and Pain. 2012;**12**(1)

[48] Nelson MR, Stepanek J, Cevette M, Covalciuc M, Hurst RT, Tajik AJ. Noninvasive measurement of central vascular pressures with arterial tonometry: Clinical revival of the pulse pressure waveform? Mayo Clinic Proceedings. 2010;**85**

[49] Peyton PJ, Wallin M, Hallbäck M. New generation continuous cardiac output monitoring from carbon dioxide elimination. BMC Anesthesiology. 2019;**19**(1)

[50] Keller M, Magunia H, Rosenberger P, Koeppen M. Echocardiography as a tool to assess cardiac function in critical care—A review. Diagnostics [Internet]. 2023;**13**(5):839. Available from: https://www.mdpi.com/2075-4418/13/5/839

[51] Myatra SN, Jagiasi BG, Singh NP, Divatia JV. Role of artificial intelligence in haemodynamic monitoring. Indian Journal of Anaesthesia [Internet]. 2024;**68**(1):93-99. Available from: https://www.ncbi.nlm.nih.gov/pmc/articles/PMC10893816/

[52] Hatib F, Jian Z, Buddi S, Lee C, Settels J, Sibert K, et al. Machine-learning algorithm to predict hypotension based on high-fidelity arterial pressure waveform analysis. Anesthesiology [Internet]. 2018;**129**(4):663-674. DOI: 10.1097/ALN.0000000000002300

[53] Smith AF, Wood J. Can some in-hospital cardio-respiratory arrests be prevented? A prospective survey. Resuscitation. 1998;**37**(3)

[54] Hyland SL, Faltys M, Hüser M, Lyu X, Gumbsch T, Esteban C, et al. Early prediction of circulatory failure in the intensive care unit using machine learning. Nature Medicine [Internet]. 2020;26(3):364-373. Available from: files/5003/Hyland et al. - 2020 - Early prediction of circulatory failure in the int.pdf

[55] Shaikh F, Kenny JE, Awan O, Markovic D, Friedman O, He T, et al. Measuring the accuracy of cardiac output using POCUS: The introduction of artificial intelligence into routine care. Ultrasound Journal. 2022;**14**(1)

[56] Mercado P, Maizel J, Beyls C, Kontar L, Orde S, Huang S, et al. Reassessment of the accuracy of cardiac Doppler pulmonary artery pressure measurements in ventilated ICU patients: A simultaneous Doppler-catheterization study. Critical Care Medicine. 2019;**47**(1)

[57] Boisson M, Poignard ME, Pontier B, Mimoz O, Debaene B, Frasca D. Cardiac output monitoring with thermodilution pulse-contour analysis vs. non-invasive pulse-contour analysis. Anaesthesia. 2019;**74**(6)

[58] Vincent JL, Michard F, Saugel B. Intensive care medicine in 2050: Towards critical care without central lines. Intensive Care Medicine [Internet]. 2018;**44**(6):922-924. Available from: http://www.ncbi.nlm.nih.gov/pubmed/29777262

[59] Joosten A, Chirnoaga D, Van der Linden P, Barvais L, Alexander B, Duranteau J, et al. Automated closed-loop versus manually controlled norepinephrine infusion in patients undergoing intermediate- to high-risk abdominal surgery: A randomised controlled trial. British Journal of Anaesthesia. 2021;**126**(1)

[60] Chen JH, Asch SM. Machine learning and prediction in medicine - beyond the peak of inflated expectations. The New England Journal of Medicine [Internet]. 2017;376(26):2507-2509. Available from: files/5024/Chen and Asch - 2017 - Machine Learning and Prediction in Medicine - Beyo.pdf

[61] Gonzalez FA, Santonocito C, Lamas T, Costa P, Vieira SM, Ferreira HA, et al. Is artificial intelligence prepared for the 24-h shifts in the ICU? Anaesthesia Critical Care & Pain Medicine [Internet]. 2024;**43**(6):101431. Available from: http://www.ncbi.nlm.nih.gov/pubmed/39368631

[62] van de Sande D, van Genderen ME, Huiskens J, Gommers D, van Bommel J. Moving from bytes to bedside: A systematic review on the use of artificial intelligence in the intensive care unit. Intensive Care Medicine [Internet]. 2021;47(7):750-760. Available from: files/5034/van de Sande et al. - 2021 - Moving from bytes to bedside a systematic review.pdf

[63] Biesheuvel LA, Dongelmans DA, Elbers PWG. Artificial intelligence to advance acute and intensive care medicine. Current Opinion in Critical Care [Internet]. 2024;**30**(3):246-250. Available from: http://www.ncbi.nlm.nih.gov/pubmed/38525882

[64] Pinsky MR, Bedoya A, Bihorac A, CeliL,ChurpekM,Economou-ZavlanosNJ, et al. Use of artificial intelligence in critical care: Opportunities and obstacles. Critical Care [Internet]. 2024;28(1):113. Available from: files/5029/Pinsky et al. - 2024 - Use of artificial intelligence in critical care o.pdf

Chapter 2

Cerebral Hemodynamics

Ali Msheik, Alaaeldin Ahmed, Omar Shihadeh and Ali Sulaiman

Abstract

Cerebral hemodynamics encompasses the regulation of blood flow within the brain to sustain oxygen and nutrient delivery while maintaining intracranial homeostasis. This chapter offers a comprehensive review of the anatomical structures and physiological mechanisms involved, including the arterial and venous systems, the protective role of the blood-brain barrier, and the metabolic demands of neural tissue. The chapter details the relationships among cerebral perfusion, arterial pressure, vascular resistance, and intracranial pressure, emphasizing how they influence cerebral blood flow. Regulatory systems such as chemical, metabolic, neurogenic, myogenic, and endothelial pathways modulate perfusion to adapt to physiological variations. Clinical monitoring techniques, including pressure measurement, ultrasound-based flow assessment, near-infrared spectroscopy for oxygenation, advanced perfusion imaging, and extracellular fluid analysis, are discussed in the context of neurocritical care and surgery. The chapter explores the pathophysiological changes associated with various neurological disorders such as ischemic stroke, hemorrhagic stroke, traumatic brain injury, subarachnoid bleeding, brain tumors, fluid accumulation disorders, and global brain ischemia. Therapeutic strategies aimed at optimizing brain perfusion, controlling intracranial pressure, modulating respiratory gases, performing surgical decompression, administering neuroprotective agents, regulating body temperature, and applying emerging treatments are reviewed. The chapter concludes by examining new technologies, including artificial intelligence, wearable noninvasive monitors, advanced imaging techniques, computer-based modeling, and personalized medical approaches. Ethical considerations surrounding invasive monitoring, interindividual variability, resource limitations, informed consent, and the role of automated decision-support systems are also addressed.

Keywords: cerebrovascular circulation, intracranial pressure, cerebral blood flow, cerebrovascular disorders, brain ischemia, traumatic brain injury, subarachnoid hemorrhage, stroke, brain neoplasms, hydrocephalus, blood-brain barrier, autoregulation, perfusion imaging, oxygen consumption, carbon dioxide, critical care, neurologic monitoring, neuroimaging, artificial intelligence, ethical issues

1. Introduction

Cerebral hemodynamics is the dynamics of blood circulation in the brain—a phenomenon that is critical for supporting cellular function, intracranial homeostasis, and the supply of oxygen as well as necessary nutrients. While the brain represents only 2% of body weight, it utilizes about 20% of the body's oxygen supply, highlighting its heavy metabolic demand and utmost dependence on uninterrupted perfusion [1].

Learning about cerebral hemodynamics is not an intellectual curiosity only; it is of immense practical importance in broad clinical settings. From acute conditions such as traumatic brain injury (TBI) and ischemic stroke to chronic illnesses like hydrocephalus or neurodegenerative conditions, cerebral perfusion status fundamentally impacts outcomes [2, 3]. Within the context of surgery, especially neurosurgery and cardiovascular operations involving cardiopulmonary bypass, close monitoring and control of cerebral blood flow can help avoid perioperative brain damage [4]. Additionally, neurocritical care units depend greatly on dynamic measurements of cerebral hemodynamics for the purpose of directing resuscitation measures [4].

This chapter offers an in-depth overview of cerebral hemodynamics with emphasis placed on the physiological and anatomical underpinnings, the physiologic principles of cerebral blood flow, control mechanisms, and clinical monitoring methods. Furthermore, the chapter discusses pathophysiologic alterations in disease conditions, contemporary therapeutic approaches, and upcoming technologies. Particular attention is devoted to the incorporation of cerebral hemodynamic information in the management of the patient, as well as the ethical implications of advanced monitoring. With this multiple-perspectival approach, the chapter strives to provide readers with both depth of knowledge as well as breadth of applicability.

2. Anatomy and physiology of cerebral circulation

A complete knowledge of cerebral hemodynamics requires an appreciation of the complex vascular structure and physiological mechanisms that control cerebral perfusion. The brain's perfusing network maintains an ongoing supply of blood, optimized for the delivery of oxygen and nutrients as well as the clearance of carbon dioxide [5].

2.1 Arterial supply and circle of Willis

The arterial supply to the brain arises from two main systems: the anterior circulation *via* the internal carotid arteries (ICAs) and the posterior circulation *via* the vertebral arteries. The ICAs enter the cranial cavity through the carotid canals and give rise to several critical branches, including the ophthalmic, anterior choroidal, anterior cerebral (ACA), and middle cerebral arteries (MCA). The ACA courses medially to supply the frontal and parietal lobes, while the MCA runs laterally into the Sylvian fissure to irrigate the lateral cerebral cortex, including motor and sensory areas [2]. The vertebral arteries ascend through the cervical vertebrae and merge to form the basilar artery, which further branches into the posterior cerebral arteries (PCAs). The PCAs supply the occipital lobes, thalamus, and parts of the temporal lobe [3]. These arterial systems are interconnected by the Circle of Willis, an anastomotic ring that provides collateral circulation, reducing the risk of ischemia during vascular compromise (**Figure 1**) [4–6].

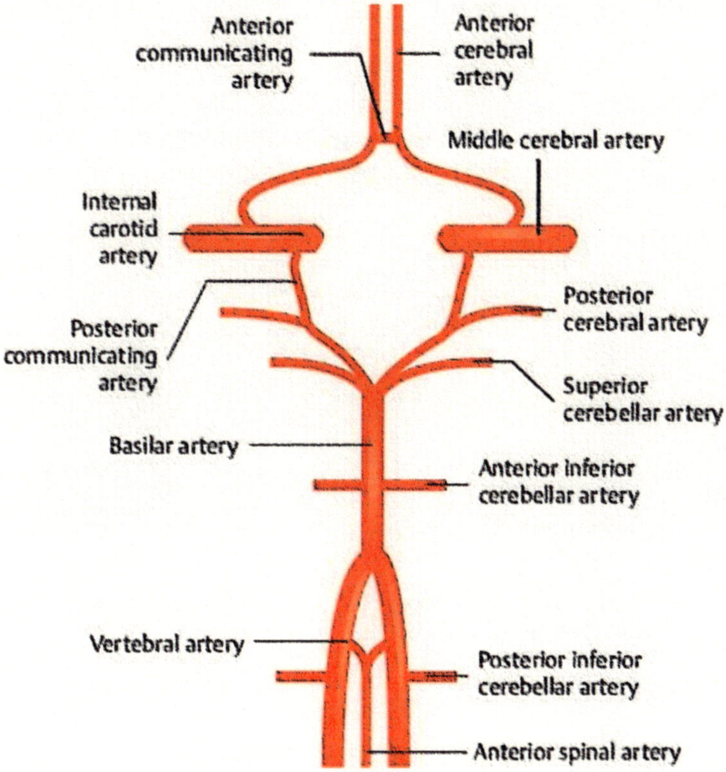

Figure 1.
Illustration of circle of Willis.

2.2 Venous drain

Venous drainage of the brain is divided into superficial and deep systems. The superficial system includes veins draining the cerebral cortex, such as the superior cerebral veins (into the superior sagittal sinus), the superficial middle cerebral vein, and the inferior cerebral veins. The deep venous system drains internal brain structures *via* the internal cerebral veins, basal veins of Rosenthal, and the great vein of Galen, which converge into the straight sinus [5]. These veins ultimately drain through the dural venous sinuses, a series of endothelial-lined channels within the dura mater. Key sinuses include the superior sagittal, straight, transverse, and sigmoid sinuses, which ultimately empty into the internal jugular veins (**Figure 2**). The cavernous sinus, with connections to facial and ophthalmic veins, is especially notable for its clinical implications in infection and thrombosis [6].

2.3 Microcirculation and exchange of capillaries

Capillaries are the primary site of gas, nutrients, and waste exchange between blood and neural tissue. Their density varies by brain region and reflects local metabolic demand. Capillary walls consist of endothelial cells with tight junctions, surrounded by astrocyte end-feet, forming the blood-brain barrier (BBB) [7].

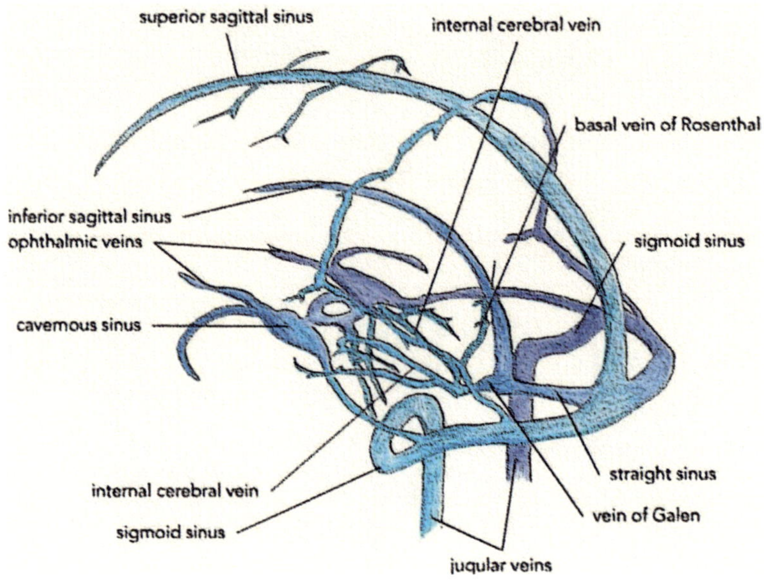

Figure 2.
Illustration of the anatomy of cerebral sinus and veins.

2.4 The blood-brain barrier (BBB)

The BBB is a permeable interface that blocks the free passage of potentially toxic materials from systemic circulation, with selective passage of necessary substances like glucose and amino acids for reaching the neuronal tissue. It consists of endothelial cell junctional tightness, basement membrane, astrocytic processes, and pericytes. The BBB is responsible for maintaining ionic equilibrium as well as protection from neurotoxins, but its function can be disrupted in the context of trauma, ischemia, infection, or malignancy, resulting in cerebral edema with raised intracranial pressure [7].

2.5 Metabolic needs and cerebral oxygen consumption

The large requirement for power of the brain makes an uninterrupted, strong blood supply necessary. Cerebral metabolic rate for oxygen ($CMRO_2$) is 3.5 mL/100 g/min, and cerebral blood flow (CBF) is tightly regulated with respect to metabolic requirements. The gray matter is perfused more than the white matter as a consequence of greater synaptic activity and density. Neurovascular coupling is such that a local rise in the activity of the neurons causes a corresponding rise in local blood flow. Abnormalities in the coupling are involved in many neurological conditions [1–3, 7].

3. Principles of cerebral hemodynamics

Cerebral hemodynamics is governed by the complex interplay among cerebral perfusion pressure (CPP), intracranial pressure (ICP), cerebrovascular resistance (CVR), blood viscosity, and vessel diameter. Knowledge of these fundamental concepts is necessary for the interpretation of blood flow alterations as well as for the formulation of appropriate therapeutic measures.

DOI: http://dx.doi.org/10.5772/intechopen.1011392

3.1 Cerebral perfusion pressure (CPP)

Cerebral perfusion pressure is the force that causes blood to perfuse the brain and can be conceived as the difference between mean arterial pressure (MAP) and intracranial pressure (ICP) [8]:

$$CCP = MAP - ICP \tag{1}$$

Under physiological conditions, CPP is regulated within the range of 60–80 mmHg. Below 60 mmHg, cerebral ischemia will ensue; above 80 mmHg, hyperemia will precipitate cerebral edema. Optimal management of CPP is key in the prevention of secondary brain injury in neurocritical care (**Figure 3**).

3.2 Cerebral blood flow (CBF) and cerebrovascular resistance

CBF is normally about 50 mL/100 g/min in adults but varies according to region and metabolic need (**Table 1**).

CBF is determined both by CPP and CVR according to Ohm's Law and the Hagen-Poiseuille equation [8].

$$CBF = CPP / CVR \tag{2}$$

Vessel diameter, length, and blood viscosity influence cerebrovascular resistance. The fourth-power relation of radius with respect to flow means that relatively small variations in vessel diameter have very large impacts on CBF. This concept is the

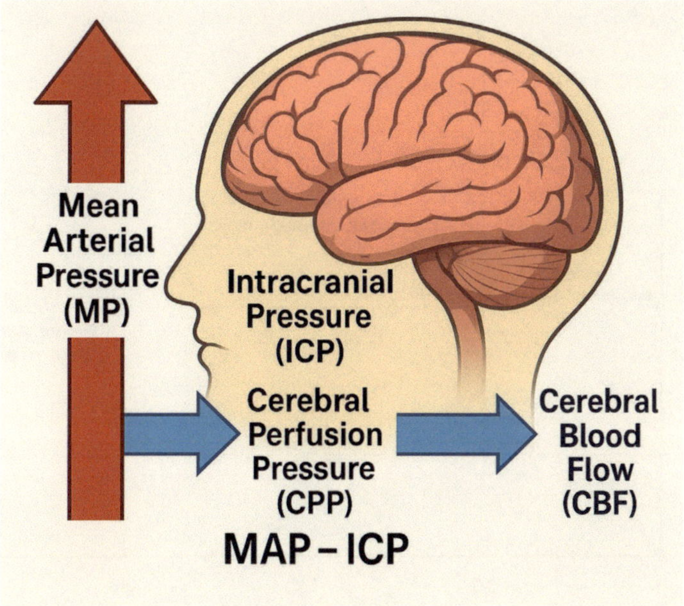

Figure 3.
Determinants of cerebral perfusion. MAP: Mean arterial pressure, ICP: Intracranial pressure, CPP: Cerebral perfusion pressure, CBF: Cerebral blood flow, CVR: Cerebrovascular resistance.

Parameter	Normal value	Description
Cerebral Blood Flow (CBF)	50 mL/100 g/min	Average perfusion to brain tissue
Cerebral metabolic rate of oxygenation ($CMRO_2$)	3.5 mL O_2/100 g/min	Oxygen consumption by neural tissue
Intracranial Pressure (ICP)	5–15 mmHg	Normal pressure within the cranial vault
Cerebral Perfusion Pressure (CPP)	60–80 mmHg	Net pressure gradient driving cerebral blood flow

Table 1.
Key cerebral hemodynamic parameters and their normal values.

foundation of physiological regulation of blood flow through vasodilation as well as vasoconstriction.

3.3 Intracranial pressure (ICP)

The pressure maintained within the cranial vault by cerebrospinal fluid (CSF), blood, and brain tissue is called ICP. ICP varies from 5 to 15 mmHg in normal adults. Any elevation of ICP may jeopardize CPP and cause ischemia of the cerebrum. Mass lesions, cerebral edema, hydrocephalus, and venous congestion are causes of increased ICP. Treatment of elevated ICP is an essential pillar of neurocritical care [8].

3.4 Autoregulation of blood flow

The brain is equipped with intrinsic mechanisms for relative constancy of CBF over a large range of MAP (usually 60–150 mmHg). Autoregulation is mediated through the capacity of cerebral blood vessels to constrict or dilate in reaction to alterations in pressure, maintaining perfusion constancy in the presence of systemic

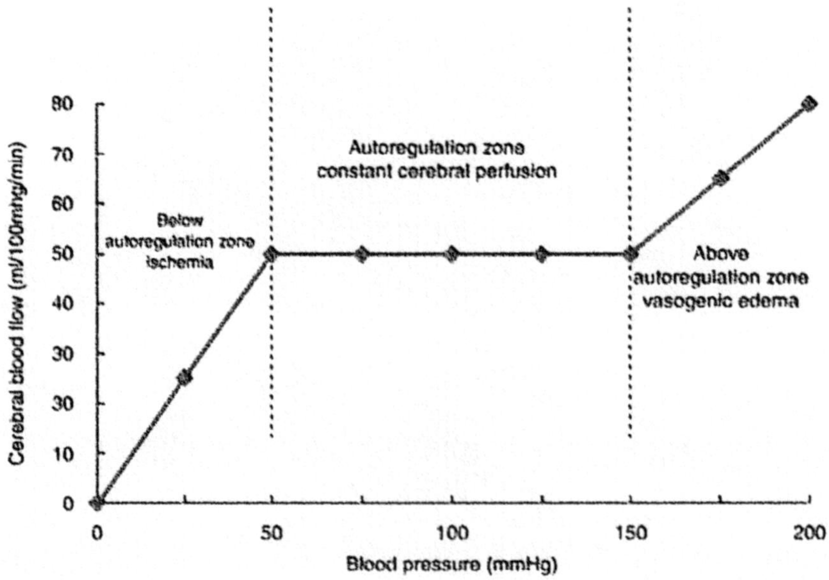

Figure 4.
Illustration of CBF autoregulation.

circulation variability. Autoregulation can be lost in TBI, stroke, as well as sepsis, leaving the brain susceptible to extremes of perfusion [9].

3.5 Blood viscosity and hematocrit

Hematocrit, temperature, as well as plasma composition affect blood viscosity, which in turn plays an ancillary role in brain hemodynamics. Although low hematocrit facilitates perfusion, it can impair oxygen delivery. Elevated hematocrit, on the other hand, causes increased viscosity and CVR that decrease CBF [8, 9]. This balance is important in the management of anemic or polycythemic patients.

3.6 Compliance and volume-pressure relationships

Compliance refers to the brain's ability to tolerate volume changes without significant increases in intracranial pressure (ICP). This compensatory buffer is lost in conditions like cerebral edema or space-occupying lesions [10]. The Monro-Kellie doctrine explains that the cranial vault has a fixed volume; thus, increases in brain tissue, blood, or cerebrospinal fluid (CSF) must be balanced by a decrease in another, or ICP will rise sharply. Understanding these dynamics is essential for diagnosing and managing intracranial hypertension (**Figure 4**).

4. Regulation of cerebral blood flow

Cerebral blood flow regulation is an intricate, dynamic process responsible for maintaining uniform perfusion in the presence of physiological variations in blood pressure, metabolic demand, and gas composition. Regulation of CBF is critical for the establishment of neural homeostasis as well as protection against ischemic or hemorrhagic damage [9–11].

4.1 Autoregulation of cerebral blood flow

Autoregulation is the inherent capacity of cerebral arteries for maintaining relatively stable CBF over an interval of mean arterial pressure (MAP), usually between 60 and 150 mmHg. The response is mediated mainly through vascular smooth muscle cells that react to variations in transmural pressure. With rising MAP, vessels constrict in order to decrease flow; with falling MAP, vessels dilate in order to restore flow [11].

Autoregulatory ability is heterogeneous from one brain region to another as well as being impaired in pathologic conditions like traumatic head injury, stroke, and sepsis. Autoregulatory loss makes CBF pressure-sensitive, with the potential for both an increased danger of hypoperfusion as well as hyperemia [10, 11].

4.2 Chemical control: CO_2 and O_2 reactivity

Cerebral blood vessels are very sensitive to variations in arterial partial pressure of carbon dioxide ($PaCO_2$). When $PaCO_2$ is increased (hypercapnia), vasodilation occurs, enhancing CBF, whereas when $PaCO_2$ is decreased (hypocapnia), vasoconstriction leads to decreased flow. The response is immediate as well as reversible and is the basis for therapeutic hyperventilation for the purpose of decreasing ICP in acute situations [7–10].

Response to oxygen (PaO_2) is weaker under conditions of normoxia. Critical hypoxia (PaO_2 < 50 mmHg) induces vasodilation in order to augment CBF. Hyperoxia is not directly associated with pronounced effects on CBF but can lead to oxidative stress.

Cerebral blood vessels are highly sensitive to fluctuations in arterial partial pressure of carbon dioxide ($PaCO_2$). Hypercapnia causes vasodilation and increases cerebral blood flow (CBF), whereas hypocapnia induces vasoconstriction, reducing CBF. These changes occur rapidly and are reversible, forming the physiological basis for therapeutic hyperventilation in acute intracranial hypertension [7–10].

The brain's response to oxygen (PaO_2) is less pronounced under normoxic conditions; however, critical hypoxia (PaO_2 < 50 mmHg) triggers vasodilation to enhance CBF. Hyperoxia, while not dramatically altering CBF, may induce oxidative stress and suppress metabolic activity.

Recent MRI-based studies have confirmed that oxygen availability directly influences cerebral metabolism and perfusion. Xu et al. demonstrated that hypoxia (14% inspired O_2) leads to a ~ 5% increase in $CMRO_2$ and a ~ 10% rise in CBF, as compensatory mechanisms attempt to preserve oxygen delivery [12]. In contrast, hyperoxia (FiO_2 50–98%) resulted in a 17% reduction in $CMRO_2$ with minimal changes in CBF. This paradoxical effect is attributed to oxygen-induced oxidative stress, which may inhibit mitochondrial metabolism and reduce neuronal activity. These findings have clinical implications: excessive oxygen supplementation, particularly in ischemic or traumatic brain injury, may depress cerebral metabolism and should be cautiously titrated [12].

4.3 Metabolic regulation

CBF is directly associated with the metabolic requirements of the neurons—a process termed metabolic or functional hyperemia. Any rise in activity of the neurons leads to the release of vasoactive metabolites, including adenosine, hydrogen ions, potassium, and nitric oxide, promoting vasodilation and increasing perfusion to the region [12].

The local regulation guarantees that areas of the brain that are being used receive comparatively increased blood supply, something used in functional neuroimaging methods like fMRI as well as PET.

4.4 Neurogenic control

Neurogenic control of cerebral circulation is conveyed through the autonomic nervous system as well as through neurotransmitters. While not as predominant as control from metabolism or chemicals, sympathetic stimulation tends generally to produce vasoconstriction, with particular emphasis in large proximal arteries, whereas parasympathetic tone yields a lesser vasodilatory action.

Neurogenic modulation is more pronounced in disease conditions like vasospasm and migraine, in which abnormal signaling in the neurons influences vascular tone.

4.5 Endothelial and myogenic mechanisms

Neurovascular coupling refers to the tight coordination between neuronal activity and local blood flow. When neurons become more active, they signal nearby blood vessels to dilate, increasing perfusion to match metabolic needs—a mechanism fundamental to both normal function and imaging techniques like fMRI. Endothelial cells of cerebral blood vessels are central in the regulation of vascular tone through the release of such substances as endothelin, prostacyclin, and nitric oxide (NO). NO is an important vasodilator with involvement in neurovascular coupling as well as autoregulation. Myogenic mechanisms react directly to mechanical stretch within the walls of blood vessels, adjusting smooth muscle contraction in order to provide uniform flow. These multifactorial mechanisms of regulation have an interactive synergy that fine-tunes perfusion in the brain. Abnormality in one or multiple pathways can predispose the brain toward ischemia, edema, or hemorrhagic complications based on the situation [13].

4.6 Integrated mechanisms and clinical assessment of autoregulation

Cerebral autoregulation refers to the brain's intrinsic ability to maintain relatively constant blood flow despite changes in cerebral perfusion pressure (CPP). This is achieved through a complex interplay of myogenic, metabolic, neurogenic, and endothelial mechanisms [11]. Myogenic responses involve vascular smooth muscle contraction in response to transmural pressure changes, while metabolic regulation is largely influenced by $PaCO_2$ and local metabolic byproducts. Neurogenic mechanisms rely on perivascular innervation and neurotransmitters like nitric oxide and serotonin, and endothelial cells release vasoactive agents such as endothelin-1 and nitric oxide. Importantly, autoregulation is frequency-sensitive—low-frequency blood pressure fluctuations (e.g., <0.4 Hz) are buffered, while higher frequencies may pass through unfiltered.

Clinically, autoregulation can be evaluated *via* dynamic techniques such as transcranial Doppler (TCD) or near-infrared spectroscopy (NIRS) by analyzing blood pressure and flow/oxygenation relationships. Techniques like pressure reactivity index (PRx), transfer function analysis, and wavelet coherence help identify individualized autoregulatory ranges. Emerging evidence suggests that deviations from a patient's personalized optimal CPP—defined by the CPP at which autoregulation is most preserved—are associated with worse outcomes in traumatic brain injury and subarachnoid hemorrhage [11]. These insights point toward a shift from static, one-size-fits-all targets to autoregulation-guided hemodynamic strategies.

5. Monitoring cerebral hemodynamics

Cerebral hemodynamic monitoring is an important foundation of contemporary neurocritical care, neurosurgery, and cerebrovascular disease management. Monitoring allows for real-time evaluation of intracranial dynamics, cerebral blood flow, and oxygenation, serving as an aid in directing intervention for maximizing outcomes as well as blocking secondary brain injury [14]. Both noninvasive and invasive methods are used, with particular indications, advantages, as well as limitations.

5.1 Invasive monitoring techniques

5.1.1 Intracranial pressure (ICP) monitoring

ICP monitoring provides continuous data on pressure within the cranial vault. It is most commonly used in patients with traumatic brain injury, hydrocephalus, or intracerebral hemorrhage. Devices include:

- External ventricular drain (EVD): Allows for both monitoring and CSF drainage. Gold standard for accuracy.

- Intraparenchymal monitors: Fiberoptic or strain gauge-based probes inserted into brain tissue, offering reliable pressure trends with minimal CSF drainage capability.

Monitoring ICP enables clinicians to calculate cerebral perfusion pressure (CPP) and respond to trends suggestive of cerebral edema, herniation risk, or impaired autoregulation [14].

5.2 Noninvasive monitoring techniques

5.2.1 Transcranial Doppler ultrasonography (TCD)

TCD is a bedside ultrasound technique used to assess blood flow velocity in major basal cerebral arteries, particularly the middle cerebral artery. It is valuable for:

- Detecting cerebral vasospasm (e.g., after subarachnoid hemorrhage)

- Assessing autoregulatory status

- Monitoring emboli or flow asymmetries.

TCD is operator-dependent and limited by skull thickness in some patients, but it remains an essential noninvasive tool [14].

5.2.2 Near-infrared spectroscopy (NIRS)

Near-Infrared Spectroscopy (NIRS) is a noninvasive method used to continuously monitor regional cerebral oxygen saturation (rSO_2), based on the differential absorption of near-infrared light (700–900 nm) by oxygenated and deoxygenated hemoglobin. Sensors placed over the forehead detect these changes, enabling real-time assessment of cerebral oxygenation, particularly in the superficial cortical regions [15]. NIRS utilizes light in the near-infrared spectrum to estimate regional cerebral oxygen saturation (rSO_2). Placed over the forehead, sensors detect changes in oxy- and deoxyhemoglobin concentrations. While NIRS offers continuous, noninvasive measurements, it is limited to superficial cortical regions and may be confounded by extracranial signals [15].

While commonly used for intraoperative monitoring during cardiovascular or neurosurgical procedures and during sedation or anesthesia in neonates and critically ill patients, the accuracy of NIRS can be influenced by several factors. These include skin pigmentation, scalp fat thickness, probe positioning, and the assumption of a constant differential path length factor (DPF), which affects inter-subject reproducibility.

Barstow's review highlights that while both hemoglobin and myoglobin contribute to NIRS signals, cerebral applications rely almost exclusively on hemoglobin-based measures [15]. NIRS can estimate tissue saturation (StO_2) and infer relative oxygen delivery and utilization. However, extracranial contamination and limited penetration depth remain challenges.

Advanced NIRS systems, such as frequency-domain and time-resolved technologies, now offer quantitative chromophore concentrations, although their clinical adoption is still limited. In cerebral hemodynamics, NIRS is increasingly employed to detect desaturation events, guide blood pressure targets, and assess neurovascular coupling, though validation against gold-standard modalities (e.g., jugular bulb oximetry or PET) remains ongoing [15].

5.2.3 Perfusion imaging

Advanced imaging modalities provide spatial and quantitative data on cerebral blood flow:

- CT perfusion: Widely used in acute stroke to distinguish infarct core from penumbra.
- MRI perfusion: Includes dynamic susceptibility contrast (DSC) and arterial spin labeling (ASL) techniques.
- PET and SPECT: Gold standard for metabolic and perfusion imaging, though less commonly used due to cost and limited availability.

Perfusion imaging is essential for preoperative planning in tumor resections and for assessing collateral circulation in chronic ischemia [16].

5.3 Multimodal neuromonitoring

Modern neurocritical care increasingly relies on integrating multiple monitoring modalities to provide a comprehensive picture of cerebral physiology. Common combinations include:

- ICP + brain tissue oxygen tension ($PbtO_2$)
- TCD + NIRS
- Microdialysis + EEG.

Multimodal monitoring allows for real-time correlation of perfusion, metabolism, and electrical activity, enabling early detection of deteriorating brain function and guiding personalized therapeutic strategies [17].

5.4 Cerebral microdialysis: A metabolic window into the injured brain

Cerebral microdialysis (CMD) is an advanced neuromonitoring technique that allows bedside, near-continuous sampling of the extracellular brain environment, offering real-time insights into energy metabolism, ischemia, excitotoxicity, and treatment efficacy in acute brain injury (ABI). As Carteron et al. emphasize, CMD—when integrated with intracranial pressure (ICP) and brain tissue oxygen ($PbtO_2$) monitoring—can be used to personalize interventions such as CPP optimization, red blood cell transfusion, oxygen therapy, and glycemic control [18]. The most clinically validated CMD biomarkers include the lactate/pyruvate (L/P) ratio and glucose. An L/P ratio > 25 signals impaired oxidative metabolism, while >40 defines an energy crisis. Simultaneously, CMD-glucose levels <0.7 mmol/L suggest cerebral hypoglycemia or metabolic dysfunction, which may be caused or worsened by tight insulin therapy or low systemic glucose.

Importantly, CMD can detect subclinical ischemia, seizure-induced metabolic stress, spreading depolarizations, and even neuroinflammation and oxidative stress using high-cutoff catheters for large molecule biomarkers (e.g., cytokines, MMPs, tau, NfL). As a physiological tool, CMD also enables real-time evaluation of emerging therapies, including hypertonic lactate, succinate, nitric oxide inhibitors, and novel sedatives. Although cost and implementation barriers remain, recent consensus recommendations support CMD as a key modality in multimodal monitoring frameworks for severe TBI, SAH, and ICH patients [18].

5.5 Combined $PbtO_2$ and ICP monitoring in severe TBI

Recent large-scale evidence underscores the growing role of combined brain tissue oxygen ($PbtO_2$) and intracranial pressure (ICP) monitoring in patients with severe traumatic brain injury (STBI). In a 2024 meta-analysis including 16 studies ($n = 2604$), Zhang et al. found that combined monitoring was associated with a 33% increase in favorable neurological outcomes at 6 months and a 28% reduction in long-term mortality compared to ICP monitoring alone ($RR = 1.33$, $P < 0.0001$; $RR = 0.72$, $P = 0.0008$, respectively) [19]. These benefits were consistent across cohort studies; however, subgroup analysis of randomized controlled trials (RCTs) showed no significant outcome benefit, highlighting ongoing controversy and the need for higher-quality evidence.

Importantly, the authors also noted that $PbtO_2$ monitoring may detect episodes of brain hypoxia not reflected by ICP—thus helping prevent occult secondary injuries. However, it may lead to longer ICU stays, increased healthcare costs, and more catheter-related complications. Probe placement accuracy and heterogeneity of monitoring protocols remain key limitations. Current trials like BOOST-III and BONANZA-GT may help clarify the role of this combined strategy. Until then, the integration of $PbtO_2$ and ICP monitoring should be personalized and embedded in multimodal neuromonitoring protocols, especially in high-risk STBI patients.

5.6 Limitations and future perspectives

Despite technological progress, there are limitations. Invasive techniques have risks of infection and hemorrhage. Depth or specificity could be lacking in noninvasive methods. Expertise is necessary for interpretation, as well as integration of clinical context, image, and neurological examination.

Future trends involve the use of wearable brain sensors, artificial intelligence-based analytics, and the incorporation of hemodynamic data in closed-loop therapy systems. These advancements will bring about increased precision, decreased harm, and better outcomes for various neurological conditions.

6. Pathophysiological alterations in cerebral hemodynamics

Disruptions in cerebral hemodynamics are key in the development and sequelae of several neurological disorders. Recognition of these changes allows for the individualization of therapies for maintaining perfusion of the brain, decreasing intracranial pressure, and maximizing oxygen delivery (**Table 2**).

Condition	Monitoring/Management tools	Therapeutic interventions
Ischemic stroke	CT/MRI perfusion imaging	Thrombolysis, mechanical thrombectomy
Hemorrhagic stroke	Transcranial Doppler (TCD), CT	Monitoring for vasospasm; supportive measures
Traumatic brain injury	ICP monitors, $PbtO_2$ probes, advanced imaging	ICP control, CPP optimization, prevention of hypoxia/hypotension
Subarachnoid hemorrhage	Serial TCDs, neurological assessments	Nimodipine, triple-H therapy, close monitoring
Brain tumors	Pre-op perfusion imaging, intraoperative mapping	Resection, antiangiogenic agents
Hydrocephalus/CSF disorders	ICP/CPP monitoring, imaging	CSF diversion *via* ventriculostomy/shunt
Global cerebral ischemia	Neurologic exams, EEG, imaging	Targeted temperature management, supportive perfusion strategies

CT—Computed Tomography; MRI—Magnetic Resonance Imaging; TCD—Transcranial Doppler; ICP—Intracranial Pressure; $PbtO_2$—Partial Pressure of Oxygen in Brain Tissue; CPP—Cerebral Perfusion Pressure; CSF—Cerebrospinal Fluid; EEG—Electroencephalography.

Table 2.
Cerebral hemodynamics in neurological conditions.

6.1 Ischemic stroke

Artery occlusion in ischemic stroke results in decreased or loss of blood supply within an area of the brain. This creates an infarct core surrounded by a penumbra—a zone of decreased perfusion that is functionally impaired but possibly salvageable [16, 17].

CBF within the infarct core tends to be <10 mL/100 g/min, resulting in permanent neuronal loss. In the penumbral area, CBF can be 10–20 mL/100 g/min, and prompt reperfusion with thrombolysis or thrombectomy will restore function [20].

Perfusion CT or MRI scans help detect the penumbra as well as therapeutic windows. Autoregulation is usually disrupted in stroke such that blood flow is strongly pressure dependent [17].

6.2 Hemorrhagic stroke

Hemorrhagic strokes, such as intracerebral and subarachnoid hemorrhages (SAH), directly cause local tissue disruption, elevation of ICP, as well as local vasoconstriction.

One of the major risks of SAH is developing secondary cerebral ischemia as a consequence of cerebral vasospasm. This can take place several days after the initial hemorrhage, producing secondary ischemic damage. TCD is frequently employed for the purpose of watching for the development of vasospasm [17, 20].

6.3 Traumatic brain injury (TBI)

TBI causes both primary mechanical trauma and secondary injuries such as cerebral edema, hemorrhage, and hypoxia. These injuries disrupt autoregulation, increase ICP, and decrease CPP, exposing patients to ischemic damage.

ICP monitors, $PbtO_2$ probes, and advanced imaging are the key management measures for TBI. Interventions target the decrease of ICP, optimization of CPP, and the avoidance of secondary injury from either hypoxia or hypotension [17, 20].

6.4 Subarachnoid hemorrhage (SAH)

Beyond contributing to acute elevation of ICP and decreased CPP, SAH is also infamous for producing cerebral vasospasm. Vasospasm peaks within days 5–7 after hemorrhage and will last for several days, contributing significantly to impaired CBF and leading to delayed ischemic neurologic deficit.

Nimodipine, the only pharmacologic agent with documented efficacy in reducing the rate of poor outcomes in SAH, may work by enhancing microcirculation. Management is guided by serial TCD examinations and frequent neurological checks [21].

6.5 Brain tumors

Tumors change local cerebral hemodynamics in several ways: mass effect, angiogenesis, and breakdown of the BBB. Abnormal, leaky blood vessels in high-grade gliomas, for example, can contribute to vasogenic edema as well as elevated ICP [22].

Preoperative perfusion imaging assists in defining tumor margins and blood supply characteristics, with intraoperative preservation of surrounding functionally important brain tissue. Antiangiogenic therapies work toward the modulation of abnormal tumor perfusion in selected cases.

6.6 Hydrocephalus and CSF disorders

Increasing CSF volume with obstructive or communicating hydrocephalus boosts ICP, decreasing CPP and impairing perfusion. Signs of clinical presentation might be altered consciousness, papilledema, and, in infancy, bulging fontanelles. CSF diversion with ventriculostomy or shunt insertion normalizes pressure dynamics. Monitoring ICP and CPP is critical for diagnosis as well as postoperative care [23].

6.7 Global cerebral ischemia

After events such as cardiac arrest, global hypoperfusion impacts the entire brain. The hippocampus, cortex, and basal ganglia are particularly sensitive. Neuronal loss results from reperfusion injury, oxidative stress, and microvascular thrombosis. Targeted temperature management and perfusion of the brain are key components of enhancing neurologic recovery following global ischemic insults. Comprehending such pathological alterations between conditions allows for specific therapeutic approaches to alleviate injury and encourage recovery.

7. Therapeutic strategies and hemodynamic targets

Effective cerebral hemodynamic management is concerned with maintaining sufficient cerebral blood flow (CBF) and optimal intracranial pressure (ICP), as well as supporting autoregulatory function. The choice of intervention is determined by the underlying pathology, the nature of neurological injury, as well as available instrumentation. This section describes the main therapeutic methods practiced in clinical management.

7.1 Intracranial pressure management

Elevated intracranial pressure is an emergent medical condition that can result in herniation of the brain, impaired perfusion of the brain (cerebral perfusion pressure), and permanent neurological loss. Treatment is with both pharmacologic and non-pharmacologic measures. Osmotic therapy with mannitol or hypertonic saline mobilizes fluid from the brain parenchyma into the intravascular compartment, thus decreasing edema of the brain; serial measurements of serum osmolality as well as sodium are important in the management [23]. Cerebrospinal fluid diversion through external ventricular drains (EVD) is both therapeutically useful in reducing pressure as well as offering real-time ICP. Elevation of the head of the bed to 30 degrees, as well as sufficient sedation, are supportive steps that facilitate increased venous outflow as well as decreased metabolic demand of the brain, respectively. When refractory intracranial hypertension is present, more intense measures like induction of coma with barbiturates or therapeutic hypothermia may be utilized, although they are associated with great potential for risk as well as an intensive level of monitoring. **Table 3** summarizes the commonly used methods for low ICP.

Monitoring tool	Invasiveness	Parameters measured	Sensitivity/ Specificity	Limitations
External Ventricular Drain (EVD)	Invasive	ICP, CSF drainage, waveform analysis	High sensitivity and specificity	Risk of infection, hemorrhage, requires surgical access
Intraparenchymal ICP probe	Invasive	ICP, waveform analysis	High for pressure, limited for location	No CSF drainage, drift over time
Transcranial Doppler (TCD)	Noninvasive	Flow velocity in basal arteries	Moderate; operator-dependent	Limited by skull thickness, poor spatial resolution
Near-Infrared Spectroscopy (NIRS)	Noninvasive	Regional cerebral oxygenation (rSO_2)	Moderate; depth-limited	Susceptible to extracranial contamination
Perfusion CT/MRI	Noninvasive	CBF, CBV, MTT, penumbra mapping	High; modality-dependent	Radiation (CT), cost, contrast use, time-consuming
Brain tissue oxygen ($PbtO_2$)	Invasive	Partial pressure of oxygen in brain tissue	High in focal measurement areas	Localized reading only, infection risk
Microdialysis	Invasive	Lactate, pyruvate, glucose, neurotransmitters	High metabolic insight	Delayed readout, highly localized

Table 3.
The commonly used cerebral monitoring tools.

7.2 Optimization of cerebral perfusion pressure (CPP)

Maintaining cerebral perfusion pressure (CPP) within a safe physiological range—typically between 60 and 80 mmHg—is essential, particularly in the management of traumatic brain injury. Achieving this balance often requires a multifaceted approach. Vasopressors, such as norepinephrine, are administered to raise mean arterial pressure (MAP) in hypotensive patients, thereby supporting CPP [22, 23]. Volume resuscitation ensures adequate intravascular volume and cardiac output, contributing to stable perfusion. Additionally, effective intracranial pressure (ICP) control enhances CPP by decreasing resistance to cerebral arterial inflow. In select cases, autoregulation-guided CPP targets may be employed, utilizing advanced neuromonitoring technologies that assess cerebral autoregulation in real-time, allowing for individualized and responsive hemodynamic management.

7.3 Control of blood gases

Carbon dioxide (CO_2) modulation is a key component in the management of elevated intracranial pressure (ICP). Mild hyperventilation, targeting a partial pressure of arterial CO_2 ($PaCO_2$) between 30 and 35 mmHg, induces cerebral vasoconstriction, thereby reducing cerebral blood volume and lowering ICP [24]. However, this intervention must be used judiciously, as prolonged hyperventilation may compromise cerebral perfusion and increase the risk of ischemia. Oxygenation management is equally critical; maintaining normoxia or mild hyperoxia helps ensure adequate oxygen delivery to brain tissue, while hypoxia must be aggressively avoided. In cases of cerebral vasospasm or systemic compromise, high-flow oxygen therapy may be warranted to optimize tissue oxygenation.

7.4 Surgical interventions

Surgical interventions play a vital role in the management of elevated intracranial pressure (ICP), particularly when medical therapies prove insufficient. Decompressive craniectomy involves the removal of a portion of the skull to alleviate mass effect and accommodate brain swelling. This procedure is typically indicated in cases of malignant cerebral edema or refractory ICP elevation unresponsive to conventional measures [23, 24]. Similarly, clot evacuation in hemorrhagic stroke or tumor resection in the presence of space-occupying lesions can significantly improve cerebral perfusion and reduce intracranial pressure by eliminating the source of compression.

7.5 Pharmacological interventions

Pharmacologic neuroprotection is a cornerstone of managing patients at risk for secondary brain injury. Nimodipine, a calcium channel blocker, has demonstrated efficacy in reducing delayed cerebral ischemic deficits following aneurysmal subarachnoid hemorrhage by improving microvascular perfusion. Anti-seizure medications are employed prophylactically or therapeutically in patients with elevated intracranial risk to prevent seizure-related metabolic surges, which can exacerbate neuronal injury. Additionally, sedatives and anesthetics serve to decrease cerebral metabolic demand, reduce sympathetic outflow, and facilitate ICP control, particularly in critically ill or mechanically ventilated patients [25, 26].

7.6 Targeted temperature management

Used post-cardiac arrest or in select cases of global cerebral ischemia. Hypothermia (32–36°C) reduces metabolic rate, mitigates excitotoxicity, and may preserve autoregulation. Requires close monitoring for arrhythmias and coagulopathies [27].

7.7 Emerging and adjunctive therapies

Advanced and investigational therapies are increasingly being explored to enhance individualized management of cerebral hemodynamics. Hyperbaric oxygen therapy has been investigated as a potential adjunct in cases of severe traumatic or ischemic brain injury, aiming to augment cerebral oxygen delivery under increased atmospheric pressure. Cerebral microdialysis enables bedside monitoring of key brain metabolites, such as lactate and pyruvate, offering real-time insights into cellular metabolism and guiding therapeutic decisions. Autoregulation-directed therapy represents a precision approach by adjusting mean arterial pressure (MAP) or cerebral perfusion pressure (CPP) targets based on continuous assessment of the brain's autoregulatory capacity [18]. Importantly, the objective of these interventions is not merely to achieve numeric normalization but to optimize cerebral oxygenation, preserve tissue viability, and prevent secondary brain injury. The integration of multimodal neuromonitoring allows for dynamic, patient-specific, physiology-driven care tailored to each individual's evolving cerebral status.

8. Emerging technologies and future directions

Advances in biomedical engineering, neuroimaging, and data science are driving rapid change in the discipline of cerebral hemodynamics. These advancements are offering more precise, noninvasive, and personalized methods to monitor as well as control cerebral blood perfusion and oxygenation in both clinical practice and in research applications (**Table 4**).

8.1 Multimodal neuromonitoring integration

The combination of several streams of data—like ICP, brain tissue oxygen tension ($PbtO_2$), cerebral microdialysis, and EEG—is being used with greater frequency in order to create an overall picture of the brain's physiology. These systems aid clinicians in being able to make more detailed assessments and provide early identification of deterioration that cannot be recognized through individual-parameter monitoring [19].

Improvements in bedside computing platforms make real-time visualization of trends, together with correlation analysis, available. For instance, plotting autoregulation indices versus time can help determine personalized targets for cerebral perfusion.

8.2 Artificial intelligence and machine learning

Artificial intelligence (AI) algorithms are being created for analyzing extensive quantities of cerebral hemodynamic data, anticipating patient deterioration, and suggesting interventions. Multimodal datasets train machine learning algorithms that

Topic	Applications	Future potential
Multimodal neuromonitoring integration	ICU bedside monitoring; autoregulation analysis	Personalized perfusion targets; early clinical intervention
Artificial intelligence and machine learning	Neuro-ICU decision support; automated alerts	Improved diagnostic precision, protocol optimization, and resource management
Wearable and noninvasive devices	Pre-hospital triage, chronic care follow-up, post-op recovery	Continuous ambulatory monitoring for epilepsy, hydrocephalus, etc.
Advanced neuroimaging and functional techniques	Mapping ischemia, tumors, vascular lesions; cellular-level neurovascular coupling research	Deeper insights into cerebrovascular physiology; enhanced diagnostics for personalized care
Computational modeling and simulation	Aneurysm surgery planning, drug delivery modeling, risk stratification	"What-if" simulations to tailor interventions and anticipate complications
Precision medicine in cerebral hemodynamics	Personalized neurocritical care	Genotype-informed therapies, real-time autoregulation-guided management, integration into clinical standards

ICU: Intensive care unit.

Table 4.
Emerging technologies and future directions in cerebral hemodynamics.

can detect intricate patterns not recognized through human knowledge, including early warning for cases of vasospasm, hypoperfusion, or impending herniation [28].

Support for these technologies can also aid in optimization of protocols as well as resource allocation, particularly in neuro-ICUs.

8.3 Wearable and noninvasive devices

Emerging wearable devices are being engineered for continual, noninvasive tracking of cerebral perfusion as well as oxygenation. Wearable NIRS headbands, helmet-based systems employing ultrasound, as well as even EEG-based smart caps, are being explored for use in ambulatory or home care environments [28].

Particularly, these devices show great potential in pre-hospital triage, post-operative management, and extended neurological observation in chronic patients with hydrocephalus or epilepsy.

8.4 Advanced neuroimaging and functional techniques

Next-generation imaging technologies are significantly enhancing the ability to assess cerebral blood flow and metabolic activity with greater precision and depth [28]. High-resolution magnetic resonance imaging (MRI), incorporating both perfusion and diffusion-weighted sequences, enables detailed mapping of ischemic territories, tumor vascularization, and perfusion heterogeneity. Arterial spin labeling (ASL) presents a noninvasive MRI-based technique for quantifying regional cerebral blood flow (CBF) without the need for contrast agents, making it especially valuable in vulnerable populations. In preclinical and translational research, optogenetics and two-photon microscopy offer unparalleled spatial and temporal resolution, allowing real-time visualization of neurovascular coupling at the cellular level [29]. Photoacoustic imaging, an emerging hybrid modality combining optical and ultrasound techniques, provides high spatial resolution and deep tissue penetration while simultaneously capturing real-time vascular and metabolic signals. Together, these innovations are broadening diagnostic and research capabilities in cerebrovascular physiology and pathology.

8.5 Computational modeling and simulation

Mathematical and computational modeling of cerebral circulation is rapidly advancing as a powerful tool for understanding and predicting cerebral hemodynamics under both physiological and pathological conditions. These models simulate complex flow dynamics and vessel behavior, offering valuable insights for surgical planning, particularly in procedures such as aneurysm clipping or carotid endarterectomy. Additionally, they are used to optimize drug delivery strategies and to support risk stratification by evaluating the potential hemodynamic impact of various interventions. By enabling clinicians to explore 'what-if' scenarios in silico, such models facilitate more precise and personalized treatment planning, enhancing the ability to anticipate patient responses and adapt therapeutic strategies accordingly [30].

8.6 Precision medicine in cerebral hemodynamics

The integration of genomics, metabolomics, and individualized physiological monitoring is driving a transformative shift toward precision medicine in neurology. Emerging evidence suggests that genetic predispositions—such as those affecting cerebrovascular autoregulation or endothelial integrity—may soon inform personalized preventive strategies and targeted therapeutic interventions. Within this evolving framework, biomarker-guided treatments, customized cerebral perfusion pressure (CPP) targets, and real-time autoregulation mapping are poised to become essential tools in optimizing cerebral hemodynamic management. These innovations reflect a broader transition toward proactive, personalized, and minimally invasive approaches to brain care. As the scientific and technological foundations continue to mature, the incorporation of precision hemodynamics into routine clinical practice is expected to redefine standards of care and enhance neurologic outcomes.

9. Challenges and ethical considerations

Despite technological progress and increasing exposure to the dynamics of the brain, some challenges in clinical work and in clinical trials continue. These challenges are not just technical in nature, as in the use of such techniques as the insertion of catheters in populations with uncertain outcomes.

9.1 Interindividual variability and monitoring limits

One of the major challenges in the management of cerebral hemodynamics is the extensive variation in autoregulatory capability, baseline CBF, as well as in response to treatments between individuals. Age, prior cerebrovascular disease, systemic comorbid conditions, as well as genetic reasons, impact the reliability of global thresholds (e.g., targets of CPP). The heterogeneity makes universal treatment algorithms difficult to apply.

Moreover, several of the available monitoring devices—though sophisticated—are of limited effectiveness. Transcranial Doppler (TCD), for example, is operator-dependent and will not necessarily yield reproducible measurements in all patients with anatomic limitations (thick skull, for example). Near-infrared spectroscopy (NIRS) is mainly sensitive to superficial cortical perfusion but is also subject to extracranial contamination. Even the invasive modalities, such as intracranial pressure (ICP) probes, involve infection hazard, hemorrhage, and technical skill [31].

9.2 Balancing benefit with risk of invasive monitoring

The most frequent use of invasive cerebral monitoring is in intensive care units, particularly in traumatic brain injury (TBI), subarachnoid hemorrhage (SAH), or hydrocephalus. Although these devices yield useful information, their benefit should be considered in relation to their risks of complications as well as their load on patients and health systems [31, 32].

In such patients with poor prognoses, for example, in cases of extensive hemorrhage or severe hypoxic brain injury, deciding on aggressive investigation and intervention is ethically problematic. Clinicians should consider whether such treatment will improve outcomes in some way or only extend suffering.

9.3 Resource allocation and equity of access

Advanced cerebral hemodynamic monitoring is associated with intense resources, such as specialized equipment, trained individuals, and critical care facilities. Limited resources in health facilities may not provide access to some of these technologies, which can pose issues regarding healthcare equity. Low-income areas are not always able to provide the same extent of monitoring or intervention as resourced areas.

Global health resources need to target the development of cost-efficient and scalable methods for cerebral monitoring. Investigations of low-cost, portable, or point-of-care diagnostic devices are picking up speed and could bridge the gap between technologically advanced settings and underserved communities.

9.4 Foretelling and obtaining consent

One other ethical dilemma is prognostication. Cerebral hemodynamic measurements—especially when interpreted in the absence of clinical context—are nonspecific. For instance, ongoing low cerebral oxygenation or impaired autoregulatory function can imply an unfavorable prognosis, but individual patient outcomes are greatly varied. This variability makes discussions with families and surrogate decision-makers difficult [5].

Ensuring that patients have informed consent for experimental therapies or invasive monitoring involves presenting uncertainties, benefits, and risks in an honest, compassionate way. Wherever patients have no capacity for decision-making, surrogate decisions must encompass known preferences of the patients and be in accord with beneficence as well as non-maleficence.

9.5 When combining AI with patient autonomy

As artificial intelligence (AI) and machine learning play more of a role in the interpretation of cerebral hemodynamic measures, several ethical issues arise. The algorithms could impact clinical decision-making or suggest treatments that are not necessarily understood by clinicians. Transparency, explainability, and accountability in AI systems must be considered to maintain trust and ensure patient autonomy.

Additionally, predictive modeling for prognostication should be treated with caution in order not to label individuals in a deterministic manner or deny them care based on algorithmic results only.

Tackling these complex challenges demands an interdisciplinary solution that integrates technological innovation with ethical awareness and dedication to just care. Protocols and guidelines should adapt to emerging technologies with the protection of human values in clinical decision-making.

10. Conclusion

Cerebral hemodynamics plays a central role in maintaining brain function by ensuring adequate delivery of oxygen and nutrients while preserving intracranial stability. Understanding the complex interplay among cerebral blood flow, vascular resistance, intracranial pressure, and perfusion pressure is essential for clinicians managing a broad spectrum of neurological conditions. Advances in monitoring techniques, both invasive and noninvasive, have greatly improved the ability to assess cerebral physiology in real time, allowing for early detection of deterioration and individualized treatment. Pathophysiological disruptions in cerebral hemodynamics contribute to various acute and chronic neurological disorders, including stroke, traumatic brain injury, subarachnoid hemorrhage, brain tumors, and hydrocephalus. Current therapeutic strategies focus on optimizing perfusion, controlling intracranial dynamics, and protecting the brain from secondary injury. Emerging technologies such as artificial intelligence, wearable monitoring devices, advanced neuroimaging, computational modeling, and precision medicine hold promise for more personalized and effective management approaches. Despite these advances, ethical challenges remain regarding invasive monitoring, resource allocation, interindividual variability, informed consent, and the integration of automated decision-support systems into clinical care. Continued research, technological innovation, and careful ethical reflection are essential to further advance the field and improve neurological outcomes.

Acknowledgements

The author gratefully acknowledges the guidance and mentorship of Dr. Nisar Shaikh, whose expertise and valuable feedback significantly contributed to the development of this chapter. Special thanks are also extended to the co-authors and collaborators for their constructive discussions, insights, and critical review during the preparation of this work. The author wishes to express appreciation to Hamad Medical Corporation for providing institutional support and access to relevant resources necessary for the completion of this chapter. The contribution of medical librarians and administrative staff who assisted in the literature search and manuscript preparation is sincerely appreciated. No external funding was received for this work.

Conflict of interest

The author declares no conflict of interest.

Notes/thanks/other declarations

The author would like to express gratitude to all colleagues and professionals who provided insightful discussions that contributed to the refinement of the chapter. Appreciation is also extended to the editorial team for their support and guidance throughout the submission process.

Author details

Ali Msheik*, Alaaeldin Ahmed, Omar Shihadeh and Ali Sulaiman
Neurological Surgery, Hamad Medical Corporation, Qatar

*Address all correspondence to: dr.alimsheik@gmail.com

References

[1] Clarke DD, Sokoloff L. Regulation of cerebral metabolic rate. In: Siegel GJ, Agranoff BW, Albers RW, et al., editors. Basic Neurochemistry: Molecular, Cellular and Medical Aspects. 6th ed. Philadelphia: Lippincott-Raven; 1999. Available from: https://www.ncbi.nlm.nih.gov/books/NBK28194/

[2] de Araújo Silva DO, Matis GK, Costa LF, Kitamura MA, de Carvalho Junior EV, de Moura SM, et al. Chronic subdural hematomas and the elderly: Surgical results from a series of 125 cases: Old "horses" are not to be shot! Surgical Neurology International. 2012;**3**:150. DOI: 10.4103/2152-7806.104744. Epub 2012 Dec 14

[3] Jha RM. Intracranial pressure monitoring in traumatic brain injury-a tool of the trade or one that betrays us? JAMA Network Open. 2023;**6**(9):e2334190. DOI: 10.1001/jamanetworkopen.2023.34190

[4] Petkar S, Chakole V, Nisal R, Priya V. Cerebral perfusion unveiled: A comprehensive review of blood pressure management in neurosurgical and endovascular aneurysm interventions. Cureus. 2024;**16**(2):e53635. DOI: 10.7759/cureus.53635

[5] Petersen NH, Silverman A, Wang A, Strander S, Kodali S, Matouk C, et al. Association of personalized blood pressure targets with hemorrhagic transformation and functional outcome after endovascular stroke therapy. JAMA Neurology. 2019;**76**(10):1256-1258. DOI: 10.1001/jamaneurol.2019.2120

[6] Purves D, Augustine GJ, Fitzpatrick D, et al. Neuroscience. In: The Blood Supply of the Brain and Spinal Cord. 2nd ed. Sunderland (MA): Sinauer Associates; 2001. Available from: https://www.ncbi.nlm.nih.gov/books/NBK11042/

[7] Dotiwala AK, McCausland C, Samra NS. Anatomy, head and neck: Blood brain barrier [Updated 2023 Apr 4]. In: StatPearls [Internet]. Treasure Island (FL): StatPearls Publishing; 2025. Available from: https://www.ncbi.nlm.nih.gov/books/NBK519556/

[8] Mount CA, Das JM. Cerebral perfusion pressure. In: StatPearls [Internet]. Treasure Island (FL): StatPearls Publishing; 2025

[9] Tong Z. A Multiscale Model of Cerebral Autoregulation in Health and Disease [Internet]. University of Oxford; 2024. Available from: https://ora.ox.ac.uk/objects/uuid:7472ed73-c6ae-4178-94c3-579e46c76554

[10] Benson JC, Madhavan AA, Cutsforth-Gregory JK, Johnson DR, Carr CM. The Monro-Kellie doctrine: A review and call for revision. AJNR. American Journal of Neuroradiology. 2023;**44**(1):2-6. DOI: 10.3174/ajnr.A7721. Epub 2022 Dec 1

[11] Silverman A, Petersen NH. Physiology, cerebral autoregulation [Updated 2023 Mar 15]. In: StatPearls [Internet]. Treasure Island (FL): StatPearls Publishing; 2025. Available from: https://www.ncbi.nlm.nih.gov/books/NBK553183/

[12] Xu F, Liu P, Pascual JM, Xiao G, Lu H. Effect of hypoxia and hyperoxia on cerebral blood flow, blood oxygenation, and oxidative metabolism. Journal of Cerebral Blood Flow and Metabolism. 2012;**32**(10):1909-1918. DOI: 10.1038/jcbfm.2012.93. Epub 2012 Jun 27

[13] Ashby JW, Mack JJ. Endothelial control of cerebral blood flow. The American Journal of Pathology. 2021;**191**(5):963-973. DOI: 10.1016/j.ajpath.2021.02.023

[14] Palavani LB, Alves Neto LB, Batista S, Ferreira MY, Emmily de Carvalho D, de Vasconcellos PG, et al. Invasive and noninvasive techniques for intracranial pressure monitoring after decompressive craniectomy: A systematic review and meta-analysis. World Neurosurgery. 2024;**190**:76-87. DOI: 10.1016/j.wneu.2024.06.118. Epub 2024 Jun 29

[15] Barstow TJ. Understanding near infrared spectroscopy and its application to skeletal muscle research. Journal of Applied Physiology. 2019;**126**(5):1360-1376. DOI: 10.1152/japplphysiol.00166.2018. Epub 2019 Mar 7

[16] Zaro-Weber O, Fleischer H, Reiblich L, Schuster A, Moeller-Hartmann W, Heiss WD. Penumbra detection in acute stroke with perfusion magnetic resonance imaging: Validation with ^{15} O-positron emission tomography. Annals of Neurology. 2019;**85**(6):875-886. DOI: 10.1002/ana.25479. Epub 2019 Apr 22

[17] Barrit S, Al Barajraji M, El Hadwe S, Niset A, Foreman B, Park S, et al. Intracranial multimodal monitoring in neurocritical care (Neurocore-iMMM): an open, decentralized consensus. Critical Care. 2024;**28**(1):427. DOI: 10.1186/s13054-024-05211-8

[18] Carteron L, Bouzat P, Oddo M. Cerebral microdialysis monitoring to improve individualized neurointensive care therapy: An update of recent clinical data. Frontiers in Neurology. 2017;**8**:601. DOI: 10.3389/fneur.2017.00601

[19] Zhang C, Zhou L, Zhang K, Huang J, Cao L, Lou Y, et al. Brain tissue oxygen pressure combined with intracranial pressure monitoring may improve clinical outcomes for patients with severe traumatic brain injury: A systemic review and meta-analysis. PeerJ. 2024;**12**:e18086. DOI: 10.7717/peerj.18086

[20] Jaffer H, Morris VB, Stewart D, Labhasetwar V. Advances in stroke therapy. Drug Delivery and Translational Research. 2011;**1**(6):409-419. DOI: 10.1007/s13346-011-0046-y

[21] de Oliveira Manoel AL, Mansur A, Murphy A, Turkel-Parrella D, Macdonald M, Macdonald RL, et al. Aneurysmal subarachnoid haemorrhage from a neuroimaging perspective. Critical Care. 2014;**18**(6):557. DOI: 10.1186/s13054-014-0557-2

[22] Arvanitis CD, Ferraro GB, Jain RK. The blood-brain barrier and blood-tumour barrier in brain tumours and metastases. Nature Reviews. Cancer. 2020;**20**(1):26-41. DOI: 10.1038/s41568-019-0205-x. Epub 2019 Oct 10

[23] Pinto VL, Tadi P, Adeyinka A. Increased intracranial pressure [Updated 2023 Jul 31]. In: StatPearls [Internet]. Treasure Island (FL): StatPearls Publishing; 2025. Available from: https://www.ncbi.nlm.nih.gov/books/NBK482119/

[24] Cardim D, Giardina A, Ciliberti P, Battaglini D, Berardino A, Uccelli A, et al. Short-term mild hyperventilation on intracranial pressure, cerebral autoregulation, and oxygenation in acute brain injury patients: A prospective observational study. Journal of Clinical Monitoring and Computing. 2024;**38**(4):753-762. DOI: 10.1007/s10877-023-01121-2. Epub 2024 Feb 4

[25] Das JM, Zito PM. Nimodipine [Updated 2024 May 7]. In: StatPearls [Internet]. Treasure Island (FL): StatPearls Publishing; 2025. Available

from: https://www.ncbi.nlm.nih.gov/books/NBK534870/

[26] Feigin VL, Rinkel GJ, Algra A, Vermeulen M, van Gijn J. Calcium antagonists in patients with aneurysmal subarachnoid hemorrhage: A systematic review. Neurology. 1998;**50**(4):876-883. DOI: 10.1212/wnl.50.4.876

[27] Omairi AM, Pandey S. Targeted temperature management [Updated 2023 Jun 25]. In: StatPearls [Internet]. Treasure Island (FL): StatPearls Publishing; 2025. Available from: https://www.ncbi.nlm.nih.gov/books/NBK556124/

[28] Pinto-Coelho L. How artificial intelligence is shaping medical imaging technology: A survey of innovations and applications. Bioengineering (Basel). 2023;**10**(12):1435. DOI: 10.3390/bioengineering10121435

[29] Hussain S, Mubeen I, Ullah N, Shah SSUD, Khan BA, Zahoor M, et al. Modern diagnostic imaging technique applications and risk factors in the medical field: A review. BioMed Research International. 2022;**2022**:5164970. DOI: 10.1155/2022/5164970

[30] Salman HE, Yalcin HC. Computational modeling of blood flow hemodynamics for biomechanical investigation of cardiac development and disease. Journal of Cardiovascular Development and Disease. 2021;**8**(2):14. DOI: 10.3390/jcdd8020014

[31] Zhou S, Gao X, Park G, Yang X, Qi B, Lin M, et al. Transcranial volumetric imaging using a conformal ultrasound patch. Nature. 2024;**629**(8013):810-818. DOI: 10.1038/s41586-024-07381-5. Epub 2024 May 22

[32] Shim Y, Kim J, Kim HS, Oh J, Lee S, Ha EJ. Intracranial pressure monitoring for acute brain injured patients: When, how, what should we monitor. Korean Journal of Neurotrauma. 2023;**19**(2):149-161. DOI: 10.13004/kjnt.2023.19.e32

Chapter 3

Clinical Monitoring of Pediatric and Adolescent Patients Undergoing Continuous Renal Replacement Therapy (CRRT)

Mohammad Mateenuddin Quadri, Bakri Alali and Nissar Shaikh

Abstract

Continuous renal replacement therapy (CRRT) is a vital life-sustaining modality for managing acute kidney injury (AKI) and fluid overload in hemodynamically unstable pediatric, adolescent, and adult patients. This comprehensive review outlines the critical aspects of CRRT monitoring, including pre-CRRT preparation, modality selection, dose calculation, vascular access, and real-time parameter tracking. The document emphasizes the importance of individualized dosing strategies tailored by age, body size, and metabolic needs, particularly in children. Detailed guidance is provided on blood flow rates, dialysate and ultrafiltration settings, anticoagulation choices, and filter selection based on patient weight and extracorporeal volume. Monitoring during CRRT includes the frequent assessment of hemodynamic status, laboratory markers, nutritional status, and infection risk. Daily interdisciplinary coordination among nephrologists, intensivists, nurses, and pharmacists is highlighted as a key component of successful CRRT implementation. Pediatric-specific considerations such as the use of pre- and post-filter weight scales and sensitivity to fluid shifts are discussed. The document provides practical strategies and checklists aimed at optimizing patient safety, therapy efficacy, and clinical outcomes in both pediatric and adult critical care settings.

Keywords: CRRT, acute kidney injury, fluid overload, pediatric dialysis, hemodynamic monitoring, extracorporeal therapy, nutrition in CRRT, anticoagulation, filter selection, ICU nephrology

1. Introduction

Since the pioneering work of Ronco and colleagues in the mid-1980s, continuous renal replacement therapy (CRRT) has evolved from an experimental and adapted treatment into a well-established standard of care in pediatric critical care nephrology [1].

Continuous renal replacement therapy (CRRT) is a life-saving modality for critically sick patients with acute kidney injury (AKI), particularly those with hemodynamic instability. Unlike intermittent hemodialysis, CRRT provides slow and continuous removal of solutes and fluids over 24 hours.

In recent years, continuous renal replacement therapy (CRRT) has been used more frequently in critically ill children thanks to better technology and easier-to-use machines. Despite these improvements, survival rates have not increased accordingly [2, 3]. Following standardized, protocol-based practices could help improve outcomes and boost survival in children receiving CRRT. Proper monitoring during CRRT is crucial for safety, efficacy, and complication prevention [4]. Monitoring must be tailored for pediatric, adolescent and adult patients, considering size, metabolic rates, and comorbid conditions.

2. CRRT in critically ill children

Continuous renal replacement therapy (CRRT) is a type of dialysis used in critically ill children, especially those who are too unstable for regular dialysis. It helps remove waste, fluid, and toxins slowly and gently.

Common indications for pediatric CRRT: Indications for renal replacement therapy (RRT) in acute kidney injury (AKI) and general indications: [5–9]. Continuous renal replacement therapy (CRRT) is indicated in several critical conditions of acute kidney injury (AKI) and other severe clinical situations. It is especially considered when fluid overload is unresponsive to medical therapy, such as in hypertension, congestive heart failure, pulmonary edema, or fluid-induced respiratory failure, particularly if cumulative fluid overload exceeds 10%.

2.1 Acute kidney injury (AKI)

AKI is common in PICUs: affects 30–60% of critically ill children. AKI increases the risk of death and long-term kidney problems. Early diagnosis is now easier using tools like KDIGO and pRIFLE. The AWARE study showed that severe AKI increases the risk of death (11% in severe AKI vs. 2.6% in mild or no AKI).

Fluid overload (FO) Fluid overload can occur with or without AKI. It is common in children with sepsis, heart surgery, and respiratory failure. Fluid overload worsens outcomes, for every 1% increase in fluid overload, the chance of death rises by 6%. Careful fluid management is essential. Measuring fluid overload exactly can be tricky.

Growing evidence shows that fluid overload in critically ill children with acute kidney injury (AKI) is linked to worse outcomes [4, 10–18]. While it is not yet proven whether fluid overload directly causes these problems, a randomized trial in hemodynamically stable patients with acute respiratory distress syndrome indicates that such a relationship may exist [4].

Acid–base and electrolyte problems: Other key indications for the CRRT include refractory hyperkalemia (especially $K > 6.5$ mmol/L), severe azotemia with symptomatic uremia (like encephalopathy), hyperphosphatemia, severe metabolic acidosis, and difficult-to-control sodium disturbances (hypo- or hypernatremia).

Non-kidney uses: CRRT additionally plays an important role in managing sepsis, septic shock, multiple organ failure—it removes inflammatory molecules (cytokines), cardiogenic shock after cardiac surgery, liver failure.

In acute liver failure—it removes harmful substances while waiting for recovery or liver transplant. Inborn errors of metabolism urea cycle defects, hyperammonemia, 45 organic acidemias, and in cases of dialyzable toxin or drug overdose.

CRRT is also used for hyperphosphatemia, tumor lysis syndrome, and crush syndrome, and to provide ultrafiltration for patients needing adequate nutrition or blood product replacement. It may also be applied in severe hyperthermia when conventional treatments are insufficient [4].

3. CRRT modalities (types of continuous renal replacement therapy)

Continuous renal replacement therapy (CRRT), also known as continuous kidney replacement therapy (CKRT), includes different methods used to support kidney function in critically ill patients, especially when the kidneys cannot remove waste or excess fluid on their own. Unlike standard dialysis, which is done only a few times per week, CRRT works continuously over 24 hours, making it gentler and better suited for unstable patients, including children.

There are three main types of CRRT, each with specific characteristics:

3.1 CVVH (continuous veno-venous hemofiltration)

This method removes waste through *convection*—pushing fluid and waste across a special filter. Since it removes a large volume of fluid, replacement fluid must be added to prevent dehydration and filter blockage.

Continuous veno-venous hemofiltration (CVVH) has the advantage of being gentle on blood pressure, making it suitable for hemodynamically unstable patients. However, one limitation is that it may not effectively clear all types of toxins compared to other dialysis modalities.

CVVHD (continuous veno-venous hemodialysis): This technique removes waste through *diffusion*, where waste moves from the blood into a dialysis fluid flowing in the opposite direction. It is especially effective for removing small waste molecules like urea.

Continuous veno-venous hemodialysis (CVVHD) is effective for removing small toxins efficiently, making it useful in many critical care situations. Its limitations include less effectiveness in fluid removal and a tendency to lower blood pressure in some patients.

CVVHDF (continuous veno-venous hemodiafiltration): This method combines *convection* and *diffusion*, making it the most effective in clearing both small and large waste molecules. It is often used in very sick patients who need strong support.

Continuous veno-venous hemodiafiltration (CVVHDF) offers powerful clearance of toxins and fluids, which helps support both heart and immune function. However, it is more complex and costly to perform, and it may also cause unwanted nutrient loss during treatment.

In addition to these, there are two other related methods:

SLED (sustained low-efficiency dialysis): This is a hybrid approach that blends features of CRRT and traditional intermittent dialysis. It typically runs for 6 to 12 hours. SLED removes both solutes (like urea and creatinine) and fluid, using standard dialysis machines with adjusted settings.

Sustained low-efficiency dialysis (SLED) is used when the patient is relatively more stable but still requires a slow and controlled dialysis treatment to maintain safety and effectiveness.

SCUF (slow continuous ultrafiltration): SCUF is used only for removing excess fluid, not waste products. It is helpful for patients with fluid overload but relatively

Goal	Description
Maintain hemodynamic stability	Continuous monitoring of blood pressure, heart rate, and perfusion to prevent hypotension or shock during CRRT.
Ensure circuit patency and effective solute clearance	Regular checks of filter function, pressures, and adequacy of solute removal (e.g., urea, creatinine, electrolytes).
Prevent and detect complications early	Vigilance for bleeding, infection, electrolyte imbalances, and clotting in the extracorporeal circuit.
Adjust therapy based on clinical progress	Modify CRRT prescription according to changes in patient condition, lab results, and fluid/electrolyte balance.
Ensure adequate nutrition and fluid balance	Maintain correct fluid removal rate while ensuring caloric and protein requirements are met.

Table 1.
Goals of CRRT monitoring.

stable kidney function. It works by removing plasma water through a filter without using dialysis or replacement fluids.

Slow continuous ultrafiltration (SCUF) is mainly used when the primary goal is gentle and continuous fluid removal, usually carried out over 24 hours or longer.

Choosing the right CRRT method depends on several factors, including the patient's blood pressure stability, the amount of fluid to be removed, and the types of waste. Products that need to be cleared and the goals of CRRT Monitoring (**Table 1**).

CRRT preparation should begin when a patient's fluid overload is more than 5% of body weight and does not improve with diuretics. If the fluid overload becomes greater than 10% of body weight, starting CRRT is strongly recommended [19].

3.2 The goals of CRRT

The main goals are to maintain hemodynamic stability, keep the circuit open for effective solute clearance, prevent and detect complications at an early stage, adjust therapy as the patient's condition changes, and ensure adequate nutrition and fluid balance throughout treatment (**Table 1**).

4. Pre-CRRT monitoring and preparation

Before initiating continuous renal replacement therapy (CRRT), a thorough pre-treatment assessment is essential to ensure patient safety and optimize treatment outcomes, especially in pediatric and adolescent patients.

In CRRT, careful monitoring is essential. Blood pressure should be checked every 15–60 minutes, with ultrafiltration adjusted as needed. Heart rate is monitored hourly, since tachycardia may suggest hypotension or low fluid levels.

Temperature is checked every 4 hours to detect hypothermia from extracorporeal circulation.

Access and return pressures are measured hourly, as high access pressure suggests clotting while low pressure points to access problems, and high return pressure may indicate filter clotting. Transmembrane pressure is also tracked hourly, with rising values signaling filter clotting.

Effluent flow is monitored hourly to ensure the prescribed dose is being delivered, while ultrafiltration volume is documented hourly to track net fluid balance. Machine alarms are continuously observed and must be investigated promptly.

Hemodynamic evaluation should include monitoring of blood pressure (BP), heart rate (HR), and an assessment of fluid responsiveness to determine the patient's cardiovascular stability (**Table 2**).

4.1 Laboratory investigations

In pediatric CRRT, lab monitoring is crucial for safety and effectiveness. Electrolytes (Na, K) are checked every 6–8 hours, BUN and creatinine daily, calcium and magnesium every 8–12 hours, and ionized calcium every 4–6 hours with citrate anticoagulation. In addition, a complete blood count (CBC) and coagulation profile (including PT, aPTT, and INR) are monitored to assess for anemia, infection risk, and bleeding tendencies (**Table 3**).

Parameters	Frequency	Notes
Blood pressure	Every 15–60 min	Adjust ultrafiltration rate accordingly
Heart Rate	Hourly	Tachycardia may indicate hypotension or hypovolemia
Temperature	4 hourly	Check for hypothermia due to extracorporeal circulation
Access pressure	Hourly	High suggests clotting; low may indicate access issues
Return pressure	Hourly	High may indicate filter clotting
Transmembrane pressure	Hourly	Increasing trend = filter clotting
Effluent flow	Hourly	Ensure dose delivery (compare prescribed vs. actual)
Ultrafiltration volume	Hourly	Document net balance, cumulative output
Machine alarm	Continuously	Investigate promptly

*Hemodynamic evaluation: monitoring of blood pressure (BP), heart rate (HR), and an assessment of fluid responsiveness —cardiovascular stability (**Table 2**).*

Table 2.
Monitoring during CRRT: Hourly monitoring (by nurses or PICU staff).

Test	Frequency	Purpose
1. Electrolytes (Na, K)	Every 6–8 hours	Potassium may drop with CRRT; sodium to assess tonicity
2. BUN, creatinine	Daily	Track renal recovery or therapy adequacy
3. Calcium, magnesium	Every 8–12 hours	Important with citrate anticoagulation
4. Ionized calcium	Every 4–6 hours (if citrate)	Monitor systemic anticoagulation effect
5. Hemoglobin, platelets	daily	Assess bleeding risk, circuit clotting
6. Coagulation panel	Daily	Esp. with heparin or liver dysfunction

Table 3.
Blood test monitoring during CRRT.

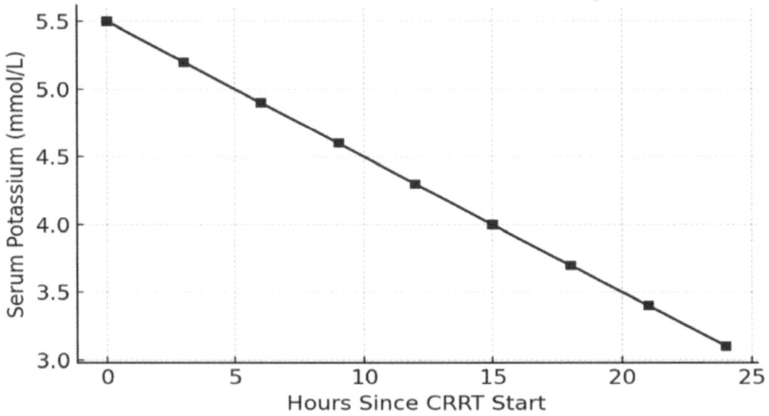

Figure 1.
Serum potassium levels during CRRT: a steady decline in serum potassium within the first 24 hours of CRRT [2, 3].

Serum potassium (K) levels during CRRT shows a steady decline within the first 24 hours of CRRT, emphasizing the need for frequent electrolyte monitoring and supplementation (**Figure 1**).

Fluid balance should be carefully evaluated, with particular attention to the percentage of fluid overload—this is especially critical in pediatric patients. A fluid overload exceeding 10–15% of body weight may indicate the need for urgent CRRT initiation [20].

Fluid overload is a key factor associated with higher mortality in children with acute kidney injury (AKI) who require CRRT. Although the exact physiological mechanism is not fully understood, research consistently demonstrates its impact [13–18].

A large multicenter prospective study showed that survivors had a significantly lower percentage of fluid overload at CRRT initiation compared to non-survivors (14.2 ± 15.9% vs. 25.4 ± 32.9%; $P < 0.03$), even after accounting for illness severity. The study also found that mortality was much higher in patients with fluid overload above 20% (58%) compared to those with less than 20% overload (40%) [16].

Another study of 297 children on renal replacement therapy (RRT) showed a clear link between fluid overload and higher mortality. Death rates increased with the degree of overload: 29.6% with less than 10, 43.1% with 10–20%, and 65.6% with more than 20% fluid overload [18].

Vascular access should be established using an appropriate central venous catheter, with the right internal jugular vein being the preferred site due to its optimal flow characteristics and lower complication rates. Use of ultrasound guidance is recommended to ensure safe and precise catheter placement.

4.2 Vascular access

Smaller vessel size demands ultrasound-guided central access. The Smaller vessel size demands ultrasound-guided central access and frequent monitoring for infection or dislodgement.

Catheter size for CRRT in children is based on weight: <3 kg needs two 5F single-lumen catheters, 3–6 kg use 6.5–7F double-lumen, 6–15 kg use 8F, 15–30 kg use 9–10F, and > 30 kg use 11.5–12.5F double-lumen catheters (**Table 4**).

Weight	Catheter size
< 3 kg	5 F - 2 separate single lumen
3–6 kg	6.5–7 F double lumen
6–15 kg	8 F double lumens
15–30 kg	9–10 F double lumen
> 30 kg	11.5–12.5 F double lumen

Table 4.
Catheter size as per body weight (Adapted from Ref. [4]).

Patient size	Catheter size
Neonate	Dual-lumen 7 French
3–6 kg	Dual-lumen 7 French
6–15 kg	Dual-lumen 8 French
15–30 kg	Dual-lumen 9–10 French
> 30 kg	Dual or triple-lumen 11.5–12.5 French

Table 5.
Catheter size according to the body weight (Adapted from Ref. [4]).

The standard temporary hemodialysis catheter sizes according to the patient's weight for CRRT are used at our hospital as mentioned below (**Table 5**).

4.3 Type and size

The choice of filter in pediatric CRRT depends on the child's weight and the priming volume of the filter. For children under 11 kg, the polysulfone HF 20 filter (60 ml priming volume) is recommended, while those over 30 kg can use the polysulfone HF 1000 (165 ml). The AN 69 M60 filter (93 ml) is suitable for children weighing 11–30 kg, and the AN 69 M100 filter (152 ml) is used for patients over 30 kg. Discontinue all ACE inhibitors if dialysis started with AN69 dialyzer. The filters we use at our hospital as mentioned below (**Tables 6** and **7**).

Extra-corporeal volume [ECV]: The extra-corporeal volume (ECV) in CRRT should be calculated carefully in children. ECV is the amount of blood that stays outside the child's body in the CRRT circuit.

Filter type – (Prismaflex)	Model	Recommended weight range	Priming volume (ml)
Polysulfone	HF 20	< 11 kg	60 ml
Polysulfone	HF 1000	>30 kg	165 ml
AN 69	M60	11–30 kg	93 ml
AN 69	M100	>30 kg	152 ml
Note: Discontinue all ACE inhibitors if dialysis started with AN69 dialyzer.			

Table 6.
Filter type, model, recommended weight, and priming volume (Adopted from Ref. [4]).

Filter set	Surface area (m^2)	Priming volume (ml)	Blood flow range (ml/min)	Max QUF** (ml/hr)	Fluid gain/loss limit (ml/3 h)	Patient's weight (kg)
HF20	0.2	58	20–100	QB 50 = 1020	60–150	0–12 kg
				QB 100 = 1440		
ST 60*	0.6	97 ml	50–180	QB100 = 2340	60–200	12–20 kg
		124 ml (with Thermax)		QB180 = 3360		
HF 1000	1.1	165	80–400	QB100 = 2640	100–400	> 20 kg
		192 (with Thermax)		QB400 = 7620		

**ST membranes are AN69 membranes that are surface coated with polyethylene imine to prevent bradykinin release syndrome). **QUF (Ultrafiltration Rate) = patient fluid removal + replacement flow rate + pre blood pump flow rate.*

Table 7.
Filter set, blood flow, ultrafiltration rate, fluid loss/gain according to the patient's age. (Adopted from Ref. [4]).

A newborn has about 100 ml of blood per kg of body weight, while infants and older children have about 80 ml/kg. To check safety, we calculate 10% of the child's total blood volume.

The ECV is then worked out by adding the volume of the filter set and any extra devices, such as a blood warmer. ECV = Filter set volume (ml) ± Hotline warmer volume (ml).

Extra-Corporeal Volume [ECV] calculations:

a. Patient's blood volume [newborn 100 ml/kg, ≥ infant 80 ml/kg] = … … . … … ml.

b. 10% of patient's blood volume = … … … … …ml.

c. ECV = [Filter set volume]. … … …ml ± [hotline warmer] … … …ml = … … … …ml.

4.4 Pediatric-specific considerations for CRRT prescription

In pediatric patients, especially neonates and infants, fluid balance is a critical aspect of CRRT prescription due to their heightened sensitivity to volume changes. Even small fluctuations in fluid volume can lead to significant clinical consequences, such as hypotension or fluid overload. Therefore, meticulous monitoring and precise fluid management are essential throughout the CRRT process.

To accurately assess fluid removal and replacement, it is important to use pre- and post-filter weight scales (**Figure 2**). These scales provide real-time measurements that help in evaluating the net fluid balance during therapy.

The pre-filter scale records the combined weight of blood and any replacement or anticoagulant fluids entering the CRRT circuit. In contrast, the post-filter scale measures the weight of the fluid and blood exiting the system. By comparing these values, clinicians can determine how much fluid has been removed or retained during the session. This method is particularly valuable in pediatric patients, where tight control of fluid status is vital to prevent complications and ensure effective therapy (**Figure 3**).

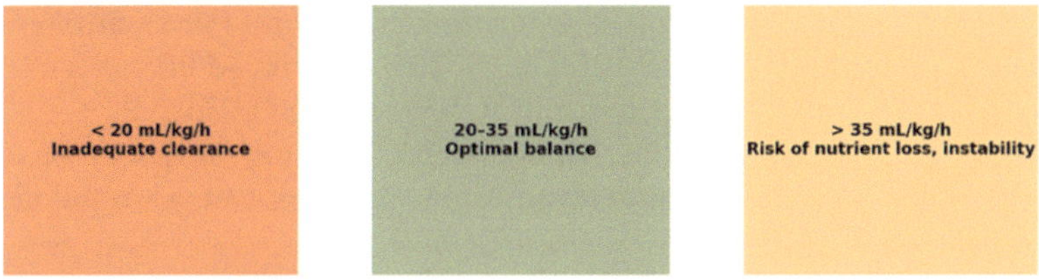

Figure 2.
CRRT dose categories in pediatric patients: The CRRT dose ranges in (mL/kg/h), how they are classified, and their clinical implications to guide appropriate dosing decisions (Adopted from Refs. [4, 12]).

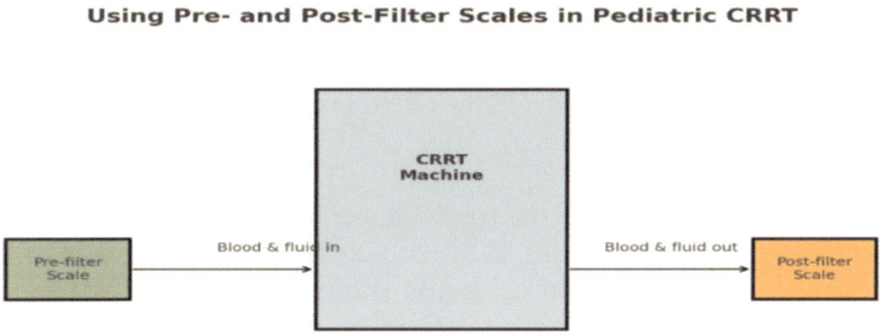

Figure 3.
The above diagram shows how pre-filter and post-filter scales are used during pediatric CRRT [9, 15].

4.5 Blood flow rate, dialysate rate, and ultrafiltration in CRRT

In pediatric CRRT, careful adjustment of blood flow rate (BFR), dialysate rate, and ultrafiltration (UF) rate is essential to ensure effective therapy while minimizing complications.

Blood flow rate (BFR):

In patients undergoing CRRT, it is crucial to adjust the blood flow rate (BFR) appropriately to ensure sufficient clearance [19, 21].

The BFR is calculated based on body weight and usually remains consistent across different CRRT modalities. It ensures sufficient solute clearance and is adjusted using standardized values (**Table 8**).

Blood flow rate (BFR) in CRRT is tailored to the patient's age and size. In practice, a simple approach is followed: Infants require 10–12 mL/kg/min, children 4–6 mL/kg/min, and adolescents 2–4 mL/kg/min. This helps ensure effective therapy while maintaining safety.

Patient weight [Kg]	Blood flow rate [mL/kg/min]
3–6 kg	8–12
6–15 kg	5–8
15–30 kg	4–6
> 30 kg	2–4

Table 8.
BFR as per body weight [4].

Writing the CRRT order sheet, BFR is written in ml/min. For example: HF 20 usually runs at 40–100 ml/min, HF 1000 at 75–200 ml/min, M 60 at 50–80 ml/min, and M 100 at 75–200 ml/min. Maximum BFR 400 ml/min/1.73 m^2.

Above are usual min/max BFR per filter specific. If using Citrate anticoagulation, minimum BFR = 40 ml/ min and maximum BFR = 100 ml/min [to avoid citrate toxicity].

4.6 CRRT dose in pediatrics

In pediatric CRRT, the "dose" refers to the rate at which solutes—such as urea and creatinine—and excess fluids are removed from the child's bloodstream using the CRRT system. This dosing parameter is essential to ensure that critically ill children receive appropriate and effective dialysis support. The prescribed dose must be individualized based on several factors, including the child's body weight, metabolic demands, degree of fluid overload, and the overall solute burden.

The CRRT dose is expressed as the total volume of effluent per kilogram of body weight per hour (mL/kg/hour). Effluent volume includes the sum of all components contributing to clearance: ultrafiltration (fluid removal), dialysate flow (used in CVVHD and CVVHDF), and replacement fluid (administered either before or after the filter). In pediatric practice, the dose is consistently measured in mL/kg/hour to accommodate variations in body size, while in adult settings, the dose may also be expressed as mL/hour or adjusted per kilogram.

Accurate measurement of the patient's body weight is crucial, as it is used to calculate the CRRT dose and guide fluid management throughout therapy.

4.7 Example calculation

A child weighs 20 kg, and the CRRT prescription is for an effluent dose of 30 mL/kg/h: Total effluent per hour = 30 × 20 = 600 mL/h.

This means the machine is set to clear 600 mL of combined waste and fluid from the blood per hour.

The recommended CRRT dose varies by age group. Neonates typically start at 20 mL/kg/h, with a range of 20–35 mL/kg/h, while children usually require 25–35 mL/kg/h due to higher catabolism. Adolescents also need 25–35 mL/kg/h, or about 2–2.5 L/h in larger teens over 50 kg, aligning with adult dosing. Adults are generally treated with 20–25 mL/kg/h (about 1.5–2.5 L/h), unless hypercatabolic (**Table 9**).

Figure 2 below shows CRRT dose categories for pediatric patients. Doses less than 20 mL/kg/h provide inadequate clearance, 20–25 mL/kg/h offer an optimal balance between effectiveness and safety, and doses above 35 mL/kg/h may cause nutrient loss and hemodynamic instability. This classification helps guide appropriate dosing decisions.

4.8 Dialysate rate in CRRT

In diffusion-based CRRT methods like CVVHD and CVVHDF, dialysate fluid helps remove waste by creating a concentration gradient across the filter membrane.

A typical dialysate flow rate of 2000 mL/1.73 m^2/hour or 20–30 mL/kg/hour is usually adequate for most pediatric patients. However, for infants weighing less than 10 kg, dosing should be based on weight to prevent excessive clearance, which can

Patient group	Typical weight-based dose	Alternative expression	Notes
Neonates	20–35 mL/kg/h	—	Start at 20 mL/kg/h and titrate
Children	25–35 mL/kg/h	—	Higher doses needed due to higher catabolism
Adolescents	25–35 mL/kg/h	OR ~ 2–2.5 L/h in large teens	Similar to adult dosing if weight > 50 kg
Adults	20–25 mL/kg/h	~1.5–2.5 L/h total	Standard dose unless hypercatabolic

Table 9.
Recommended CRRT dose by age group (Adopted from Refs. [4, 22]).

lead to nutrient and electrolyte loss. For example, a child with a body surface area of 0.6 m^2 would require a dialysate rate of around 690 mL/hour [4].

Example: If the patient is 0.6 m^2, dialysis rate = 2000 X 0.6/1.73 = 693 » 690 mL/hour.

In cases like drug poisoning or metabolic coma with high ammonia levels, higher dialysate rates (up to 8000 mL/1.73 m^2/hour or 40–60 mL/kg/hour) may be required for faster toxin removal. Adding albumin (2–4 g/dL) to the dialysate can enhance clearance of protein-bound toxins [23–26].

In small children, the use of high-flow dialysate can lead to rapid solute removal, which may increase the risk of electrolyte disturbances. To minimize such risks, medium-flow hemofiltration is generally preferred in the absence of urgent clinical indications for rapid clearance [27, 28]. This approach provides a more controlled and safer therapy, supporting electrolyte stability while ensuring effective solute removal [22, 29].

4.9 Clearance dose in pediatric CRRT

In CVVH, solute clearance is achieved mainly by convection using pre- or post-dilution replacement fluids. In CVVHD, diffusion is the key mechanism, relying on a dialysis fluid flow. CVVHDF combines both convection and diffusion, using replacement fluids (pre- and/or post-dilution) along with dialysis fluid, providing the most efficient clearance. The choice depends on the patient's clinical condition and treatment goals (**Figure 4**).

In CRRT, pre- and post-dilution refer to where the replacement fluid is given in relation to the filter. In pre-dilution, fluid is added before the filter, which helps prevent clotting and prolongs filter life but slightly reduces solute clearance. In post-dilution, fluid is given after the filter, providing better clearance but with a higher risk of filter clotting. CVVH and CVVHDF can use either or both methods, while CVVHD relies only on dialysate flow and does not use dilution (**Figure 4**).

In children receiving CRRT, the clearance (effluent) dose is based on the total effluent volume and adjusted for the child's body surface area (BSA). In CRRT, adjusting the effluent dose to the child's BSA ensures safe and effective solute clearance.

The calculation differs depending on the CRRT modality (CVVH, CVVHD or CVVHDF): Using standardized doses helps tailor therapy to the child's size and clinical needs (**Table 10**).

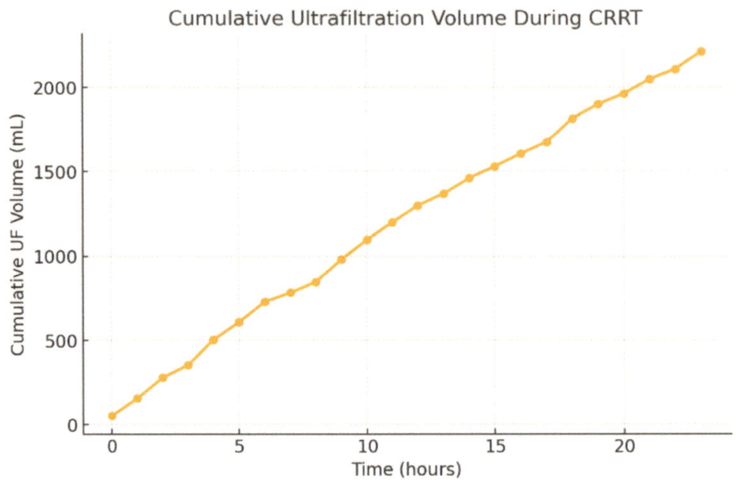

Figure 4.
A graph showing cumulative ultrafiltration volume during CRRT over 24 hours. It demonstrates how fluid removal adds up over time, helping evaluate fluid balance and patient volume status [1, 12].

CRRT modality	Clearance mechanism	Dose (mL/hr)	Standardized dose (mL/hr./m^2)	Target dose in children
CVVH	Convection (replacement fluid)	Replacement fluid rate	Replacement fluid rate ÷ BSA	~2000 mL/1.73 m^2/hr. (~35–40 mL/kg/hr)
CVVHD	Diffusion (dialysate flow)	Dialysate flow rate	Dialysate flow rate ÷ BSA	~2000 mL/1.73 m^2/hr. (~35–40 mL/kg/hr)
CVVHDF	Convection + Diffusion	Replacement fluid rate + Dialysate flow rate	(Replacement fluid rate + Dialysate flow rate) ÷ BSA	~2000 mL/1.73 m^2/hr. (~35–40 mL/kg/hr), split equally between replacement fluid and dialysate

Table 10.
CRRT clearance dose calculation in pediatric patients (Adopted from Ref. [4]).

Table 10 summarizes CRRT clearance dosing for pediatric patients. This table makes it easy to quickly identify the clearance mechanism and how to calculate the dose for each CRRT modality.

Standard dose $= 2000$ ml$/1.73\,m^2$ BSA/hr $= (2000\ X\ \text{BSA})/1{,}73\,m^2 =$ … … … … … .ml/hr.

Recommended CRRT type in pediatric is CVVHDF (dose =50% dialysis and 50% replacement fluid).

5. Dialysis and replacement fluid

In citrate anticoagulation, calcium is removed from the dialysis/replacement fluid to allow citrate to bind calcium effectively and prevent clotting in the extracorporeal circuit (**Figure 5**). Since this lowers systemic calcium, patients require a separate calcium infusion to maintain normal blood calcium levels (**Table 11**).

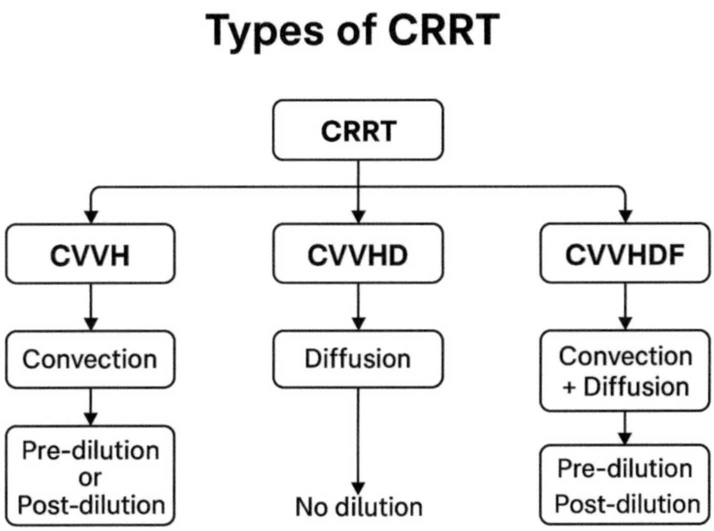

Figure 5.
The main CRRT modalities and method of solute clearance using pre- or post- dilution replacement fluids [3, 6].

Anticoagulation method	Fluid type	Composition (mmol)
Heparin/heparin-free	Hemosol BO	Na 140, K 0, Cl 109.5, HCO_3 32, Ca 1.75, PO_4 0, Mg 0.5
Citrate anticoagulation	PrismaOcal	Na 140, K 0, Cl 109.5, HCO_3 32, Ca 0, PO_4 0, Mg 0.5
Key difference	—	Calcium present in Hemosol BO (1.75 mmol) but absent in PrismaOcal

Table 11.
Dialysis and replacement fluids used in CRRT.

Anticoagulation is necessary to maintain circuit patency; regional citrate anticoagulation is preferred for patients at higher risk of bleeding, while unfractionated heparin may be used in others. A coagulation profile (including PT, aPTT, and INR) is monitored to assess for anemia and bleeding tendencies (**Table 12**).

Type	Monitoring parameter	Comments
Heparin	aPTT, ACT	Risk of bleeding; monitor daily
Citrate	Ionized Ca (systemic and post-filter)	Maintain systemic iCa >1.1 mmol/L
No anticoagulation	Visual inspection	Shorter circuit life; reserved for high bleed risk

Table 12.
Anticoagulation monitoring.

Additive	Amount to add	Instructions/notes	Maximum in bag (per L)
Phosphate (PO_4)	... ... mmol	Add to 5 L bag of dialysis or replacement fluid	1.5 mmol/L
Potassium (K)	... ... mmol	Add to 5 L bag of dialysis or replacement fluid	5 mmol/L
Sodium (Na)	... ... mmol	Add to 5 L bag of dialysis or replacement fluid	5 mmol/L

Note: If mixing phosphate to Ca++ containing solution, mixing of PO4 should be done before starting CRRT [within < 2 hours] to avoid precipitation. Additives should be the same in both dialysate and replacement fluid. Correct low serum Mg, PO4 or K [despite additives] with an IV infusion or TPN.

Table 13.
Additives for dialysis/replacement fluids in CRRT [23].

5.1 Additives

Additives like phosphate, potassium, and sodium are added to dialysis or replacement fluids to maintain the patient's normal blood levels during CRRT. The maximum limits are important to prevent complications such as high potassium (hyperkaliemia) or high phosphate, which can be harmful. Careful adjustment ensures safe and effective therapy (**Table 13**).

6. Clinical importance, monitoring, and adjustment of CRRT dose

The clinical effectiveness of CRRT in pediatric patients depends heavily on delivering an appropriate dose. An insufficient (under-dosed) CRRT prescription may lead to inadequate clearance of metabolic waste products, such as azotemia, metabolic acidosis, or persistent fluid overload.

On the other hand, excessive (over-dosed) therapy can result in unwanted complications, including the loss of essential nutrients, electrolyte disturbances such as hypophosphatemia, and hemodynamic instability due to rapid fluid shifts.

To maintain therapeutic effectiveness and minimize adverse effects, continuous monitoring and timely adjustment of the CRRT dose are essential. The dose should be reassessed regularly based on three key factors: (a) the degree of metabolic control, assessed through laboratory parameters such as urea, creatinine, and lactate levels; (b) the patient's fluid balance, including the degree of fluid overload or dehydration; and (c) the overall clinical condition of the patient, including hemodynamic stability and the level of catabolism. This individualized approach ensures that CRRT remains both safe and effective across the dynamic clinical course of critically ill pediatric patients.

Finally, ultrafiltration targets should be individualized according to the degree of fluid overload and the patient's hemodynamic tolerance. Slow and controlled fluid removal is recommended to avoid hypotension and other complications during therapy.

6.1 Ultrafiltration (UF) rate in CRRT

Ultrafiltration (UF) in a child on CRRT refers to the process of removing excess fluid from the blood through the dialysis filter. It works by applying pressure across the filter membrane, which pushes water (and some dissolved solutes) out of the blood into the effluent.

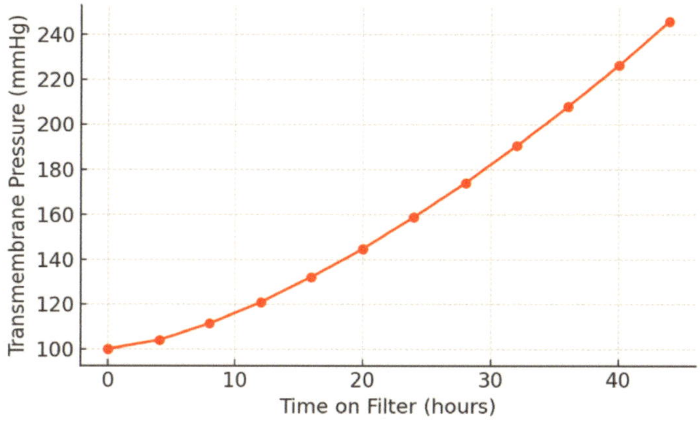

Figure 6.
Filter life vs. transmembrane pressure (TMP): Demonstrates how TMP increases with time, indicating progressive filter clotting [4, 18].

In pediatric patients, UF is carefully prescribed based on the child's weight, hemodynamic status, and fluid overload. The goal is to restore and maintain the right fluid balance—removing extra fluid to relieve edema, control blood pressure, and improve breathing, while avoiding dehydration or low blood pressure.

Monitoring UF rate (mL/kg/hr) and cumulative UF volume over time helps ensure safe and effective therapy.

Cumulative ultrafiltration volume represents the total fluid removed over time during CRRT. Tracking it on a graph provides a clear picture of the patient's fluid removal trend, helping clinicians assess volume status and maintain appropriate fluid balance. It is clearly illustrated in the graph below (**Figure 6**).

CRRT enables effective fluid removal (UF) due to two main factors: continuous operation and the use of highly permeable membranes (**Figure 6**). In pediatric ICU settings, the target UF rate is 1–2 mL/kg/h, which can be increased in stable patients with fluid overload.

The UF rate must also account for ongoing fluid intake and urine output. For example, a 30 kg child receiving 80 mL/h fluid and producing urine at 1 mL/kg/h would require a UF rate of 110 mL/h to maintain fluid balance.

When increasing the UF rate, especially in small children, it is important not to exceed the filtration fraction (FF) limit of 0.35–0.4 to avoid filter clotting.

FF is calculated as the UF rate divided by plasma flow rate. Plasma flow rate depends on BFR and hematocrit:

$$\text{Plasma flow rate} = \text{BFR} \times (1\text{–haematocrit})$$

For instance, in a 10 kg child with BFR of 60 mL/min and hematocrit of 30%, the plasma flow rate is 2520 mL/h, and the maximum safe UF rate would be about 882 mL/h (or ~ 88 mL/kg/h) [4].

For the above example of a 10 kg child with a blood flow rate (BFR) of 60 mL/min and hematocrit of 30%, the plasma flow is calculated as BFR × (1 − Hct), giving 3600 × 0.7 = 2520 mL/h. The maximum safe ultrafiltration (UF) rate depends on the filtration fraction (FF), which is the portion of plasma removed as fluid. For pre-dilution or mixed dilution, FF can go up to 35%, so the maximum UF = 0.35 × 2520 ≈ 882 mL/h (~88 mL/kg/h). In post-dilution only, FF is usually

Scenario	Desired net removal (mL/hr)	Calculation (mL/hr)	UF set (mL/hr)	UF per kg (mL/kg/hr)
Maintain balance	0	80–30 + 0 = 50	50	50 ÷ 30 = 1.7
Gentle removal	10	80–30 + 10 = 60	60	60 ÷ 30 = 2.0
Aggressive removal	60	80–30 + 60 = 110	110	110 ÷ 30 = 3.7

Table 14.
With 3 scenarios for a 30 kg child (Adopted from Refs. [2, 4, 16]).

limited to 20–25%, giving a UF of 630 mL/h (~63 mL/kg/h). These calculations are correct and help ensure safe fluid removal while minimizing the risk of clotting (**Figure 4**).

For another example, for a 30 kg child, fluid removal during CRRT can be tailored based on the clinical goal. To maintain fluid balance, the ultrafiltration (UF) rate is set at 50 mL/hr. (1.7 mL/kg/hr). For gentle fluid removal, the UF is increased to 60 mL/hr. (2.0 mL/kg/hr), and for aggressive removal, it rises to 110 mL/hr. (3.7 mL/kg/hr). These rates are calculated by adjusting the net desired removal along with ongoing fluid intake and urine output.

One-line formula and three different clinical scenarios are shown below (for a 30 kg child) with clear numbers and per-kg rates (**Table 14**)

$$\text{UF (mL/hr)} = \text{Fluid input (mL/hr)} - \text{Urine output (mL/hr)} + \text{Desired net removal (mL/hr)}.$$

(If your goal is simply to maintain balance, set Desired net removal = 0.)

Example with the baseline values (used in **Table 14**): For a 30 kg child receiving 80 mL/hr. of fluids and producing 30 mL/hr. of urine (1 mL/kg/hr), the net positive fluid balance is 50 mL/hr.

With the three clinical scenarios for the same child the net balance guides the ultrafiltration rate during CRRT depending on the desired fluid removal goal as shown below in **Table 14**.

Importantly for a 30 kg child on CRRT, the usual fluid removal rate is about 1–2 mL/kg/hr. Gentle removal at 2 mL/kg/hr. is at the higher end of this range, while aggressive removal at 3.7 mL/kg/hr. is high and should only be done if the child is stable, with careful monitoring of blood pressure, circulation, and electrolytes. Remember to include other fluid losses, like drains or sweating, when deciding the ultrafiltration rate (**Table 14**).

7. Access issues, filter clotting, low BP, and machine alarms during CRRT

During CRRT, common problems include filter clotting, access issues, low blood pressure, electrolyte imbalances, bleeding, and machine alarms. Filter clotting shows as rising pressures and is managed by changing the filter and checking anticoagulation.

Access problems cause low flow and frequent alarms, requiring catheter repositioning or new access. Hypotension is treated by stopping ultrafiltration, giving fluids, and using vasopressors if needed. Electrolyte problems are corrected by adjusting dialysate or replacement fluids, while bleeding may require holding anticoagulation and transfusion. Any machine alarm, like air or blood leak, needs immediate attention following the device protocol (**Table 15**).

Problem	Signs	Action
Filter clotting	↑ TMP, ↑ return pressure	Change filter, check anticoagulation
Access dysfunction	↓ access flow, frequent alarms	Reposition catheter, consider new access
Hypotension	↓ BP, ↑ HR	Stop ultrafiltration, give fluids, vasopressors if needed
Electrolyte imbalance	Muscle twitching, cardiac arrhythmias	Adjust dialysate/replacement fluids
Bleeding	↑ PT/APTT, ↓ Hb	Hold anticoagulation, transfuse if needed
Alarms (air, blood leak)	Audible/visual alarm	Immediate attention; follow machine protocol

Table 15.
Troubleshooting during CRRT.

7.1 Transmembrane pressure (TMP)

TMP gradually rises over time during CRRT, which shows that the filter is starting to clot. By monitoring TMP, clinicians can recognize this change early and decide the right time to replace the filter.

7.2 Nutritional and infection control monitoring in CRRT

Nutritional monitoring is an essential part of managing pediatric patients on CRRT, as the therapy results in ongoing losses of vital nutrients such as amino acids, glucose, and trace elements. Regular assessment of serum protein markers, including albumin and prealbumin, is recommended on a weekly basis to guide nutritional support.

When enteral nutrition is insufficient, parenteral nutrition should be considered to meet the caloric and metabolic demands. Electrolytes like phosphate and potassium, which may be significantly depleted during CRRT, must be closely monitored and supplemented as needed to avoid complications such as hypophosphatemia and hypokalemia.

A proactive and individualized approach helps prevent malnutrition and improves clinical outcomes.

Infection control is equally important during CRRT, particularly in critically ill pediatric patients who are at increased risk of catheter-related bloodstream infections. Daily inspection of the catheter site is important to identify early signs of infection, as prolonged use of central lines and continuous blood circulation through CRRT increases the risk of hospital-acquired infections.

Strict aseptic techniques must be followed during all CRRT-related procedures, including catheter care and filter changes. If sepsis is suspected, cultures from the catheter and CRRT system components should be obtained promptly to identify the infection source and guide appropriate antimicrobial therapy. Early detection and timely intervention are critical to preventing serious, potentially life-threatening infections in.

Daily review and team coordination in CRRT management: The successful management of continuous renal replacement therapy (CRRT) in critically ill pediatric patients depends on regular assessment and strong teamwork among healthcare professionals. A daily, structured review during pediatric intensive care unit (PICU) or intensive care unit (ICU) rounds is crucial to monitor the effectiveness of CRRT, detect complications early, and make timely adjustments based on the patient's changing condition (**Table 16**).

This process requires close coordination between nephrologists, intensivists, critical care nurses, and clinical pharmacists. Each member plays a key role: Nephrologists manage the dialysis prescription and fluid balance; intensivists monitor the patient's overall stability and organ function; nurses maintain the CRRT circuit, monitor patient comfort, and report any concerns, while pharmacists help adjust medication doses considering the continuous clearance by CRRT.

During these reviews, the CRRT prescription—including flow rates, anticoagulation strategy, and replacement fluid volume—should be carefully re-evaluated and modified as needed, based on current lab values, vital signs, and fluid status. This multidisciplinary, patient-centered approach ensures safe and effective CRRT delivery, supports rapid clinical decision-making, and ultimately improves outcomes in critically ill pediatric patients.

In prescribing CRRT for critically ill children, it is important to consider not only fluid and solute removal but also the clearance of medications, antibiotics, and essential nutrients. Because CRRT can significantly alter drug levels and nutritional balance, a multidisciplinary approach involving intensivists, nephrologists, pharmacists, and dietitians is essential to ensure safe drug dosing and adequate nutrition support.

CRRT outcomes are monitored using key targets. Fluid balance is assessed by net ultrafiltration, aiming to restore normal fluid status (euvolemia). Solute control is tracked with BUN, creatinine, and electrolytes, which should remain stable or improve (**Table 16**).

Hemodynamic tolerance is measured by blood pressure and heart rate, with the goal of stability and minimal need for pressors. Circuit patency is checked through transmembrane pressure and alarms, aiming for a filter life of at least 24–48 hours. Finally, kidney recovery is monitored by urine output and creatinine, with improvement indicating return of function (**Table 16**).

The CRRT follow-up chart described by Köker et al. in the *CRRT Protocol in Critically Ill Children* (with permission from Demet Demirkol) serves as a structured tool for systematic monitoring during continuous renal replacement therapy in pediatric patients. It outlines essential parameters such as hemodynamic status, fluid

Target outcome	Parameter	Goal
Fluid balance	Net ultrafiltration	Return to euvolemia
Solute control	BUN, creatinine, electrolytes	Stable or improving values
Hemodynamic tolerance	MAP, HR	Stable with minimal pressor support
Circuit patency	TMP, alarm frequency	≥ 24–48 hours filter life
Recovery of kidney	UOP, creatinine	Spontaneous UOP increase, creatinine improvement

Table 16.
Monitoring outcome.

balance, solute clearance, anticoagulation, and circuit function, ensuring early detection of complications and timely therapy adjustments. This standardized approach promotes safe, effective, and individualized CRRT management in critically ill children.

The chart below demonstrates how to calculate the total fluid removal during CRRT. The total amount of fluid to be extracted is obtained by subtracting the sum of all inputs (column 2, e.g., fluids administered) from the sum of all fluid accumulations or targets (column 1, e.g., excess fluid or desired removal). This simple method provides a structured way to guide ultrafiltration, ensuring accurate fluid balance management.

This simplified workflow illustrates the stepwise approach to CRRT monitoring, beginning with initial patient assessment (hemodynamic status, fluid needs, and lab values), followed by prescription setup (dose, modality, and anticoagulation). It then emphasizes ongoing monitoring of circuit function, solute clearance, and fluid balance, with adjustments based on clinical progress. Finally, daily evaluation ensures therapy goals are met, complications are detected early, and weaning readiness is assessed.

7.3 Weaning of CRRT

Weaning from CRRT depends on several factors, including stable blood pressure, good fluid balance, controlled solute levels, and reduced daily fluid needs. CRRT is often continued in patients needing vasopressors since it is better tolerated for fluid removal than other dialysis methods. Assessing kidney recovery, especially urine output, is central to deciding when to stop CRRT. Although no standard guidelines exist, studies show that higher urine output before stopping CRRT is a strong predictor of success. In adults, a daily urine output of at least 400 mL (or $\sim$ 8.5 mL/kg/24 h) without diuretics and urine output measured shortly after stopping CRRT are good indicators of successful weaning [30]. Outcomes: Successful weaning is linked to improved kidney function, reduced need for ongoing dialysis, and better overall recovery, though close monitoring remains essential [31].

CRRT with extracorporeal membrane oxygenation (ECMO): CRRT can be combined with extracorporeal membrane oxygenation (ECMO) in critically ill children, mainly to prevent or treat fluid overload and to keep solute levels balanced. Acute kidney injury (AKI) occurs in about 40% of children on ECMO, and around 5% may require renal replacement therapy. When CRRT is used with ECMO, the blood flow rate of the CRRT machine should remain independent from the ECMO device, and the arterial access of the CRRT must be adjusted to tolerate positive pressure, as ECMO provides a low-resistance circuit compared to the usual negative pressure setting [4, 16].

8. Conclusion

Monitoring during CRRT is an interdisciplinary effort requiring real-time vigilance and proactive management. Pediatric patients need closer fluid and access monitoring due to their size and fragility. Whether in pediatric-PICU, adolescent and adult ICUs, structured and simplified protocols, and continuous training ensure CRRT remains safe and effective.

Abbreviations

AKI	acute kidney injury
BFR	blood flow rate
CRRT	continuous renal replacement therapy
CVVH	continuous venou-venous hemofiltration
CVVHD	continuous venou venous hemodialysis
CVVHDF	Continuous venou venous hemodiafiltration
ECMO	extra-corporeal membrane oxygenation
ECV	extra-corporeal volume
FO	fluid overload
FF	filtration fraction
HF	hemofiltration
SCUF	slow continuous ultrafiltration
SLED	sustained low-efficiency dialysis
TMP	transmembrane pressure
UF	ultrafiltration

Author details

Mohammad Mateenuddin Quadri[1], Bakri Alali[2] and Nissar Shaikh[2]*

1 Pediatric Nephrology Division, Department of Pediatric, Mubarak Al Kabeer Hospital, Kuwait

2 Surgical Intensive Care, Hamad Medical Corporation, Doha, Qatar

*Address all correspondence to: nissatfirdous99@gmail.com

References

[1] Ronco C, Brendolan A, Bragantini L, et al. Treatment of acute renal failure in newborns by continuous arteriovenous hemofiltration. Kidney International. 1986;**29**:908-915

[2] Bellomo R, Ronco C. Continuous haemofiltration in the intensive care unit. Critical Care. 2000;**4**:339-345

[3] Brush KA, Bilodeau ML. Continuous renal replacement therapy. International Anesthesiology Clinics. 2001;**39**:111-125

[4] Köker A, Yaman A, Akkuzu E, Duyu M, Akçay N, Dalkıran T, et al. Continuous renal replacement therapy (CRRT) protocol in critically ill children. Journal of Pediatric Emergency and Intensive Care Medicine (Turkey). 2024; **11**(1):29-56. DOI: 10.4274/cayd. galenos.2023.71677

[5] Goldstein SL. Overview of pediatric renal replacement therapy in acute renal failure. Artifical Organs. 2003;**27**:781-785

[6] D'Intini V, Ronco C, Bonello M, Bellomo R. Renal replacement therapy in acute renal failure. Best Practice & Research: Clinical Anaesthesiology. 2004;**18**:145-157

[7] Bock KR. Renal replacement therapy in pediatric critical care medicine. Current Opinion in Pediatrics. 2005;**17**: 368-371

[8] Goldstein SL. Continuous renal replacement therapy: Mechanism of clearence, fluid removal, indications and outcomes. Current Opinion in Pediatrics. 2011;**23**:181-185

[9] Kornecki A, Tauman R, Lubetzky L, Sivan Y. Continuous renal replacement therapy for non-renal indications: Experience in children. The Israel Medical Association Journal. 2012;**4**: 345-348

[10] Bouchard J, Soroko SB, Chertow GM, et al. Fluid accumulation, survival and recovery of kidney function in critically ill patients with acute kidney injury. Kidney International. 2009;**76**: 422-427

[11] Payen D, de Pont AC, Sakr Y, et al. A positive fluid balance is associated with a worse outcome in patients with acute renal failure. Critical Care. 2008;**12**: R74

[12] Brandstrup B, Tonnesen H, Beier-Holgersen R, et al. Effects of intravenous fluid restriction on postoperative complications: Comparison of two perioperative fluid regimens: A randomized assessor-blinded multicenter trial. Annals of Surgery. 2003;**238**:641-648

[13] Foland JA, Fortenberry JD, Warshaw BL, et al. Fluid overload before continuous hemofiltration and survival in critically ill children: A retrospective analysis. Critical Care Medicine. 2004; **32**:1771-1776

[14] Gillespie RS, Seidel K, Symons JM. Effect of fluid overload and dose of replacement fluid on survival in hemofiltration. Pediatric Nephrology. 2004;**19**:1394-1399

[15] Goldstein SL, Currier H, Graf C, et al. Outcome in children receiving continuous venovenous hemofiltration. Pediatrics. 2001;**107**:1309-1312

[16] Goldstein SL, Somers MJ, Baum MA, et al. Pediatric patients with multiorgan dysfunction syndrome receiving continuous renal replacement therapy. Kidney International. 2005;**67**:653-658

[17] Hayes LW, Oster RA, Tofil NM, et al. Outcomes of critically ill children requiring continuous renal replacement therapy. Journal of Critical Care. 2009; **24**:394-400

[18] Sutherland SM, Zappitelli M, Alexander SR, et al. Fluid overload and mortality in children receiving continuous renal replacement therapy: The prospective pediatric continuous renal replacement therapy registry. American Journal of Kidney Diseases. 2010;**55**:316-325

[19] Pedersen O, Jepsen SB, Toft P. Continuous renal replacement therapy for critically ill infants and children. Danish Medical Journal. 2012; **59**:A4385

[20] Khwaja A. KDIGO clinical practice guidelines for acute kidney injury. Nephron Clinical Practice. 2012;**120**(4): c179-c184. DOI: 10.1159/000339789

[21] Sutherland SM, Alexander SM. Continuous renal replacement therapy in children. Pediatric Nephrology. 2012;**27**: 2007-2016

[22] Askenazi DJ, Goldstein SL, Koralkar R, Frontberry J, Baum M, et al. Continuous renal replacement therapy for children ≤10 kg: A report from the prospective pediatric continuous renal replacement registry. The Journal of Pediatrics. 2013;**162**:587-92. e3

[23] McBryde KD, Kershaw DB, Bunchman TE, Maxvold NJ, Mottes TA, et al. Renal replacement therapy in the treatment of confirmed or suspected inborn errors of metabolism. The Journal of Pediatrics. 2006;**148**:7708

[24] Demirkol D, Aktuğlu ZÇ, Karacabey BN, Cesur Y, Ataman Y, et al. The role of supportive treatment in the management of hyperammonemia in neonates and infants. Blood Purification. 2019;**48**:150-157

[25] Eminoğlu TF, Öncül Ü, Kahveci F, Okulu E, Kraja E, et al. Characteristics of continuous venovenous hemodiafiltration in the acute treatment of inherited metabolic disorders. Pediatric Nephrology. 2022;**37**:1387-1397

[26] Aygün F, Kıykım E, Aktuğlu-Zeybek Ç, Zubarioğlu T, Cam H. Treatment of maple syrup urine disease with high-flow hemodialysis in a neonate. The Turkish Journal of Pediatrics. 2019;**61**: 107-110

[27] Santiago MJ, López-Herce J, Urbano J, Solana MJ, del Castillo J, et al. Complications of continuous renal replacement therapy in critically ill children: A prospective observational evaluation study. Critical Care. 2009;**13**: R184

[28] Palmieri TL. Complications of continuous renal replacement therapy in children are all created equal. Critical Care. 2010;**14**:105

[29] Gün E, Gurbanov A, Nakip ÖS, Yöntem A, Aslan AD, et al. Clinical characteristics, and outcomes of continuous renal replacement therapy performed on young children weighing up to 10 kg. Turkish Journal of Medical Sciences. 2023;**53**:791-802

[30] Gautam SC, Srialluri N, Jaar BG. Strategies for continuous renal replacement therapy de-escalation. Kidney360. 2021;**2**(7):1166-1169

[31] Haddad M, Butani L. Continuous renal replacement therapy in children. Indian Pediatrics. 2025;**62**:295-299. DOI: 10.1007/s13312-025-00026-4 [Accessed: March 21, 2025]

Chapter 4

Hemodynamic Challenges in Critically Ill Patients with Cirrhosis

Aanchal Kapoor

Abstract

Cirrhosis profoundly alters cardiovascular physiology, creating unique challenges in diagnosis and treatment circulatory shock. In patients with advanced liver disease, portal hypertension, splanchnic vasodilation, and hyperdynamic circulation reduce effective arterial blood volume, while cirrhotic cardiomyopathy limits cardiac reserve. Together, these changes complicate hemodynamic assessment and undermine the applicability of standard sepsis algorithms. Conventional markers of shock, including targeted mean arterial pressure and serum lactate levels, can be misleading because cirrhotic patients often tolerate lower baseline pressures and exhibit impaired lactate clearance. Fluid resuscitation carries a high risk of volume overload; albumin has demonstrated improvements in short-term hemodynamic parameters but not consistent survival benefits. Norepinephrine is the first-line vasopressor, while vasopressin analogues are considered in refractory cases or when hepatorenal physiology predominates. Emerging tools such as bedside ultrasound and the Venous Excess Ultrasound (VExUS) score may aid in differentiating hypovolemia from venous congestion. Acute-on-chronic liver failure, frequently precipitated by infection, exemplifies the complex interplay of systemic inflammation, circulatory collapse, and multiorgan failure in this population. Optimal management therefore requires an individualized, physiology-driven approach emphasizing cautious fluid administration, tailored vasopressor use, and serial assessment of tissue perfusion. Future trials focused on cirrhotic populations are essential to refine resuscitation targets and improve survival outcomes.

Keywords: cirrhosis, advanced liver disease, chronic liver failure, portal hypertension, systemic vascular resistance (SVR), cirrhotic cardiomyopathy, hyperdynamic circulation, vasodilatation, multiorgan failure

1. Introduction

Cirrhosis and advanced liver disease remain major global health burdens, representing the final stage of diverse hepatic injuries including viral hepatitis, alcohol-associated liver disease, and metabolic dysfunction-associated steatohepatitis (MASH). Recent data from the United States Nationwide Inpatient Sample highlights the growing prevalence and impact of this critical care challenge [1, 2]. Worldwide, cirrhosis contributes to substantial morbidity and mortality, accounting for an estimated 1.3–1.5 million deaths annually, ranking it among the top 15 causes of death globally [3].

Chronic liver disease leads to approximately 700,000 hospitalizations and 44,000 deaths each year. Among those admitted for cirrhosis-related complications, about 10% require intensive care unit (ICU) admission. Mortality among critically ill patients with cirrhosis remain high, with reported ICU-related death rates ranging from 29 to 87% [4].

Cirrhosis is a systemic disease with profound cardiovascular consequences. Portal hypertension, splanchnic vasodilation, hyperdynamic circulation, and cirrhotic cardiomyopathy interact to create a hemodynamic state that complicates both diagnosis and management of circulatory shock. Bacterial translocation from the gut, impaired reticuloendothelial clearance, and immune dysfunction create a "cirrhosis-associated immunodeficiency" [5]. Because of this immunocompromised state, these patients remain at high risk for developing infections in their hospital course.

Sepsis is the leading trigger of acute decompensation in cirrhosis and is responsible for up to 40% of hospitalizations [6]. Mortality rates for septic shock exceed 50% in this group, far higher than in the general ICU population, in part because of the overlapping pathophysiology of cirrhosis and sepsis, and also because of limitations of conventional diagnostic and therapeutic strategies when applied to this population [7].

Acute-on-chronic liver failure (ACLF) is a distinct clinical syndrome that develops in patients with underlying cirrhosis, most commonly following an infectious trigger. It is characterized by rapid development of multiorgan failure and carries a high short-term mortality, often exceeding 40% at 28 days [8–10]. Standard septic shock definitions and management protocols have been derived from non-cirrhotic populations and may not adequately account for these unique physiological alterations. This review synthesizes the current evidence on the pathophysiology of hemodynamic changes in cirrhosis, highlights diagnostic pitfalls in recognizing shock, and discusses management strategies tailored to cirrhotic physiology.

2. Pathophysiology of hemodynamic alterations in cirrhosis

The hemodynamic disturbances in cirrhosis arise from two interrelated mechanisms: increased intrahepatic resistance to portal blood flow and a hyperdynamic circulatory state driven by splanchnic vasodilation. This dual process sustains and perpetuates portal hypertension, driving the development of gastroesophageal varices, ascites, and other key manifestations of decompensated state as described below.

2.1 Portal hypertension and increased resistance

Portal hypertension, a defining feature of cirrhosis, develops from both structural changes, such as fibrosis, sinusoidal capillarization, and dynamic alterations within the hepatic vasculature resulting from sinusoidal endothelial dysfunction and increased intrahepatic vascular tone. Endothelial cell dysfunction leads to decreased production and bioavailability of nitric oxide (NO) and increased production of vasoconstrictors such as thromboxane A_2 and endothelin-1. In parallel, activation of hepatic stellate cells (HSCs) drives phenotypic and cellular changes that promote fibrosis and angiogenesis [11]. Conversely, splanchnic vasodilation reduces effective circulatory blood volume, triggering the activation of renin-angiotensin-aldosterone system (RAAS) and increased secretion of antidiuretic hormone (ADH). These responses promote sodium and water retention further augmenting portal blood flow. The combination of increased flow and resistant results in portal hypertension as shown in **Figure 1**.

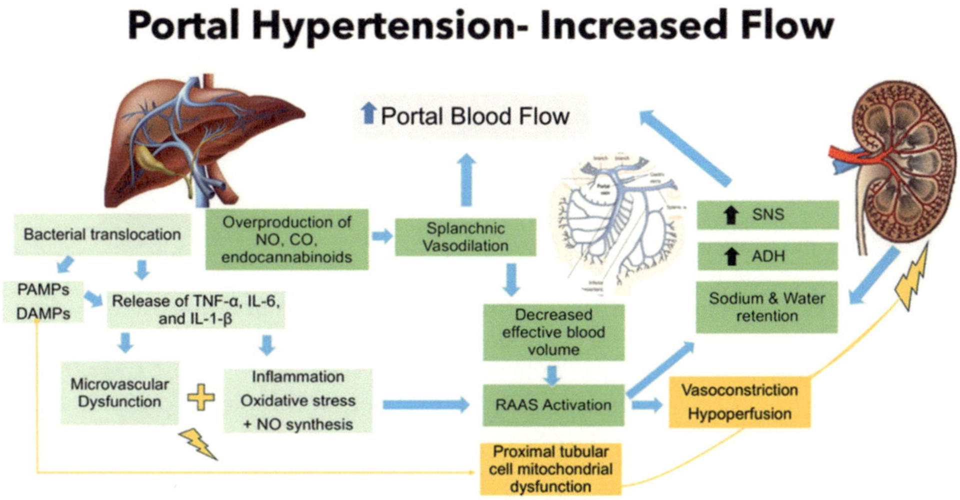

Figure 1.
Mechanisms leading to increase in portal flow (Designed by the author).

Together, these processes increase intrahepatic resistance to portal blood flow, ultimately fostering collateral vessel formation and portosystemic shunting [12].

2.2 Hyperdynamic circulation

Patients with cirrhosis frequently develop a hyperdynamic circulatory state. Hyperdynamic circulation was first described in 1953 when investigators noted that patients with cirrhosis had cardiac outputs 50–75% above normal at rest [12]. This hyperdynamic condition is characterized by elevated heart rate and cardiac output accompanied by a reduction in systemic vascular resistance (SVR) [13].

Hyperdynamic circulation develops because of systemic vasodilation, particularly within splanchnic circulation. This splanchnic vasodilatation is driven by several vasoactive substances, including NO, carbon monoxide, endocannabinoids, and other vasoactive mediators. As a result, there is an increase in venous capacitance and expansion of the unstressed venous volume, which reduces mean systemic filling pressure (MSFP). Peripheral vasodilation and portosystemic shunting decrease afterload, while activation of neurohormonal activation including RAAS and sympathetic nervous system promote sodium and water retention. Arteriovenous shunting increases blood flow per unit time but does not necessarily improve tissue oxygen delivery. Although initially compensatory, this state becomes maladaptive as the cardiovascular system has little reserve to increase output further when faced with sepsis or hemorrhage.

Venous return to the heart depends on the gradient between MSFP and right atrial pressure (RAP) determines venous return to the heart as depicted in the equation.

$$\mathrm{MSFP} - \mathrm{RAP} = \mathrm{CO} \times \mathrm{VR} \tag{1}$$

where CO In this equation is venous return and VR is venous resistance.

In cirrhosis, this gradient narrows, impairing preload despite extracellular volume expansion. This pattern predisposes to reduced effective arterial blood volume despite expanded total body water and increased extracellular fluid. This results in hypotension, renal hypoperfusion, and difficulty in maintaining effective arterial blood volume.

Clinically, this explains the paradox of patients presenting with tense ascites and peripheral edema but remaining intravascularly depleted and highly preload responsive.

2.3 Cirrhotic cardiomyopathy (CCM)

Cirrhotic cardiomyopathy (CCM) is characterized by a triad of impaired cardiac contractility in response to stress, diastolic dysfunction, and electrophysiologic abnormalities, arising within the setting of a hyperdynamic state [14]. CCM often remains asymptomatic for years, as resting cardiac output is typically preserved and the disease progresses slowly. It comes to clinical attention during the decompensation stage of cirrhosis with features of diastolic dysfunction. This makes it difficult to accurately determine the true prevalence of CCM. However, it is estimated that about 50% of patients with cirrhosis do have underlying CCM. The impaired cardiac performance likely reflects a blunted chronotropic response to exercise and reduced myocardial contractile reserve, while concomitant skeletal muscle wasting further limits peripheral oxygen extraction and effective oxygen utilization.

2.3.1 Systolic dysfunction

Pathophysiologically, splanchnic vasodilatation reduced central and arterial blood volume leading to deactivation of arterial baroreceptors and increased sympathetic activity. Chronic overstimulation results in desensitization of β-adrenergic receptors through uncoupling of G proteins, down-regulation of β-adrenergic receptors and altered β-adrenergic signaling. In addition, up-regulation of cardio depressant cannabinoid 1-receptors, along with increase cardio-inhibitory effect of mediators like hemoxygenase (HO), carbon monoxide (CO), nitric oxide synthase (NOS)-induced NO release, and tumor necrosis factor-α (TNF-α) contributes to systolic dysfunction and poor cardiac response to stress [15].

2.3.2 Diastolic dysfunction

Diastolic dysfunction in CCM results from structural and molecular alterations, including an increased proportion of stiffer collagen type I, and reduction in the more compliant collagen III, decreased phosphorylation of protein titin which is a scaffold protein essential for myofibrillar elasticity, cardiomyocyte hypertrophy, cardiac fibroblast proliferation, and fibrosis driven by sodium retention and activation of RAAS [16].

2.3.3 Electrophysiological abnormalities

Prolongation of QT interval is observed in approximately 40–50% patients with advanced cirrhosis. Studies have shown that its prevalence increases substantially with disease severity, rising from Child-Pugh class A to B [17]. Clinically, cardiac dysfunction is observed in up to 50% of patients following liver transplantation, with peri-transplant heart failure contributing to mortality in approximately 7–21% of cases [18]. **Figure 2** summarizes mechanisms involved in cardiac dysfunction in cirrhosis.

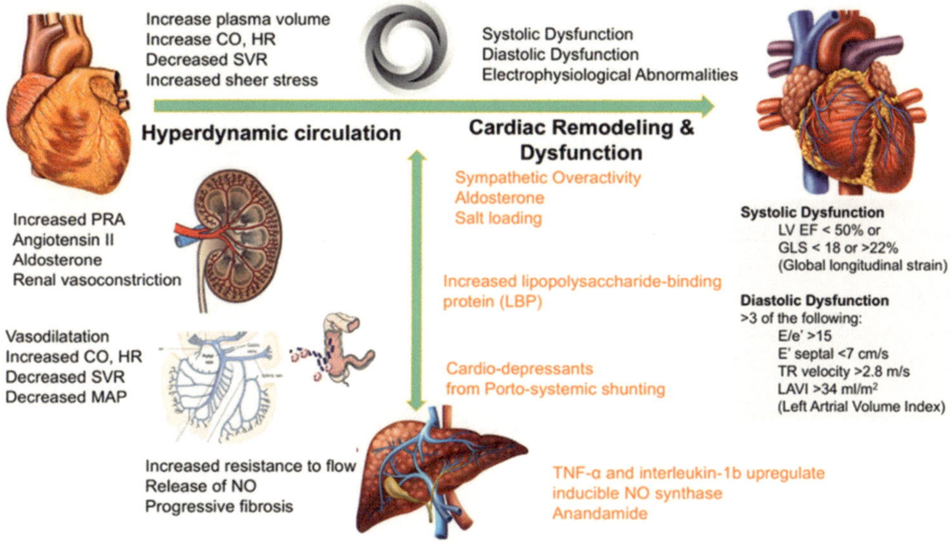

Figure 2.
Summarizing mechanisms causing cardiac dysfunction in cirrhosis (designed by the author).

These factors shift baseline hemodynamics: cirrhotic patients often tolerate MAPs of 55–60 mmHg chronically, have elevated lactate at baseline, and manifest fluid overload sometimes even before resuscitation. In septic shock, cirrhotic cardiomyopathy blunts the ability to augment contractility in response to vasopressor-induced afterload, further complicating management. Standard septic shock algorithms, including the use of a 30 mL/kg crystalloid bolus and targeting a mean arterial pressure of 65 mmHg, were developed based on studies conducted in the general intensive care unit (ICU) population. When applied unmodified to cirrhotic patients, these recommendations may result in harmful fluid overload, inadequate recognition of hypoperfusion, or inappropriate escalation of vasopressor therapy.

3. Diagnostic challenges in assessing shock in cirrhosis

Standard hemodynamic indices in use to assess circulatory shock in non-cirrhotic population may mislead the approach to diagnosis and hence the therapeutic strategies.

3.1 Definition of septic shock

International guidelines for management of sepsis and septic shock defines septic shock as hypotension that persists after adequate fluid resuscitation accompanied by a serum lactate concentration greater than 2 mmol/L [19]. However, applying these criteria in patients with cirrhosis could be challenging. Many patients live chronically with mean arterial pressures of 55–60 mmHg without overt hypoperfusion, raising uncertainty over which blood pressure thresholds indicate shock. The TARGET-C randomized trial evaluated the effects of higher mean arterial pressure targets (80–85 mmHg) compared with standard targets (65–70 mmHg) in patients with cirrhosis experiencing septic shock. Although higher targets improved renal outcomes in some subgroups, no mortality benefit was observed, suggesting that MAP thresholds should be individualized rather than universally raised above 65 [20].

3.2 Interpretation of serum lactate and designing interventions accordingly

Septic shock is defined using lactate levels and is also used as a resuscitation target [21]. Lactate is elevated in cirrhosis even without hypoperfusion due to decreased hepatic clearance and increased splanchnic production. Studies show that lactate rises after meals or galactose challenge in cirrhotic, independent of hypoxia [22] While elevated lactate retains sensitivity for detecting severe illness, its specificity for tissue hypoxia and mortality prediction is reduced. Interpretation should therefore emphasize trends and clearance over absolute cut-offs [23].

3.3 Challenges with hemodynamic concepts: Mean systemic filling pressure and stressed volume

3.3.1 Mean systemic filling pressure and stressed volume

Advanced hemodynamic concepts—particularly mean systemic filling pressure (MSFP) and stressed volume—provide important insights into why assessing volume responsiveness in cirrhosis is uniquely challenging. MSFP represents the equilibrium pressure in the systemic circulation when cardiac activity ceases. It is determined by both venous tone and the volume of blood actively contributing to generate circulatory pressure, known as the stressed volume [24].

Traditional concepts of preload/afterload can be refined using Guyton's venous return model. According to this model, venous return is governed by the pressure gradient between MSFP and RAP, with the rate of return further modulated by resistance to venous flow, as described before.

$$\text{MSFP} - \text{RAP} = \text{CO} \times \text{VR} \tag{2}$$

In cirrhosis, profound changes in vascular compliance and blood volume distribution alter this relationship. Splanchnic vasodilation increases the proportion of unstressed volume (blood contained in compliant venous reservoirs that does not generate pressure), thereby lowering effective MSFP even when total blood volume is normal or increased. RAP, in turn, functions as a backpressure to venous return. A combination of reduced MSFP and elevated RAP impairs the pressure gradient for venous return, thereby limiting cardiac output.

Clinically, this explains the paradox frequently observed in cirrhotic patients: they may appear "volume-overloaded" on examination, with ascites and peripheral edema, yet remain hypotensive and preload-responsive. Attempts to increase stressed volume by fluid resuscitation often fail to raise MSFP effectively because the infused fluid preferentially redistributes into the splanchnic venous reservoir or the extravascular space rather than augmenting effective circulating volume (**Figure 3**). As a result, cirrhotic patients may not respond to fluids as predicted by standard preload concepts, underscoring the importance of cautious resuscitation and reliance on advanced hemodynamic monitoring to guide therapy.

Operating point A of Guyton's curve (Orange-Guyton venous return and Red-Starling cardiac function curve) indicates normal physiology in compensated cirrhosis. Point B (Blue-Guyton venous return and Red-Starling cardiac function

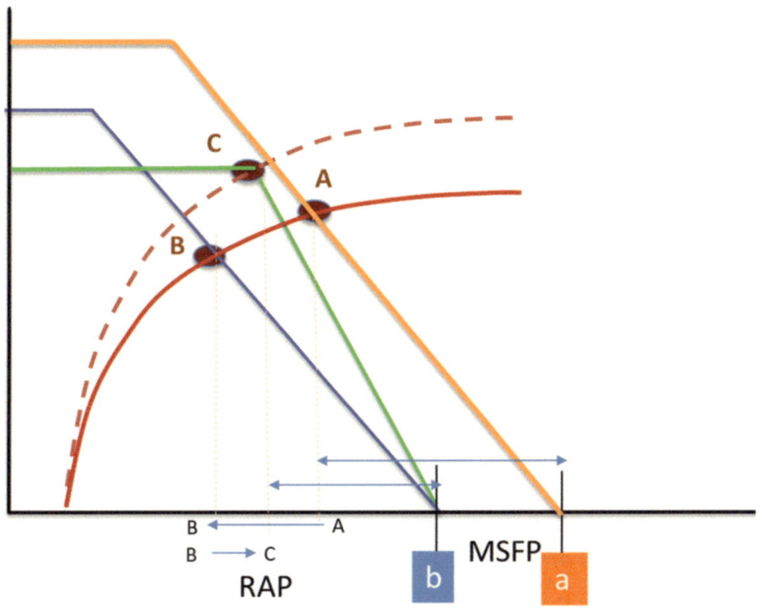

Figure 3.
Altered physiology in cirrhosis depicted by venous return and cardiac function curves (designed by the author).

curve) indicates a drop in MSFP from A to B, with the same cardiac output. This decrease in MSFP is because of splanchnic vasodilatation and decreased effective circulating volume, causing decrease in RAP from A to B. Point C (Green-Guyton venous return and Dotted-red-Starling cardiac function curve) indicates an increase in the cardiac output with the same MSFP but with increased slope of venous return. This change is due to a decrease in afterload and increase in water retention with activation of RAAS and sympathetic stimulation. This results in an increase in RAP from B to C, thus decreasing the gradient between MSFP and RAP causing a decrease in venous return.

MSFP = mean systemic filling pressure, RAP = right atrial pressure, RAAS = renin-angiotensin-aldosterone system.

3.3.2 Critical closing pressure (Pcrit)

Pcrit is the arterial pressure at which vessels collapse, and flow ceases. As the blood flows down the arterial tree towards the terminal arterioles, flow velocity increases, while the vessel diameter decreases, resulting in rapid drop in pressure due to rising resistance. Once the local arteriolar pressure falls below the level required to overcome vasomotor tone, the vessel collapses, and blood flow stops. This closing pressure is defined as Pcrit. Pcrit is usually higher than MSFP. Standard SVR calculations that use CVP as downstream pressure may therefore underestimate true afterload.

$$\text{SVR} = \text{MAP} - \text{CVP}/\text{CO} \text{ instead of } \text{SVR} = \text{MAP} - \text{Pcrit}/\text{CO} \qquad (3)$$

Tissue perfusion pressure is better represented by (MAP – Pcrit) rather than (MAP – CVP) [25].

In patients with cirrhosis, global Pcrit is lower because of peripheral vasodilatation. Although it theoretically should increase local tissue perfusion, it also causes a proportional decrease in MAP, and autoregulation of blood flow to the tissue is blunted [26].

These concepts explain why standard formulas for SVR and preload often mislead in cirrhotic patients.

3.4 Alternative strategies to diagnose shock in patients with end stage liver disease

Diagnosing shock in patients with advanced cirrhosis poses unique challenges because the conventional criteria used in critical care do not reliably capture the altered physiology of this population. As discussed above, MAP thresholds are problematic as many cirrhotic patients live chronically with MAPs in the range of 55–60 mmHg without overt tissue hypoperfusion. Similarly, lactate levels are frequently elevated due to impaired hepatic clearance and increased splanchnic production, even in the absence of systemic hypoxia. Central venous pressure, long used as a surrogate for preload, is often misleading because intra-abdominal hypertension, altered venous compliance, and redistribution of blood volume distort its relationship with effective circulating volume. Given these limitations, alternate diagnostic strategies are increasingly necessary. A few of them are listed below.

Capillary refill time and Mottling score: Bedside clinical perfusion markers may offer more reliable guidance. The ANDROMEDA-SHOCK trial demonstrated that targeting resuscitation to peripheral perfusion indices, particularly capillary refill time, improved organ dysfunction compared with lactate-targeted resuscitation [27]. The mottling score, a semiquantitative measure of cutaneous hypoperfusion, has been shown to be a strong predictor of short-term mortality independent of vasopressor dose [28].

These markers, together with urine output and mental status, are valuable adjuncts in cirrhotic patients where traditional biochemical markers may mislead.

Invasive hemodynamic monitoring: Use of arterial catheters for continuous blood pressure monitoring and frequent blood sampling for lactate and gases can provide dynamic assessment. Central venous catheters allow the measurement of central venous oxygen saturation (ScVO2) and central venous-arterial CO_2 gap, both of which can provide valuable insights into adequacy of tissue perfusion [29]. However, central venous pressure alone is of limited value in cirrhosis given altered vascular compliance and elevated abdominal pressure with ascites.

Point-of-care ultrasound (POC): Cardiac function including contractility and volume status can be assessed at bedside by point of care echocardiography. Assessment of intravascular volume, by estimating RAP from inferior venous cava (IVC) collapsibility index, can help guide fluid management. Lung ultrasound is particularly useful for detecting pulmonary edema. Building on these assessments, the venous excess ultrasound (VExUS) grading system offers a more advanced and integrative approach to venous congestion. VExUS combines IVC assessment with Doppler waveforms analysis of hepatic, portal, and intrarenal veins to quantify venous congestion. Higher VExUS scores have been associated with increased degree of venous overload. Higher VExUS scores have been correlated with elevated venous pressures and with increased risk of developing acute kidney injury (AKI). This is especially relevant in patients with cirrhosis, where distinguishing between hypovolemia and venous congestion can be challenging. Early studies suggest that VExUS not only correlates with AKI risk but may also help identify fluid intolerance, providing a valuable non-invasive tool to guide hemodynamic and fluid management in cirrhosis-associated AKI [30].

Ventriculo-arterial coupling: It is a dynamic assessment with the use of pressors and inotropes. Ventriculo-arterial coupling (the ratio of arterial elastance to ventricular elastance, Ea/Ees) refers to assessment of energy transfer between cardiac pump and downstream arterial tree. Septic patients often show ventriculo-arterial decoupling [31]. Arterial elastance reflects left ventricular (LV) afterload, whereas ventricular elastance serves as an index of myocardial contractility. Ea/Ees represents the relationship between arterial elastance (Ea) and end systolic elastance of LV (Ees). For bedside measurement, single beat method is used [32]. Ees can be estimated noninvasively using systolic and diastolic blood pressure measurements in conjunction with echocardiographic parameters, including stroke volume (SV), ejection fraction (EF), pre-ejection time, and total ejection time. Ea is derived by dividing 90% of the systolic blood pressure (SBP) by SV according to the formula:

$$\mathrm{Ea} = (0.9 \times \mathrm{SBP}) / \mathrm{SV}. \tag{4}$$

An optimal Ea/Ees ratio indicates effective energy transfer from the ventricle to the arterial system, whereas an increased ratio suggests impaired coupling due to either reduced contractility or elevated afterload. Ventriculo-arterial decoupling may be accentuated in patients with CCM. Systemic vasodilatation and hence low SVR altered vascular compliance, and blunted myocardial contractile reserve can alter this relationship and limit the heart's ability to respond to hemodynamic and physiological stress. A high left ventricular ejection fraction (LVEF) and low Ea is indicative of hyperdynamic circulatory state, a pattern commonly observed in patients with advanced cirrhosis. In such cases, if clinical signs of poor perfusion are present, vasopressor therapy might be warranted to restore vascular tone and improve perfusion. However, increasing Ea with vasopressor use may lead to reduction in LVEF in patients with underlying CCM. Under these circumstances, the addition of an inotrope agent may be necessary to support cardiac output [33].

4. Management of shock in cirrhosis

In cirrhosis, the constellation of splanchnic vasodilation, activation of RAAS, and reduced systemic vascular resistance leads to sequestration of circulating blood volume within the splanchnic bed. This pathophysiology, coupled with a chronic hyperdynamic circulation that can evolve into cirrhotic cardiomyopathy, complicates the prediction of hemodynamic responses to interventions such as fluid resuscitation and vasopressor therapy. Standard septic shock algorithms, recommending resuscitation with 30 mL/kg crystalloid bolus and targeting a MAP of 65 mmHg, were studied in general ICU populations. Applied unmodified to patients with cirrhosis, these protocols may result in detrimental fluid overload, delayed recognition of tissue hypoperfusion, or inappropriate escalation of vasopressors. Consequently, management strategies in cirrhotic patients require individualized assessment of volume status, perfusion, and cardiac function to optimize outcomes.

4.1 MAP targets

Evidence on optimal MAP in cirrhosis is evolving. The TARGET-C randomized trial compared higher (80–85 mmHg) vs. standard (65–70 mm Hg) MAP targets in patients with cirrhosis and septic shock. While routine use of higher MAP goal did not confer a survival benefit, certain subgroups such as patients with severe renal hypoperfusion or HRS physiology may experience transient hemodynamic improvement with higher perfusion pressures [21]. However, the benefit must be weighed against the risk of excessive vasoconstriction and peripheral ischemia. Current practice is to individualize MAP targets (e.g., consider higher targets for renal protection if signs of ongoing renal hypoperfusion, while monitoring for harms from excessive vasoconstriction).

4.2 Fluid resuscitation

The Surviving Sepsis Campaign recommends an initial 30 mL/kg crystalloid bolus for patients with septic shock [20]. However, in patients with cirrhosis, aggressive crystalloid resuscitation carries a heightened risk of fluid overload, worsening ascites, and developing pulmonary edema. The positive cumulative fluid balance is strongly associated with mortality [34, 35]. A more conservative approach using small boluses of 250–500 mL with frequent reassessment (clinical perfusion markers, ultrasound, and dynamic hemodynamic tests) is prudent.

Albumin has theoretical advantages in cirrhosis (oncotic effect, anti-inflammatory properties, and improved endothelial function). A randomized trial with comparing 5% albumin with saline (FRISC trial) demonstrated that albumin administration improved MAP, enhanced lactate clearance, increased urine output, and better short-term survival compared to saline [36]. Similarly, the ALPS trial, which evaluated 20% albumin, showed earlier vasopressor independence, faster hemodynamic improvements, and lactate clearance; however, no significant 28-day survival benefit was observed. The albumin group experienced higher rates of pulmonary complications [37] in the albumin arm. These data support considering albumin as part of resuscitation in selected cirrhotic patients but emphasize close monitoring for pulmonary complications and individualized decision-making (**Table 1**).

4.3 Vasopressor support

As indicated before, fluid resuscitation might not assist in increasing MSFP and can result in fluid overload in patients with cirrhosis, and a careful assessment should

Trial	Population	Intervention	Main findings	Notes
FRISC [36]	Cirrhosis + septic shock	5% albumin vs saline	↑ MAP, lactate clearance, short-term survival	Pulmonary edema rare
ALPS [37]	Cirrhosis + sepsis hypotension	20% albumin vs plasmalyte	↑ vasopressor-free at 6h, no survival difference	Pulmonary complications higher in albumin

Table 1.
Summary of key fluid resuscitation trials in cirrhosis and shock.

be performed to initiate pressors early. Early initiation of vasopressor therapy has been shown to accelerate resolution of shock [38], whereas delayed administration is associated with increased mortality. In fact, each hour of delay is estimated to increase the risk of death by approximately 5.3% [39]. Based on head-to-head randomized controlled trials (RCTs) comparing adrenergic vasopressors, the Surviving Sepsis Campaign (SSC) recommends norepinephrine as the first-line agent for the management of septic shock [19]. However, most of these RCTs included fewer than 10% of patients with underlying liver disease.

Norepinephrine remains the first-line vasopressor for septic shock, but cirrhotic patients with cirrhosis may demonstrate an enhanced response to vasopressin or terlipressin due to preserved vascular V1 receptor sensitivity [40]. Terlipressin, a selective V1 receptor agonist, has been proposed as an alternative vasopressor in this patient population with septic shock. In a small RCT, terlipressin showed comparable efficacy to norepinephrine in patients with cirrhosis and septic shock [41] and appeared to improve renal perfusion in the setting of hepatorenal physiology. However, both terlipressin and high doses of vasopressors are associated with significant adverse reactions, including ischemia and respiratory failure, and current evidence does not demonstrate a clear survival benefit. Early addition of vasopressin for norepinephrine-refractory hypotension is considered [42]. Tailoring therapy requires consideration of ventriculo-arterial coupling to balance cardiac performance with vascular tone [31].

5. Special considerations: Acute-on-chronic liver failure (ACLF)

ACLF is a distinct syndrome characterized by acute decompensation, multi-organ failure and markedly elevated 28-day mortality [8]. ACLF affects 24–40% of hospitalized patients with cirrhosis and is associated with rapid progression to multiorgan failure and high short-term mortality. Hemodynamic instability is common and often multifactorial, requiring early identification, aggressive supportive care and expedited transplant evaluation.

6. Conclusion

Cirrhotic patients with circulatory shock present unique diagnostic and therapeutic challenges due to profound and dynamic changes in vascular tone, cardiac function, and fluid distribution. Clinicians should adopt an individualized approach incorporating advanced hemodynamic assessment, cautious fluid resuscitation with consideration of albumin, and early and tailored vasopressor therapy. Further research is needed to refine MAP targets, optimize monitoring, and improve outcomes in this high-risk population.

Conflict of interest

None.

Author details

Aanchal Kapoor
Cleveland Clinic, Cleveland, Ohio, USA

*Address all correspondence to: kapoora@ccf.org

References

[1] Xiao S, Xie W, Zhang Y, Lei L, Pan Y. Changing epidemiology of cirrhosis from 2010 to 2019: Results from the global burden disease study 2019. Annals of Medicine. 2023;**55**(2):2252326

[2] Garg SK, Goyal H, Obaitan I, Shah PA, Sarvepalli S, Jophlin LL, et al. Incidence and predictors of 30-day hospital readmissions for liver cirrhosis: Insights from the United States National Readmissions Database. Annals of Translational Medicine. 2021;**9**(13):1052

[3] GBD 2017 Cirrhosis Collaborators. The global, regional, and national burden of cirrhosis by cause in 195 countries and territories, 1990-2017: A systematic analysis for the global burden of disease study 2017. The Lancet Gastroenterology & Hepatology. 2020;**5**(3):245-266

[4] Goble SR, Ismail AS, Debes JD, Leventhal TM. Critical care outcomes in decompensated cirrhosis: A United States national inpatient sample cross-sectional study. Critical Care (London, England). 2024;**28**(1):150

[5] Albillos A, Lario M, Álvarez-Mon M. Cirrhosis-associated immune dysfunction: Distinctive features and clinical relevance. Journal of Hepatology. 2014;**61**(6):1385-1396

[6] Piano S, Singh V, Caraceni P, Maiwall R, Alessandria C, Fernandez J, et al. Epidemiology and effects of bacterial infections in patients with cirrhosis worldwide. Gastroenterology. 2019;**156**(5):1368-1380.e10

[7] Gustot T, Felleiter P, Pickkers P, Sakr Y, Rello J, Velissaris D, et al. Impact of infection on the prognosis of critically ill cirrhotic patients: Results from a large worldwide study. Liver International: Official Journal of the International Association for the Study of the Liver. 2014;**34**(10):1496-1503

[8] Moreau R, Jalan R, Gines P, Pavesi M, Angeli P, Cordoba J, et al. Acute-on-chronic liver failure is a distinct syndrome that develops in patients with acute decompensation of cirrhosis. Gastroenterology. 2013;**144**(7):1426-1437.e1-9

[9] Allen AM, Kim WR, Moriarty JP, Shah ND, Larson JJ, Kamath PS. Time trends in the health care burden and mortality of acute on chronic liver failure in the United States. Hepatology (Baltimore, Md.). 2016;**64**(6):2165-2172

[10] Trebicka J, Fernandez J, Papp M, Caraceni P, Laleman W, Gambino C, et al. PREDICT identifies precipitating events associated with the clinical course of acutely decompensated cirrhosis. Journal of Hepatology. 2021;**74**(5):1097-1108

[11] Thabut D, Shah V. Intrahepatic angiogenesis and sinusoidal remodeling in chronic liver disease: New targets for the treatment of portal hypertension? Journal of Hepatology. 2010;**53**(5):976-980

[12] Kowalski HJ, Abelmann WH. The cardiac output at rest in Laennec's cirrhosis. The Journal of Clinical Investigation. 1953;**32**(10):1025-1033

[13] Blendis L, Wong F. The hyperdynamic circulation in cirrhosis: An overview. Pharmacology & Therapeutics. 2001;**89**(3):221-231

[14] Zardi EM, Abbate A, Zardi DM, Dobrina A, Margiotta D, Van Tassell BW, et al. Cirrhotic cardiomyopathy. Journal of the American College of Cardiology. 2010;**56**(7):539-549

[15] Chayanupatkul M, Liangpunsakul S. Cirrhotic cardiomyopathy: Review of pathophysiology and treatment. Hepatology International. 2014;**8**(3):308-315

[16] Wong F. Cirrhotic cardiomyopathy. Hepatology International. 2009;**3**(1):294-304

[17] Møller S, Bernardi M. Interactions of the heart and the liver. European Heart Journal. 2013;**34**(36):2804-2811

[18] Kwon HM, Moon YJ, Jung KW, Park YS, Kim KS, Jun IG, et al. Appraisal of cardiac ejection fraction with liver disease severity: Implication in post-liver transplantation mortality. Hepatology (Baltimore, Md.). 2020;**71**(4):1364-1380

[19] Evans L, Rhodes A, Alhazzani W, Antonelli M, Coopersmith CM, French C, et al. Surviving sepsis campaign: International Guidelines for Management of Sepsis and Septic Shock 2021. Critical Care Medicine. 2021;**49**(11):e1063-e1143

[20] Maiwall R, Rao Pasupuleti SS, Hidam AK, Kumar A, Tevethia HV, Vijayaraghavan R, et al. A randomised-controlled trial (TARGET-C) of high vs. low target mean arterial pressure in patients with cirrhosis and septic shock. Journal of Hepatology. 2023;**79**(2):349-361

[21] Lee SM, An WS. New clinical criteria for septic shock: Serum lactate level as new emerging vital sign. Journal of Thoracic Disease. 2016;**8**(7):1388-1390

[22] Jeppesen JB, Mortensen C, Bendtsen F, Møller S. Lactate metabolism in chronic liver disease. Scandinavian Journal of Clinical and Laboratory Investigation. 2013;**73**(4):293-299

[23] Cheng CY, Kung CT, Wu KH, Chen FC, Cheng HH, Cheng FJ, et al. Liver cirrhosis affects serum lactate level measurement while assessing disease severity in patients with sepsis. European Journal of Gastroenterology & Hepatology. 2021;**33**(9):1201-1208

[24] Persichini R, Lai C, Teboul JL, Adda I, Guérin L, Monnet X. Venous return and mean systemic filling pressure: Physiology and clinical applications. Critical Care (London, England). 2022;**26**(1):150

[25] Kottenberg-Assenmacher E, Aleksic I, Eckholt M, Lehmann N, Peters J. Critical closing pressure as the arterial downstream pressure with the heart beating and during circulatory arrest. Anesthesiology. 2009;**110**(2):370-379

[26] Pinsky MR, García MIM, Dubin A. Significance of critical closing pressures (starling resistors) in arterial circulation. Critical Care. 2024;**28**:127

[27] Hernández G, Ospina-Tascón GA, Damiani LP, Estenssoro E, Dubin A, Hurtado J, et al. Effect of a resuscitation strategy targeting peripheral perfusion status vs serum lactate levels on 28-day mortality among patients with septic shock: The ANDROMEDA-SHOCK randomized clinical trial. Journal of the American Medical Association. 2019;**321**(7):654-664

[28] Dumas G, Lavillegrand JR, Joffre J, Bigé N, de Moura EB, Baudel JL, et al. Mottling score is a strong predictor of 14-day mortality in septic patients whatever vasopressor doses and other tissue perfusion parameters. Critical Care (London, England). 2019;**23**(1):211

[29] Vallée F, Vallet B, Mathe O, Parraguette J, Mari A, Silva S, et al. Central venous-to-arterial carbon dioxide difference: An additional target for goal-directed therapy in

septic shock? Intensive Care Medicine. 2008;**34**(12):2218-2225

[30] Koratala A, Romero-González G, Soliman-Aboumarie H, Kazory A. Unlocking the potential of VExUS in assessing venous congestion: The art of doing it right. Cardiorenal Medicine. 2024;**14**(1):350-374

[31] Guarracino F, Ferro B, Morelli A, Bertini P, Baldassarri R, Pinsky MR. Ventriculoarterial decoupling in human septic shock. Critical Care (London, England). 2014;**18**(2):R80

[32] Chen CH, Fetics B, Nevo E, Rochitte CE, Chiou KR, Ding PA, et al. Noninvasive single-beat determination of left ventricular end-systolic elastance in humans. Journal of the American College of Cardiology. 2001;**38**(7):2028-2034

[33] Pinsky MR, Guarracino F. Pathophysiological implications of ventriculoarterial coupling in septic shock. Intensive Care Medicine Experimental. 2023;**11**:87

[34] Messmer AS, Zingg C, Müller M, Gerber JL, Schefold JC, Pfortmueller CA. Fluid overload and mortality in adult critical care patients - A systematic review and meta-analysis of observational studies. Critical Care Medicine. 2020;**48**(12):1862-1870

[35] Boyd JH, Forbes J, Nakada T, Walley KR, Russell JA. Fluid resuscitation in septic shock: A positive fluid balance and elevated central venous pressure are associated with increased mortality. Critical Care Medicine. 2011;**39**(2):259-265

[36] Philips CA, Maiwall R, Sharma MK, Jindal A, Choudhury AK, Kumar G, et al. Comparison of 5% human albumin and normal saline for fluid resuscitation in sepsis induced hypotension among patients with cirrhosis (FRISC study): A randomized controlled trial. Hepatology International. 2021;**15**(4):983-994

[37] Maiwall R, Kumar A, Pasupuleti SSR, Hidam AK, Tevethia H, Kumar G, et al. A randomized-controlled trial comparing 20% albumin to plasmalyte in patients with cirrhosis and sepsis-induced hypotension [ALPS trial]. Journal of Hepatology. 2022;**77**(3):670-682

[38] Permpikul C, Tongyoo S, Viarasilpa T, Trainarongsakul T, Chakorn T, Udompanturak S. Early use of norepinephrine in septic shock resuscitation (CENSER). A randomized trial. American Journal of Respiratory and Critical Care Medicine. 2019;**199**(9):1097-1105

[39] Beck V, Chateau D, Bryson GL, Pisipati A, Zanotti S, Parrillo JE, et al. Timing of vasopressor initiation and mortality in septic shock: A cohort study. Critical Care (London, England). 2014;**18**(3):R97

[40] Jimenez JV, Garcia-Tsao G, Saffo S. Emerging concepts in the care of patients with cirrhosis and septic shock. World Journal of Hepatology. 2023;**15**(4):497-514

[41] Choudhury A, Kedarisetty CK, Vashishtha C, Saini D, Kumar S, Maiwall R, et al. A randomized trial comparing terlipressin and noradrenaline in patients with cirrhosis and septic shock. Liver International: Official Journal of the International Association for the Study of the Liver. 2017;**37**(4):552-561

[42] Ukor IF, Walley KR. Vasopressin in vasodilatory shock. Critical Care Clinics. 2019;**35**(2):247-261

Chapter 5

Maintaining Peripheral Circulation in the Surgical Patient: A Narrative Review of the Importance of Near-Infrared Spectroscopy

Henning Bay Nielsen

Abstract

Since Cushing described heart rate and blood pressure as the variables regularly recorded during surgery, the advancement of devices to record beat-to-beat changes in cardiac stroke volume has provided additional opportunities for perioperative monitoring. While such monitoring focuses on central parameters, as they are derived from the pressure curve, peripheral circulation has received little attention. Secondly, traditional monitoring does not reflect changes in cerebral blood flow, which needs to be considered in frail elderly patients who, due to conditions such as atherosclerosis, are vulnerable to hypotension secondary to impaired cerebral autoregulation. Here, near-infrared spectroscopy, and particularly cerebral oximetry, seem relevant to include in the toolbox for perioperative monitoring. For high-risk surgical patients, it is paramount to assess peripheral circulation during anesthesia. This chapter provides a narrative review of the relevance of the use of NIRS in the perioperative setting.

Keywords: brain, cerebral autoregulation, cerebral oximetry, hypotension, muscle oximetry, orthopedics, vascular surgery

1. Introduction

Maintaining adequate tissue oxygenation is critical for optimizing surgical outcomes and preventing complications during major procedures [1]. Near-infrared spectroscopy (NIRS) has emerged as a noninvasive tool for continuously monitoring regional oxygen saturation (rSO_2) in tissues such as the brain and skeletal muscle [2]. By providing real-time monitoring, NIRS enables early detection of hypoxemia, guiding perioperative management strategies to limit the risk of deteriorated regional perfusion. In fact, lowered organ blood supply remains key factor for most cases of perioperative complications [1].

While NIRS is well-established in cardiac surgery [3–7], its application in noncardiac procedures is increasingly recognized as a mean to enhance patient safety and improve clinical outcomes [8]. In various noncardiac surgeries, specific procedures impact regional O_2 delivery, particularly in conditions where patient positioning, vascular occlusion, or hemodynamic instability compromise regional tissue perfusion. Carotid endarterectomy (CEA), for example, carries the risk of cerebral ischemia during carotid cross-clamping, which can lead to postoperative neurological deficits [9]. In this situation, monitoring cerebral oxygenation with NIRS provides insight into changes in cerebral perfusion, which assist for decisions related to interventions such as selective shunting or blood pressure optimization [10–12]. Another example relates to reconstructive surgery where a free flap of tissue anatomical is repositioned to cover for removal of cancer in e.g. breast. Here, NIRS is reported to be superior to clinical monitoring for identifying a change in perfusion in the free flap [13–16].

Similarly, lower extremity bypass surgery involves prolonged ischemic periods due to vascular clamping and potential graft-related complications. The ability to assess muscle tissue perfusion using NIRS may aid the surgeon to evaluate the time with limb ischemia, and during the reperfusion period, graft patency may be assessed using changes in the NIRS signal [17]. Concerning the influence of patient position, robotic-assisted laparoscopic surgery performed in the Trendelenburg position, with patients placed in a head-down tilt to optimize surgical view, challenges cardiac preload and its afterload [18]. Due to potential hindered venous return in the jugular vein [19] as well as affected leg blood flow in the leg-up head-down position, regional tissue oxygenation may be impaired [20]. Here, NIRS-based monitoring may help clinicians implement strategies such as adjusting ventilation parameters, modifying patient positioning, or administering vasoactive agents to maintain adequate tissue O_2 delivery.

Given the increasing number of aging and frail patients in the surgical population [21] also considering the diabetes epidemic, there is need for individualized assessment of changes in regional oxygenation due to the vulnerability of microvascular function of such patients. While advancement of devices to record beat-to-beat changes in cardiac stroke volume have provided additional opportunities for perioperative monitoring [22], such monitoring offers a reflection of central parameters only without knowledge of what is distributed to peripheral circulation. Furthermore, in many institutions and surgeries, the blood pressure measurements remain the most frequent recorded variables as also noted by Cushing in 1903 [23]. Now, the use of NIRS is expanded beyond cardiac surgery, and it continues to receive attention in how the technology can be incorporated in managing regional circulation with potential impact on patient outcome [8]. Recently, the relevance of using cerebral oximetry in high-risk surgical patients has been highlighted and an algorithm for treatment of adverse cerebral oxygenation has been presented [24].

This narrative review explores the clinical relevance, potential benefits, and limitations of using NIRS to monitor tissue oxygenation during selected examples of noncardiac surgeries, underscoring its potential impact on decision-making in the perioperative setting.

2. Short history of NIRS development

Development of optical technologies in last century inspired further use of NIRS as a noninvasive tool for monitoring changes in tissue oxygenation [2]. One of the first papers on changes in NIRS-determined muscle oxygenation in humans was published by Wilson et al. [25], and shortly thereafter, Britton Chance further published the effect of rowing [26]. These initial reports were followed by studies on tissue oxygenation in models of hypovolemia shock [27, 28] and maximal physical exertion [29]. Over the past 30 years, the literature on NIRS in clinical settings has exploded [8, 24]. Thus, it is clear the NIRS technology is relevant for physiological assessments.

The principle of NIRS relies on light absorption by oxyhemoglobin (HbO_2) and deoxyhemoglobin (HHb) [2]. These spectral differences were employed in blood gas analyzers, and such devices, the so-called ABL analyzers of which the Danish company Radiometer markets several types, are now standard of care equipment at most operation theater and intensive care units. Building on NIRS principles, the first pulse oximeter as a noninvasive method for monitoring arterial O_2 saturation (SpO_2) was developed in 1972 by Japanese bioengineers at an electronic equipment manufacturer. Pulse oximetry devices typically incorporate two wavelengths of light. These are usually red light (660 nm) and near-infrared light (940 nm). These wavelengths help differentiate between HbO_2 and HHb. The typical location of measurement is the finger pulp or the earlobe. Such allows to track changes in transmitted light during pulsatile arterial flow to estimate O_2 saturation. However, pulse oximetry reflects only arterial blood.

To address a more diverse purpose, NIRS was further developed for continuous monitoring of tissue oxygenation, particularly in brain and muscle. Modern NIRS-systems use multiple source-detectors to differentiate between superficial and deep tissue signals. Today, NIRS is widely used in clinical and research settings to monitor changes in tissue oxygenation in various tissues. Key applications include:

- Cerebral oximetry: Seems preferred in cardiac surgery although noncardiac surgery such as CEA also has relevance. For other noncardiac surgeries, cerebral oximetry can be incorporated in anesthetic care to monitor cerebral oxygenation that may signal regional hypoperfusion.

- Muscle oximetry: Mostly employed in exercise physiology to assess balance between O_2 extraction and O_2 demand under various conditions and experimental models.

- Pediatric oximetry: Used to monitor care in preterm infants.

3. Technology of NIRS for tissue oxygenation

This technique utilizes near-infrared light (typically 650–950 nm), which penetrates biological tissues and interacts with chromophores that absorbs light. Such chromophores include hemoglobin (and myoglobin) that absorbs light in the near-infrared spectra, and through the reflected light, absorption can be determined.

The fundamental principle for use of NIRS to determine tissue oxygenation is that both HbO_2 and HHb absorb light in the near-infra spectra, but they do so at different wavelengths as reviewed more than 25 years ago by Madsen and Secher [2] and summarized below. The HbO_2 absorbs more light at higher NIR wavelengths (around 850–940 nm), whereas HHb absorbs more light at lower wavelengths (around 660–760 nm). The traditional NIRS device allows light transmission at two or four (or multiple) specific NIR wavelengths *via* diodes or a specifically designed sensor. The concept is that light enters the tissue through the sensor applied to the skin (e.g., on the forehead or muscle). As light passes through the tissue, it is scattered and partially absorbed by predominantly HbO_2 and HHb depending on the local hemoglobin distribution in the tissue beneath the sensor. Here, hemoglobin resides in blood vessels with capillaries representing the largest area where hemoglobin can be exposed to near-infrared light. The near-infra light also passes through skin, fat, muscle, while none-absorbed light is scattered back to the skin surface. The back-scattered is detected by diodes (integrated in the system sensor) that are separated from the light source. Most commercially available NIRS devices use a sensor with a light transmission source and two diodes each separated by app. 1 cm. The light source is separated from the light collecting diodes. Increasing the distance between the diodes allows for signal detection of deeper tissue. The intensity of the returning light is inversely related to the amount of absorption. This means that with greater light absorption, it equals to that less light is detected by the collecting photodiodes.

Using a modification of the Beer-Lambert law, which accounts for both absorption and scattering in tissue, the relative concentrations of HbO_2 and HHb can be calculated depending on some assumptions. Such calculations are usually integrated in the commercial NiRS-devices without user access to the computation. Usually, algorithms are considered under some sort of patent protection and therefore unavailable. The key assumptions for using a modified Beer-Lambert in NIRS devices are *(i)* HbO_2 and HHb are the main light absorbers, *(ii)* Extinction coefficients for HbO_2 and HHb are known, *(iii)* Scattering is constant during the measurement, and *(iv)* Optical pathlength can be estimated. Some NIRS devices use several wavelengths to improve accuracy, and such also allows for a differentiation of, for instance, cytochrome oxidase.

In some commercially available NIRS devices, the Beer-Lambert Law allows for quantification of the relative concentration changes in μmol. The advantage of the unit μmol/L is that it resembles the unit for hemoglobin concentration in blood, but the approximation between mmol and μmol may be difficult to apply in clinical work. Alternatively, based on data for optical densities, an NIRS device may calculate rSO_2 using the formula $[(HbO_2/(HbO_2 + HHb)) \times 100]$ providing simplicity as the influence of absolute pathlength and varying baseline concentrations is excluded. Secondly, rSO_2 depends only on the ratio of two hemoglobin types, not on absolute values or exact pathlengths. The unit % resembles the unit used for the pulse oximetry determined SpO_2. Thus, a value for rSO_2 like "70%" allows use of trigger alarms for interventions. Importantly, rSO_2 appears clinical feasible as the rSO_2 value is under the influence of factors impacting microvasculature blood flow such as cardiac output, blood pressure, and CO_2. Thus, a drop in SrO_2 reflects decrease in regional perfusion. This qualifies for its feasibly as a clinical tool reflecting the impact of systemic hemodynamic on regional blood flow. That is why Murkin described cerebral oximetry as the index organ for systemic organ blood flow [4].

In summary, with a pulse oximeter attached to finger or the ear lobe, a pulse oximetry determined SpO_2 provides a measure of O_2 hemoglobin saturation in arterial blood. The NIRS determined rSO_2 is an estimate of O_2 hemoglobin saturation in the microvasculature beneath the NIRS sensor; the value represents a summation of light absorption by hemoglobin in arterioles, capillaries, and venules. This rSO_2 estimate is not the total amount of hemoglobin or O_2 delivered to the tissue; however, with a drop in rSO_2, it may relate to a decrease in local perfusion reflecting less hemoglobin is being delivered. Thus, changes in rSO_2 mirror changes in regional blood supply, and it also mirrors the balance between O_2 supply and O_2 demand.

4. Relevance of NIRS in the operating theater

For the clinician interested in monitoring regional tissue oxygenation and the impact of conditions on regional perfusion, NIRS is considered an invaluable tool. None of the traditional or modern devices to track central hemodynamics or the pulse oximetry perfusion index can deliver insight into regional tissue perfusion. This is highly relevant to consider in patients who may have deteriorated capacity for blood flow regulation. Such patients include but is not limited to frail patients or elderly patients with atherosclerosis, heart failure, or just diabetes. Other concerns relate to surgical positions that hinders or could influence the integrity of regional blood flow homeostasis. It needs to be considered that the proportion of elderly patients with multimorbidity requiring polypharmaceutical treatment is in dramatic increase throughout the Western hemisphere.

The risk for elderly frail patient in general anesthesia (GA) is difficult to ignore especially in complicated surgeries under prolonged time for intervention. In these patients, the risk for development of postoperative cognitive decline is significant [30]. Therefore, lowered cerebral perfusion even locally should be avoided [31]. The potential for an impact of anesthesia on regional blood flow in certain areas of the brain is also difficult to exclude. Importantly, low preoperative ScO_2 associates with 30-day all-cause mortality in elderly patients undergoing surgery for hip fracture [32]. The frail elderly patients should be offered the opportunity to have their brain monitored for adequate O_2 supply. Cerebral oximetry is easy to apply on the forehead below the hairline and above the expected location of the frontal sinuses.

In the operating theater with patients in GA, physiological parameters usually rapidly change in a hyperdynamic environment. Although the use of pulse oximetry failed to impact outcome in large clinical trials in the 1990s [33] later confirmed in Cochrane review papers [34, 35], most patients now have their finger pulp fixed for SpO_2 monitoring in the operating theater. Therefore, the vast amount of literature supporting use of NIRS in the operating theater is difficult to ignore as otherwise assessment of the anesthetized brain in most cases is done using clinical eyeballing. Thus, during cardiac surgery involving on-pump low-pressure circulation, cerebral oximetry assisted management of circulation is associated with better outcome as compared to no-brain assisted circulatory management [7]. Furthermore, Casati et al. [36, 37] explored the effects during major abdominal surgery, and already in 2009, it was noted that cerebral oxygen desaturation predicts cognitive decline and longer hospital stay [38]. In addition, Heringlake et al. [39] suggest preoperative rSO_2 below 50% should prompt concern for systemic hypoperfusion. The association between changes in cerebral oxygenation intraoperatively and postoperative cognitive decline supports the use of cerebral oximetry as a standard of care procedure in vulnerable patients [31]. A recent meta-analysis has underscored the need to incorporate NIRS in the monitoring toolbox for anesthetic care of high-risk surgical patients [24].

The usual argument for ignoring the potential of NIRS to track changes in regional perfusion is based on uncertainty for what NIRS estimates and how to intervene if the recording for rSO_2 drops. When NIRS is applied on the forehead before anesthesia is delivered, the value for rSO_2 in the frontal lobe is 40–90% with highly individual variations in an unselected pool of noncardiac vascular surgical patients [40]. Of interest, a value below 50% is reported to be associated with higher risk for development of postoperative complications following cardiac surgery [39]. Furthermore, with an abrupt change in systemic blood flow, regional perfusion in the tissue beneath an NIRS sensor becomes lowered as visualized by sudden drop in tissue oxygenation (see **Figure 1**). Furthermore, the rSO_2 value reflecting brain oxygenation in the frontal lobe is responsive to changes in CO_2 [2, 41, 42]. Only the brain vasculature or the chemoreceptors controlling the cerebral vascular bed demonstrates significant CO_2 reactivity [41, 42]. The traditional view is that neither the skin nor the skeletal muscle has capacity to regulate regional perfusion upon changes in arterial CO_2 levels. In contrast, the level of O_2 transport capacity influences the NIRS signal. This is shown by increasing the arterial hemoglobin concentration through blood transfusion [43–46]. Furthermore, breathing oxygen enriched atmospheric raises the level of not only physical dissolved O_2 in blood but also SaO_2 and in turn, the NIRS determined muscle oxygenation by 5% and the frontal lobe oxygenation by 10% [40]. The reason may be that oxygen levels on the venous side of capillaries are slightly higher and as such sensed by NIRS.

Figure 1 shows the rSO_2 responses for rSO_2 of skeletal muscle (SmO_2) and for rSO_2 of the frontal lobe (ScO_2) in patient under GA for open surgical repair of abdominal aortic aneurysm. As shown in the figure, the sudden downslope drop of the curves coincides with cardiac arrest induced by ventricular tachycardia. In principle, such condition

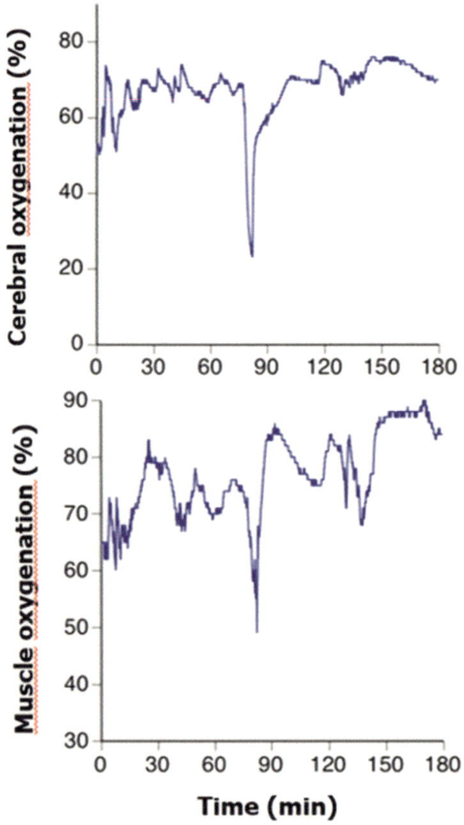

Figure 1.
Lower panel shows in skeletal muscle oxygenation with a NIRS sensor placed on the middle part of the biceps muscle and upper panel is cerebral oxygenation determined by a NIRS sensor placed unilateral on the forehead in patient undergoing open surgical repair of an abdominal aortic aneurysm. As shown in the figure, the sudden downslope drop of the curves coincides with cardiac arrest induced by ventricular tachycardia. As systemic circulation was restored, the values for tissue oxygenation in brain and skeletal muscle gained pre-arrest levels. After the cardiac arrest, blood loss necessitated blood transfusion creating up-slope of the curves for tissue oxygenation.

provokes zero systemic perfusion. As cardiac output was restored, the values for tissue oxygenation in brain and skeletal muscle gained pre-arrest levels. The figure illustrates the close relationship between systemic flow and NIRS determined tissue oxygenation.

Although the values for SmO_2 and ScO_2 may respond in parallel, the responses depend on autoregulation and the influence of the sympathetic nervous system. In hypovolemia that can be graduated progressively in the head-up tilt model in healthy humans, SmO_2 is reduced with a gradual reduction in central blood volume while an increase in heart rate attempts to maintain blood pressure [27, 28, 47, 48]. As central blood volume becomes depleted, blood pressure is maintained through increased activity of sympathetic activity that raises heart rate [49]. However, syncope occurs when sympathetic drive abruptly loses its activity whereby parasympathetic probably gets an overhand [50, 51]. This may be seen as decrease in blood pressure that affects blood supply to the brain. The increased vasodilatory component in skeletal muscle is noted by an increase in SmO_2 that comes few seconds before the drop ScO_2 [48]. This

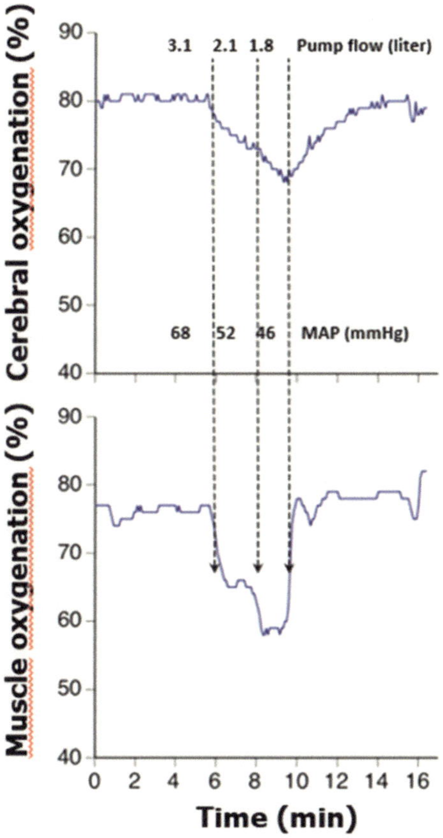

Figure 2.
The panels show tissue oxygenation (lower panel is oxygenation the biceps skeletal and upper panel is the frontal lobe) in a patient with severe heart failure (due to left ventricular ejection fraction below 10%) that was supported by an external ventricular assist device. As part of the medical treatment, it was needed to observe whether the patient could manage own circulation with limited external assist support. Thus, the external pump flow was reduced gradually (from 3.1 to 1.8 L) without changes in the administered doses of vasoactive medication whereby mean arterial pressure (MAP) decreased. While muscle oxygenation responded rapidly to the changes in systemic flow, the frontal lobe oxygenation response appeared slower.

coincides with development of syncopal symptoms like nausea, dizziness, blurred vision, and eventual loss of consciousness.

The different response of SmO_2 and ScO_2 to gradual systemic flow by hypovolemia can also be visualized by limiting the level of cardiac output. **Figure 2** shows tissue oxygenation in a patient with severe heart failure (due to left ventricular ejection fraction below 10%) that was supported by an external ventricular assist device. As part of the medical treatment, it was needed to observe whether the patient could manage own circulation with limited external assist support. Thus, the external pump flow was reduced gradually without changes in the administered doses of vasoactive medication. While SmO_2 responded rapidly to the changes in systemic flow, the ScO_2 response appeared slower. It could be that cerebral autoregulation attempted to regulate perfusion for the new systemic situation of flow and pressure.

5. Specific noncardiac surgeries and NIRS

This is a broad category covering abdominal, orthopedic, neurological, urological, and other procedures as well as vascular surgery where various arteries may be clamped to allow for the surgical repair. Such could involve the carotid, mesenteric, and femoral artery as well as the abdominal aorta. Secondly, in noncardiac surgery, the patient may be exposed to a variability of positions depending on the intended surgery. Most commonly, patients are supine, but a prone position could come in use in certain rectal procedures. The Trendelenburg is used to enhance surgical field visibility. A steep Trendelenburg position (STP) may be applied in urology and gynecology, while a head-up position could come in use for shoulder surgery. Each position could include a specific risk for regional tissue oxygenation. A direct impact on the brain is when a longitudinal incision is made along the anterior border of the sternocleidomastoid muscle to expose the common carotid artery, carotid bifurcation, and internal carotid artery and external carotid artery during vascular surgery.

5.1 Carotid endarterectomy

For patients undergoing CEA, the surgery should not be done without some sort of monitoring of changes of brain perfusion even if the surgery is done solely by use of local anesthesia (LA). The debate is not new. Thus, CEA may be executed using LA or GA [52]. In both situations the concern is what happens when the carotid artery is clamped. The advantage of LA is that the level of consciousness of the patient is easy to monitor, and it speaks for use of LA [53]. Here, a simple routine is that the patient is asked to squeeze a hand. If hand force drops or the level of consciousness fades, then it is likely cerebral perfusion is inadequate to maintain specific tasks of neurons. Then, concern is raised on whether it is needed to insert a shunt or to finish surgery in a hurry. With the patient in GA, a change in the level of consciousness is difficult to monitor. Here, the surgeon must rely on stump pressure measurements for assessment of the integrity of the Circle of Willis [54]. In principle, it is unknown whether atherosclerosis is manifested in main cerebral arteries besides the internal carotid artery of interest for surgery. Thus, recordings of ScO_2 by NIRS provide an opportunity for a keyhole view of changes in global cerebral blood flow during CEA [55–59].

The experience is that a rapid drop in the ScO_2 recording occurs ahead of loss of consciousness (**Figure 3**). Thus, when the internal carotid artery is clamped,

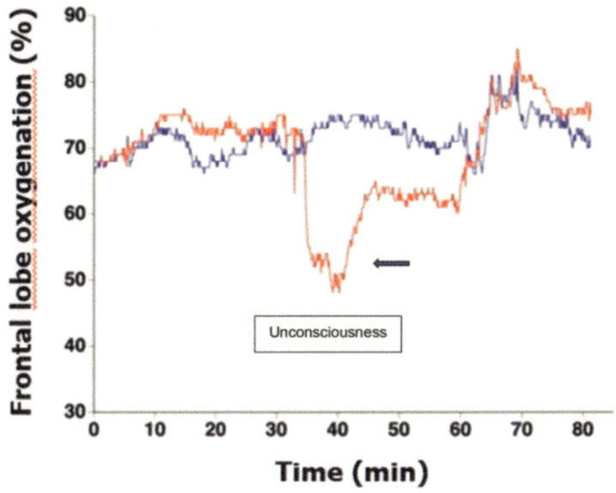

Figure 3.
The figure demonstrates changes in frontal lobe oxygenation before, during and after carotid endarterectomy. The red line represents the NIRS signal for the right frontal lobe, while the blue line is the NIRS signal from the left frontal lobe. It can be seen with a cross-clamp on the right internal carotid artery, the frontal lobe oxygenation (same side as surgery) demonstrated a marked and rapid down-hill slope corresponding to an absolute 20–25% drop or a relative reduction by ~30%. It is clearly visualized that the frontal lobe oxygenation opposite to the surgical side was remarkable unchanged by carotid endarterectomy. With the red line reaching a minimum, it coincided with that the patient became unconsciousness. The anesthetist administered vasoactive therapy intravenously to allow for a rapid increase in blood pressure. Such initiated increase in frontal lobe oxygenation probably due to an increase in cerebral blood flow following change in systolic blood pressure from ~120 to ~170 mmHg. The patient regained consciousness (indicated by horizontal arrow) that allowed the surgeon to terminate CEA that resulted in successful outcome. The sudden up-slope of the red curve at the time point 60 minutes indicates when the cross-clamp was released to allow for a marked increase in frontal lobe oxygenation that stabilized when antihypertensive medication was administered. The up-slope of the curves illustrates the potential of NIRS to unmask episodes of cerebral hyperperfusion after surgery.

ScO_2 may decrease on same side as surgery. The contralateral ScO_2, however, usually remains unchanged. In the case presented, ~10–20 seconds after the artery was clamped, ScO_2 reached a minimum coinciding with that the patient became unconsciousness. The anesthetist administered vasoactive therapy intravenously to allow for a rapid increase in blood pressure. Then, ScO_2 increased to a plateau probably due to an increase in cerebral blood flow following change in systolic blood pressure from ~120 to ~170 mmHg. The patient regained consciousness which allowed the surgeon to terminate CEA that resulted in successful outcome.

When CEA is performed using GA, the state of patient following carotid cross clamp is difficult to monitor. In this situation, other precautions are needed. The surgeon may rely on stump pressure measurements to evaluate whether other cerebral arteries are able to supply the circle of wills. Low stump pressure may support a decision to insert a shunt to secure blood supply to the brain while internal artery is clamped [54]. The advantage of GA is that the metabolic rate of neurons is lowered.

When surgery is terminated, then the neurological state of the awake patient becomes of interest. Such is a concern when CEA is done in GA. Carotid clamping and shunt placement could provoke mobilization of small arteriosclerotic plaque that in turn may impact blood flow in small arteries of the brain with potential to form a blood clot. Following reperfusion after cross clamp is released, there is a risk of cerebral hyperperfusion due to impaired cerebral autoregulation [9] and greater intraoperative variability in blood pressures associates with a higher risk of headache after CEA [60]. The risk remains for several days after surgery and blood pressure reduction therapy is usually proactive. The predominant symptom is neurological deficits or even just headache complaints. Thus, monitoring cerebral oxygenation may be considered also in the recovery phase following CEA [61]. In summary, NIRS is highly relevant for the anesthetic care of the patient undergoing CEA.

5.2 Head down position

Certain surgical interventions in gynecology and urology may require Trendelenburg position to optimize visualization of the surgical field, a process further supported by intraperitoneal gas insufflation (IGI). The robot-assisted laparoscopic prostatectomy may use STP characterized by 30–40-degree head down. Patients generally tolerate robot-assisted surgery similar to open surgery [62, 63], and laparoscopic surgery seems not associated with an increased risk of venous thromboembolism and cardiac complications [64]. However, the combined effect of STP and IGI challenges the cardiovascular integrity and in turn neurocognitive recovery [18]. Also, intracranial pressure may increase during STP [65] with consequence for intraocular pressure [66, 67]. Thus, the integrity of cerebral blood flow is likely affected although the NIRS determined cerebral oxygenation remains remarkable stable during STP [68, 69]. However, ScO_2 may decrease in the elderly [20] as cerebral autoregulation of the brain of elderly patient seems impaired [70]. Here, an NIRS device would be feasible to record changes of cerebral oxygenation especially with patients in prolonged STP.

Another argument for inclusion of NIRS in the monitoring package for surgery in STP with IGI is the reported cardiovascular changes: blood pressure increases by ~35%, cardiac stroke volume and cardiac output decrease by ~20%, central venous pressure increases to app. 20 mmHg, and pulmonary capillary pressure is raised 2–3 fold [18, 71, 72] with significant overall increase in cardiac afterload [73]. In fact, the perioperative changes reflect a hyperdynamic situation [74] although little effect on cardiac workload and cardiac performance also is reported [75, 76]. The affected cardiovascular integrity remains when the patient is returned to the supine position as hypotension occurs in up to 20% of patients [77]. Even brief episodes of hypotension are associated with an increased risk of end-organ injury [1, 78] supporting the use of brain as the index organ for systemic flow [4].

Recently, it has been reported that the combined effects of IGI and STP may damage venous endothelium secondary to lowered venous blood flow in the lower limbs predisposing for deep venous thrombosis [19]. In fact, the diameter of the femoral vein becomes enlarged as also femoral venous bloods flow drops [19]. Thus, development of compartment syndrome in the lower limbs is reported [79] and lower limb perfusion evaluated by NIRS could be considered for patients undergoing surgery in STP. Such may contribute to assist anesthetic care of the patient.

5.3 Head up position: Beach chair

The beach chair position (also known as sitting of semi-sitting) may find its use in certain areas of surgical interventions in the orthopedic and neurosurgical specialities. In the orthopedic surgery, the beach chair may be considered for shoulder arthroscopy or even more complicated repair. It is chosen to facilitate better surgical view of the field of interest, but specific risks need to be considered such as the level of comorbidities of the patient. Secondly, the beach chair position may challenge circulatory integrity with potential impact on the brain [80]. Thus, complications such as cerebral hypotension, infarction, cutaneous facial nerve neuropraxia, hypoglossal nerve injury, and blindness are all rare but seen only in beach chair positioning [81]. Thus, when using the beach chair, specific attention needs to be devoted to the brain. The reason is that in GA, normal compensatory mechanisms for central blood volume depletion (due to that legs may be positioned below the heart) is inadequate as they rely on sympathetic nervous activity. As mentioned in previous sections, depletion of central blood volume challenges the normal compensatory mechanisms and occurrence of hypotension may have consequence for the ability of circulation to supply the brain with blood. Thus, during beach chair, ScO_2 may become dramatically reduced even in healthy subjects [82, 83]. In such case, interventions need to be established to protect the cerebral perfusion as guided by changes in ScO_2 [80].

5.4 Frail patients

It is suggested that especially elderly patients and those with impaired myocardial contractility are at risk for development of adverse cardiovascular effects following robot-assisted surgery in STP [18]. In particular, cardiovascular disease, such as heart failure, atherosclerosis, and diabetic cardiomyopathy, is associated with impaired autonomic dynamics, and patients presenting such disease may be vulnerable to the physiological abnormalities induced by anesthesia.

For certain surgeries, there might be an option to choose between the use of spinal anesthesia (SP) or GA. Interesting, SP is associated with a favorable hemodynamic profile compared to GA [84]. Presence of hypotension may disrupt blood flow autoregulation with potential consequences for oxygenation in local tissue and organs (eq the brain) in vulnerable individuals [85]. Frailty determines the outcome after surgery [86], and especially patients with urine bladder cancer are often elderly with multiple comorbidities [87]. In these patients, increasing frailty is associated with a higher risk of discharge to assisted living facilities after surgery [88]. Furthermore, they have higher risk of cancer recurrence [89].

Frailty is associated with raised levels of C-reactive protein with inflammation playing a role in aging [90] and cardiovascular disease [91] due to the impact of inflammation on endothelial function. Thus, circulatory integrity is likely less adaptable to abrupt vasodilatory challenge by anesthesia that may have consequence for the brain. While SP seems to benefit the hemodynamic profile in certain patients [84], SP may be associated with more frequent episodes of lowered ScO_2 in elderly patients [92]. As the brain serves as the index organ for detecting systemic hypoperfusion [4], low cerebral oxygenation associates with cognitive decline after GA in elderly patients [8, 31]. Monitoring the brain is recommended for high-risk surgical patients [24], and such should include the frail who may be more intolerable to even low to modest change in cerebral oxygenation.

5.5 Hypotensive anesthesia

A specific use of NIRS may be in spine surgery where controlled hypotension is often used to reduce blood loss [93]. During such procedure, cerebral hypoperfusion is a risk [94], especially in vulnerable patients. Thus, during hypotensive anesthesia, NIRS provides a practical tool to guide safe lower blood pressure limits in accordance with the cerebral autoregulation [95]. This would allow the anesthetist to adjust blood pressure targets, to optimize oxygen delivery, and to minimize the risk of neurologic complications using the ScO_2 cuff-off values suggesting regional hypoperfusion of the brain in clinical practice.

5.6 Is monitoring of muscle oxygenation relevant during surgery?

The NIRS determined SmO_2 may be a valuable adjunct in perioperative monitoring. By providing continuous measurements of SmO_2, NIRS enables early detection of muscle hypoperfusion in consequence of specific surgical procedures that could impact regional blood supply.

In noncardiac vascular surgery, use of NIRS was probably first described by Eiberg et al. more than 25 years ago in patients undergoing infrainguinal bypass procedures [17]. In this study, SmO_2 on the dorsum of the foot dropped significantly during femoral artery clamping and then rose sharply after revascularization. Others have used NIRS in lower-limb revascularization, with sensors placed over the gastrocnemius or tibialis anterior may help to detect graft occlusion or thrombosis [96]. In endovascular aortic repair, Taudorf et al. [97] demonstrated that gluteal SmO_2 becomes lowered following hypogastric artery occlusion, with prolonged recovery times linked to symptomatic gluteal claudication.

In orthopedic surgery, particularly those involving pneumatic tourniquet use, NIRS may help to diagnose tissue ischemia. With sensors placed on the vastus lateralis muscle distal to the cuff, NIRS may help to guide earlier cuff deflation or pressure adjustments. In reconstructive microsurgery, including use of free-flap in breast reconstruction, NIRS offers a monitoring of flap viability. Sustained reductions in SmO_2 are associated with venous or arterial compromise [98]. Such should prompt re-exploration.

Finally, in major abdominal and high-risk general surgery, monitoring of peripheral muscle such is reported to uncover hypoperfusion despite normal systemic hemodynamics, enabling targeted fluid or vasopressor therapy [99]. Furthermore, during abdominal surgery or gynecological interventions with application of the lithotomy (Steinschnittlage) position, compression of the leg muscle may cause a risk for hypoperfusion and pressure-related tissue injury. Thus, Svendsen et al. [100] applied NIRS to the medial gastrocnemius during surgery in the lithotomy position and observed a significant decline in SmO_2 during leg elevation for ~25 minutes, corresponding with a marked drop in perfusion pressure. Further emphasizing the clinical relevance, crural compartment syndrome is associated with the lithotomy positioning [101] and patients with acute compartment syndrome have lower SmO_2 as compared to the healthy limb [102].

The NIRS determined SmO_2 complements traditional monitoring by providing a window into the adequacy of perfusion at the tissue level. In these settings, the ability to detect ischemia early and intervene promptly has the potential to improve surgical outcomes and reduce complications.

6. Pitfalls for use of NIRS

When an NIRS sensor is intended for recording of ScO_2, the sensor placement on the forehead needs to take few issues into consideration that could impact the quality of the backscattered light and in turn the level of tissue oxygenation. First, in most cases, the orientation of the frontal sinuses is unknown. Usually, the frontal sinuses typically lie around 1.5 cm above the eyebrow, though the exact location can vary between individuals. Thus, care should be taken to place the NIRS sensor at least 3 cm above the upper level the eyebrow [103]. In addition, the NIRS sensor should be placed as lateral as possible and avoidance of central placement on the forehead.

The extensive venous drainage of the brain is also an issue. Here, the veins are collected in the sagittal sinuses justifying the lateral position of NIRS sensor on the forehead. In most patients, an artery exits from the orbital cave almost at the midline of the eyebrow. This artery (the supraorbital artery) supplies the skin around the eyebrow and the lower part of the forehead with oxygen. The hairline is an issue as signal handling by most commercial NIRS devices could be influenced by hair and its color as is the case with the impact of nail polish on pulse oximetry recordings. The influence of skin on the NIRS recording is a topic. For most humans, however, the skin including its different layers on the forehead is ~1.0 mm thick [104]. Therefore, the contribution of skin to the overall light absorption seems almost trivial. With extensive accumulation of bilirubin in skin, however, NIRS readings seem complicated [105, 106].

The thickness of the scull bone varies by location and individual, but on average, it ranges from 5.5 to 8.2 mm. The occipital and frontal bones are typically thicker than the parietal and temporal bones. Studies show that women's sculls tend to be thicker than men's. Bone is usually rather less obstructive to light. Bone is relatively easy to pass for near-infra light without much absorption unless hemoglobin is trapped in the bone. As light is considered to penetrate tissue to a depth of 3–4 cm, the brain tissue seems likely to contribute most to light absorption.

Changes of CO_2 could impact the level of vasoconstriction in the skin. The traditional view, however, is that skin possesses little CO_2 reactivity while cerebral perfusion is under the influence of CO_2. Thus, hyperventilation-induced hypocapnia decreases ScO_2 [2] with little effect on SmO_2, and ScO_2 helps to identify the lower limit of the cerebral autoregulation [95]. Such needs to be considered with the patient in GA as ventilatory settings usually follows standard guideline in accordance to age and weight of the patient. The capnography measurement of expired CO_2 reflects the arterial levels but not to a 1:1 equation.

Vasoactive drugs may be administered to compensate for anesthesia-induced vasodilatation that may result in lowered blood pressure. The anesthetist may use noradrenaline, ephedrine, and phenylephrine to stimulate alpha- and beta-adrenergic receptors. These drugs deliver increase in blood pressure by vasoconstriction and increase in heart rate although the response on tissue oxygenation depends on the vasoactive agent used [107–109]. While most vessels present responsiveness to adrenergic stimulation, the brain seem without such mechanisms. Furthermore, genetic variability of the adrenergic receptors [110, 111] may determine the response to vasoactive drugs and in turn the impact on ScO_2. Use of calcium as a vasoactive drug does not affect the level of ScO_2 when calcium is used to treat anesthetic induced hypotension [112]. In addition, in most cases, even 30% drop in mean arterial pressure at the induction of anesthesia has little effect on cerebral oxygenation [113].

The different NIRS devices may not report similar values for tissue oxygenation. Different devices seem to be influenced differently by extracerebral components [114]. One NIRS device may use a spatially resolved NIRS-technology where two light detectors provide a signal that appears to be a combination of cerebral and extracerebral components. Other devices use a technology aiming for ScO_2 estimates from deeper tissue. As the skin perfusion also reflects changes in systemic perfusion, it seems a matter of temper which company brand to use for tracking changes in regional tissue oxygenation in the perioperative setting.

7. Recommended actions

When planning anesthetic care, it is recommended to consider risk factors for the development of perioperative hypoperfusion such as hypotension, hypovolemia, and anemia, also considering an influence of hypocapnia. This is important in patients with severe arteriosclerosis who suffer from impaired autoregulation. Preexisting cerebrovascular disease should be considered as well.

The intended surgery is always an issue when anesthetic care of the patient is planned. Thus, based on this narrative review, cerebral oximetry should be considered for major abdominal surgery, specific orthopedic surgeries involving the elderly, neurosurgery when feasible, and particularly in vascular surgery and in surgery involving frail patients. The anesthetic considerations involve the capacity to provide vasopressor therapy and the ability to adjust for ventilation as well as knowledge on how to administer fluid in a goal-directed manner using cardiac stroke volume. For practical purposes, a baseline NIRS recording before anesthesia is considered an advantage. Attention is devoted to that movement of the head, for example, in response to orotracheal intubation, affects the pathway of light into the brain. Also, movement of the NIRS sensor is considered to affect the baseline recording. An algorithm or a guideline may help to support the decision-making strategy as supplemented by NIRS recordings [8, 24].

8. Conclusion

Cerebral oximetry is considered a valuable tool as a monitoring device to record changes in frontal lobe oxygenation during noncardiac surgery to reduce the risk of perioperative complications. Implementing targeted interventions in response to change in cerebral oxygenation may improve the patient's postoperative outcome. Further research is needed to establish standardized protocols and ensure broader clinical adoption. Secondly, newer NIRS devices offering insight into whole brain oxygenation may be on the doorstep as next generation for perioperative monitoring.

Author details

Henning Bay Nielsen
Department of Anesthesia and Intensive Care, Zealand University Hospital, University of Copenhagen, Denmark

*Address all correspondence to: hennin@regionsjaelland.dk

References

[1] Vincent JL, Pelosi P, Pearse R, Payen D, Perel A, Hoeft A, et al. Perioperative cardiovascular monitoring of high-risk patients: A consensus of 12. Critical Care. 2015;**19**:224. DOI: 10.1186/s13054-015-0932-7

[2] Madsen PL, Secher NH. Near-infrared oximetry of the brain. Progress in Neurobiology. 1999;**58**:541-560. DOI: 10.1016/s0301-0082(98)00093-8

[3] Murkin JM. Is it better to shine a light, or rather to curse the darkness? Cerebral near-infrared spectroscopy and cardiac surgery. European Journal of Cardio-Thoracic Surgery. 2013;**43**:1081-1083. DOI: 10.1093/ejcts/ezt186

[4] Murkin JM. Cerebral oximetry: Monitoring the brain as the index organ. Anesthesiology. 2011;**114**:12-13. DOI: 10.1097/ALN.0b013e3181fef5d2

[5] Murkin JM, Arango M. Near-infrared spectroscopy as an index of brain and tissue oxygenation. British Journal of Anaesthesia. 2009;**103**(Suppl 1):i3-i13. DOI: 10.1093/bja/aep299

[6] Murkin JM, Adams SJ, Pardy E, Quantz M, McKenzie FN, Guo L. Monitoring brain oxygen saturation during coronary bypass surgery improves outcomes in diabetic patients: A post hoc analysis. The Heart Surgery Forum. 2011;**14**:E1-E6. DOI: 10.1532/HSF98.20101065

[7] Murkin JM, Adams SJ, Novick RJ, Quantz M, Bainbridge D, Iglesias I, et al. Monitoring brain oxygen saturation during coronary bypass surgery: A randomized, prospective study. Anesthesia and Analgesia. 2007;**104**:51-58

[8] Nielsen HB. Systematic review of near-infrared spectroscopy determined cerebral oxygenation during non-cardiac surgery. Frontiers in Physiology. 2014;**5**:93. DOI: 10.3389/fphys.2014.00093

[9] Galyfos G, Sianou A, Filis K. Cerebral hyperperfusion syndrome and intracranial hemorrhage after carotid endarterectomy or carotid stenting: A meta-analysis. Journal of the Neurological Sciences. 2017;**381**:74-82. DOI: 10.1016/j.jns.2017.08.020

[10] Duarte-Gamas L, Fragão-Marques M, Zlatanovic P, Andrade JP, Rocha-Neves J. The diagnostic accuracy of intraoperative near-infrared spectroscopy in carotid artery endarterectomy under general anesthesia: A systematic review with meta-analysis. Scandinavian Journal of Surgery. 2025;**114**:84-94. DOI: 10.1177/14574969241282611

[11] Duarte-Gamas L, Pereira-Neves A, Sousa J, Sousa-Pinto B, Rocha-Neves J. The diagnostic accuracy of intra-operative near infrared spectroscopy in carotid artery endarterectomy under regional anaesthesia: Systematic review and meta-analysis. European Journal of Vascular and Endovascular Surgery. 2021;**62**:522-f31. DOI: 10.1016/j.ejvs.2021.05.042

[12] Alhaizaey A, Yousif M, Azazy A, Saber A, Safan M, Elgamal GA, et al. Prospective single-center study on the reliability of ipsilateral cerebral oximetry using near-infrared spectroscopy as a predictor for selective shunting during carotid endarterectomy. Vascular. 2024;**32**(6):1304-1308. DOI: 10.1177/17085381231214596

[13] Hill WF, Kinaschuk K, Temple-Oberle C. Intraoperative near-infrared

spectroscopy can predict skin flap necrosis. Plastic and Reconstructive Surgery. Global Open. 2024;**12**(3):e5669. DOI: 10.1097/GOX.0000000000005669

[14] Chan SS, Pek CH, Wu Y, Kong Y, Ho WM, Hwee JJ. Near-infrared spectroscopy-guided flap delay: For flap training and timing of pedicle division. Journal of Plastic and Reconstructive Surgery. 2024;**4**:57-60. DOI: 10.53045/jprs.2023-0063

[15] Kagaya Y, Miyamoto S. A systematic review of near-infrared spectroscopy in flap monitoring: Current basic and clinical evidence and prospects. Journal of Plastic, Reconstructive & Aesthetic Surgery. 2018;**71**:246-257. DOI: 10.1016/j.bjps.2017.10.020

[16] Hill WF, Webb C, Monument M, McKinnon G, Hayward V, Temple-Oberle C. Intraoperative near-infrared spectroscopy correlates with skin flap necrosis: A prospective cohort study. Plastic and Reconstructive Surgery. Global Open. 2020;**8**(4):e2742. DOI: 10.1097/GOX.000000000000274

[17] Eiberg JP, Schroeder TV, Vogt KC, Secher NH. Near-infrared spectroscopy during peripheral vascular surgery. Cardiovascular Surgery. 1997;**5**:304-308. DOI: 10.1016/s0967-2109(97)00015-x

[18] Aceto P, Galletta C, Cambise C, Punzo G, Luca E, Schipa C, et al. Challenges for anaesthesia for robotic-assisted surgery in the elderly: A narrative review. European Journal of Anaesthesiology and Intensive Care. 2023;**2**:e0019. DOI: 10.1097/EA9.0000000000000019

[19] Wang Z, Wang X, Yu X. The effects of different positions on lower extremity hemodynamics during robot-assisted laparoscopic radical prostatectomy for prostate cancer. BMC Urology. 2024;**24**:92. DOI: 10.1186/s12894-024-01462-3

[20] Özgün A, Sargin A, Karaman S, Günüşen İ, Alper I, Aşkar FZ. The relationship between the Trendelenburg position and cerebral hypoxia inpatients who have undergone robot-assisted hysterectomy and prostatectomy. Turkish Journal of Medical Sciences. 2017;**47**:1797-1803. DOI: 10.3906/sag-1704-159

[21] Brincat SD, Caruana C, Mukherjee R. Frailty status as a predictor of outcomes in emergency surgeries for older adults: A systematic review and meta-analysis. Cureus. 2025;**17**:e84160. DOI: 10.7759/cureus.84160

[22] Kan CFK, Skaggs JD. Current commonly used dynamic parameters and monitoring systems for perioperative goal-directed fluid therapy: A review. The Yale Journal of Biology and Medicine. 2023;**96**:107-123. DOI: 10.59249/JOAP6662

[23] Cushing H. On routine determinations of arterial tension in operating room and clinic. The Boston Medical and Surgical Journal. 1903;**48**:250-256

[24] Navarro-Perez R, Romero-García N, Paolessi C, Robba C, Badenes R. Cerebral oximetry in high-risk surgical patients: Where are we? Current Opinion in Critical Care. 2024;**30**:672-678. DOI: 10.1097/MCC.0000000000001204

[25] Wilson JR, Mancini DM, McCully K, Ferraro N, Lanoce V, Chance B. Noninvasive detection of skeletal muscle underperfusion with near-infrared spectroscopy in patients with heart failure. Circulation. 1989;**80**:1668-1674. DOI: 10.1161/01.cir.80.6.1668

[26] Chance B, Dait MT, Zhang C, Hamaoka T, Hagerman F. Recovery from exercise-induced desaturation in the quadriceps muscles of elite competitive rowers. The American Journal of Physiology. 1992;**262**(3 Pt 1):C766-C775. DOI: 10.1152/ajpcell.1992.262.3.C766

[27] Madsen P, Olesen HL, Klokker M, Secher NH. Peripheral venous oxygen saturation during head-up tilt induced hypovolaemic shock in humans. Scandinavian Journal of Clinical and Laboratory Investigation. 1993;**53**:411-416. DOI: 10.3109/00365519309086634

[28] Madsen P, Lyck F, Pedersen M, Olesen HL, Nielsen HB, Secher NH. Brain and muscle oxygen saturation during head-up-tilt-induced central hypovolemia in humans. Clinical Physiology. 1995;**15**:523-533. DOI: 10.1111/j.1475-097x.1995.tb00541.x

[29] Nielsen HB, Boushel R, Madsen P, Secher NH. Cerebral desaturation during exercise reversed by O_2 supplementation. American Journal of Physiology. Heart and Circulatory Physiology. 1999;**277**(3):H1045-H1052. DOI: 10.1152/ajpheart.1999.277.3.H1045

[30] Rasmussen LS. Postoperative cognitive dysfunction: Incidence and prevention. Best Practice & Research. Clinical Anaesthesiology. 2006;**20**:315-330. DOI: 10.1016/j.bpa.2005.10.011

[31] Wong ZZ, Chiong XH, Chaw SH, Hashim NHBM, Abidin MFBZ, Yunus SNB, et al. The use of cerebral oximetry in surgery: A systematic review and meta-analysis of randomized controlled trials. Journal of Cardiothoracic and Vascular Anesthesia. 2022;**36**:2002-2011. DOI: 10.1053/j.jvca.2021.09.046

[32] Clemmesen CG, Pedersen LM, Hougaard S, Andersson ML, Rosenkvist V, Nielsen HB, et al. Cerebral oximetry during preoperative resuscitation in elderly patients with hip fracture: A prospective observational study. Journal of Clinical Monitoring and Computing. 2018;**32**(6):1033-1040. DOI: 10.1007/s10877-018-0107-6

[33] Moller JT, Johannessen NW, Espersen K, Ravlo O, Pedersen BD, Jensen PF, et al. Randomized evaluation of pulse oximetry in 20,802 patients: II. Perioperative events and postoperative complications. Anesthesiology. 1993;**78**:445-453. DOI:10.1097/00000542-199303000-00007

[34] Pedersen T, Dyrlund Pedersen B, Møller AM. Pulse oximetry for perioperative monitoring. Cochrane Database of Systematic Reviews. 2003;(3):CD002013. DOI: 10.1002/14651858.CD002013

[35] Pedersen T, Nicholson A, Hovhannisyan K, Møller AM, Smith AF, Lewis SR. Pulse oximetry for perioperative monitoring. Cochrane Database of Systematic Reviews. 2014;**2014**:CD002013. DOI: 10.1002/14651858.CD002013

[36] Casati A, Fanelli G, Pietropaoli P, Proietti R, Tufano R, Montanini S, et al. Monitoring cerebral oxygen saturation in elderly patients undergoing general abdominal surgery: A prospective cohort study. European Journal of Anaesthesiology. 2007;**24**:59-65. DOI: 10.1017/S0265021506001025

[37] Casati A, Fanelli G, Pietropaoli P, Proietti R, Tufano R, Danelli G, et al. Continuous monitoring of cerebral oxygen saturation in elderly patients undergoing major abdominal surgery minimizes brain exposure to potential hypoxia. Anesthesia and Analgesia. 2005;**101**:740-747. DOI: 10.1213/01.ane.0000166974.96219.cd

[38] Slater JP, Guarino T, Stack J, Vinod K, Bustami RT, Brown JM, et al. Cerebral oxygen desaturation predicts cognitive decline and longer hospital stay after cardiac surgery. The Annals of Thoracic Surgery. 2009;**87**:36-44. DOI: 10.1016/j.athoracsur.2008.08.070

[39] Heringlake M, Garbers C, Käbler JH, Anderson I, Heinze H, Schön J, et al. Preoperative cerebral oxygen saturation and clinical outcomes in cardiac surgery. Anesthesiology. 2011;**114**:58-69. DOI: 10.1097/ALN.0b013e3181fef34e

[40] Rokamp KZ, Secher NH, Eiberg J, Lønn L, Nielsen HB. O_2 supplementation to secure the near-infrared spectroscopy determined brain and muscle oxygenation in vascular surgical patients: A presentation of 100 cases. Frontiers in Physiology. 2014;**5**:66. DOI: 10.3389/fphys.2014.00066

[41] Moreira TS, Mulkey DK, Takakura AC. Update on vascular control of central chemoreceptors. Experimental Physiology. 2024;**109**:1837-1843. DOI: 10.1113/EP091329

[42] Jørgensen LG. Transcranial Doppler ultrasound for cerebral perfusion. Acta Physiologica Scandinavica. Supplementum. 1995;**625**:1-44

[43] Garcia AV, Velez AK, Surma V, Jager LR, Bembea MM. Impact of red blood cell transfusion on regional cerebral oxygen saturation during pediatric ECMO. Transfusion (Paris). 2023;**63**:942-951. DOI: 10.1111/trf.17317

[44] Yee MEMP, Fasano RM. Novel approaches to measure transfusion effectiveness. Current Opinion in Hematology. 2023;**30**(6):230-236. DOI: 10.1097/MOH.0000000000000783

[45] Torella F, McCollum C. Regional haemoglobin oxygen saturation during surgical haemorrhage. Minerva Medica. 2004;**95**(5):461-467

[46] Møller A, Wetterslev J, Shahidi S, Hellemann D, Secher NH, Pedersen OB, et al. Effect of low vs high haemoglobin transfusion trigger on cardiac output in patients undergoing elective vascular surgery: Post-hoc analysis of a randomized trial. Acta Anaesthesiologica Scandinavica. 2021;**65**:302-312. DOI: 10.1111/aas.13733

[47] Madsen P, Iversen H, Secher NH. Central venous oxygen saturation during hypovolaemic shock in humans. Scandinavian Journal of Clinical and Laboratory Investigation. 1993;**53**:67-72. DOI: 10.1080/00365519309092533

[48] Lund A, Sørensen H, Jensen TW, Niemann MJ, Olesen ND, Nielsen HB, et al. Muscle oxygen saturation increases during head-up tilt-induced (pre)syncope. Acta Physiologica (Oxford, England). 2017;**221**(1):74-80. DOI: 10.1111/apha.12863

[49] Pedersen M, Madsen P, Klokker M, Olesen HL, Secher NH. Sympathetic influence on cardiovascular responses to sustained head-up tilt in humans. Acta Physiologica Scandinavica. 1995;**155**:435-444. DOI: 10.1111/j.1748-1716.1995.tb09993.x

[50] Van Lieshout JJ, Secher NH. Reflex control of sympathetic vasoconstrictor activity in vasovagal syncope. Clinical Autonomic Research. 2003;**13**:175-177. DOI: 10.1007/s10286-003-0094-6

[51] Wasmund SL, Smith ML, Takata TS, Joglar JA, Li JM, Kowal RC, et al. Sympathoexcitation is attenuated during low level lower body negative pressure in subjects who develop pre-syncope. Clinical Autonomic Research. 2003;**13**(3):208-213. DOI: 10.1007/s10286-003-0093-7

[52] Licker M. Regional or general anaesthesia for carotid endarterectomy. Does it matter? European Journal of Anaesthesiology. 2016;**33**:241-243. DOI: 10.1097/EJA.0000000000000376

[53] Cedergreen P, Swiatek F, Nielsen HB. Local anaesthesia for carotid endarterectomy: Pro: Protect the brain. European Journal of Anaesthesiology. 2016;**33**:236-237. DOI: 10.1097/EJA.0000000000000370

[54] Czinege Z, Sándor ÁD, Gyürki D, Varga A, Csípő T, Székely A, et al. Understanding perioperative risk determinants in carotid endarterectomy: The impact of compromised circle of Willis morphology on inter-hemispheric blood flow indices based on intraoperative internal carotid artery stump pulse pressure and backflow patterns. Geroscience. 2025;**47**:2159-2177. DOI: 10.1007/s11357-024-01390-y

[55] Pennekamp CWA, Moll FL, De Borst GJ. The potential benefits and the role of cerebral monitoring in carotid endarterectomy. Current Opinion in Anaesthesiology. 2011;**24**:693-697. DOI: 10.1097/ACO.0b013e32834c7aa1

[56] Pennekamp CWA, Bots ML, Kappelle LJ, Moll FL, de Borst GJ. The value of near-infrared spectroscopy measured cerebral oximetry during carotid endarterectomy in perioperative stroke prevention. A review. European Journal of Vascular and Endovascular Surgery. 2009;**38**(5):539-545. DOI: 10.1016/j.ejvs.2009.07.008

[57] Pennekamp CWA, Immink RV, Den Ruijter HM, Kappelle LJ, Bots ML, Buhre WF, et al. Near-infrared spectroscopy to indicate selective shunt use during carotid endarterectomy. European Journal of Vascular and Endovascular Surgery. 2013;**46**(4):397-403. DOI: 10.1016/j.ejvs.2013.07.007

[58] Li M, Ma T, Yin X, Zhang X, Long T, Zeng M, et al. Cerebral oximetry index indicates delirium or stroke after carotid endarterectomy: An observational study. Journal of Clinical Anesthesia. 2025;**101**:111733. DOI: 10.1016/j.jclinane.2024.111733

[59] Zipfel J, Bantle SJ, Magunia H, Schlensak C, Neunhoeffer F, Schuhmann MU, et al. Non-invasive cerebral autoregulation monitoring during awake carotid endarterectomy identifies clinically significant brain ischaemia. European Journal of Vascular and Endovascular Surgery. 2020;**60**(5):647-654. DOI: 10.1016/j.ejvs.2020.07.076

[60] Lee D, Batista PM, McMackin KK, Ha A, Trani J, Carpenter JP, et al. Intraoperative blood pressure lability carries a higher risk of headache after carotid endarterectomy. Journal of Vascular Surgery. 2022;**75**:592-598.e1. DOI: 10.1016/j.jvs.2021.08.070

[61] Togashi S, Shimizu H, Suda Y. Utility of near-infrared spectroscopy monitoring in the management of hyperperfusion syndrome after intracranial carotid artery stenting. NMC Case Report Journal. 2020;**7**:223-227. DOI: 10.2176/nmccrj.cr.2020-0003

[62] Lavoue V, Zeng X, Lau S, Press JZ, Abitbol J, Gotlieb R, et al. Impact of robotics on the outcome of elderly patients with endometrial cancer. Gynecologic Oncology. 2014;**133**(3):556-562. DOI: 10.1016/j.ygyno.2014.03.572

[63] Vejlgaard M, Maibom SL, Joensen UN, Thind PO, Rohrsted M, Aasvang EK, et al. Quality of life and secondary outcomes for open versus robot-assisted radical cystectomy: A double-blinded, randomised feasibility trial. World Journal of Urology. 2022;**40**:1669-1677. DOI: 10.1007/s00345-022-04029-9

[64] Katayama S, Mori K, Pradere B, Yanagisawa T, Mostafaei H, Quhal F, et al. Influence of steep Trendelenburg position on postoperative complications: A systematic review and meta-analysis. Journal of Robotic Surgery. 2022;**16**:1233-1247. DOI: 10.1007/s11701-021-01361-x

[65] Robba C, Cardim D, Donnelly J, Bertuccio A, Bacigaluppi S, Bragazzi N, et al. Effects of pneumoperitoneum and Trendelenburg position on intracranial pressure assessed using different non-invasive methods. British Journal of Anaesthesia. 2016;**117**(6):783-791. DOI: 10.1093/bja/aew356

[66] Blecha S, Harth M, Schlachetzki F, Zeman F, Blecha C, Flora P, et al. Changes in intraocular pressure and optic nerve sheath diameter in patients undergoing robotic-assisted laparoscopic prostatectomy in steep 45° Trendelenburg position. BMC Anesthesiology. 2017;**17**(1):40. DOI: 10.1186/s12871-017-0333-3

[67] Ripa M, Schipa C, Kopsacheilis N, Nomikarios M, Perrotta G, De Rosa C, et al. The impact of steep Trendelenburg position on intraocular pressure. Journal of Clinical Medicine. 2022;**11**:2844. DOI: 10.3390/jcm11102844

[68] Karaveli A, Kavakli AS, Özçelik M, Ateş M, İnanoğlu K, Özmen S. The effect of different levels of pneumoperitoneum pressures on regional cerebral oxygenation during robotic assisted laparoscopic prostatectomy. Turkish Journal of Medical Sciences. 2021;**51**:1136-1145. DOI: 10.3906/sag-2005-368

[69] Wiesinger C, Schoeb DS, Stockhammer M, Mirtezani E, Mitterschiffthaler L, Wagner H, et al. Cerebral oxygenation in 45-degree trendelenburg position for robot-assisted radical prostatectomy: A single-center, open, controlled pilot study. BMC Urology. 2020;**20**(1):198. DOI: 10.1186/s12894-020-00774-4

[70] Schramm P, Treiber AH, Berres M, Pestel G, Engelhard K, Werner C, et al. Time course of cerebrovascular autoregulation during extreme Trendelenburg position for robotic-assisted prostatic surgery. Anaesthesia. 2014;**69**:58-63. DOI: 10.1111/anae.12477

[71] Lestar M, Gunnarsson L, Lagerstrand L, Wiklund P, Odeberg-Wernerman S. Hemodynamic perturbations during robot-assisted laparoscopic radical prostatectomy in 45° Trendelenburg position. Anesthesia and Analgesia. 2011;**113**:1069-1075. DOI: 10.1213/ANE.0b013e3182075d1f

[72] Darlong V, Garg R, Kumar R, Kunhabdulla NP, Pandey R, Chandralekha, et al. Hemodynamic changes during robotic radical prostatectomy. Saudi Journal of Anaesthesia. 2012;**6**:213-218. DOI: 10.4103/1658-354X.101210

[73] Rosendal C, Markin S, Hien MD, Motsch J, Roggenbach J. Cardiac and hemodynamic consequences during capnoperitoneum and steep Trendelenburg positioning: Lessons learned from robot-assisted laparoscopic prostatectomy. Journal of Clinical Anesthesia. 2014;**26**:383-389. DOI: 10.1016/j.jclinane.2014.01.014

[74] Pawlik MT, Prasser C, Zeman F, Harth M, Burger M, Denzinger S, et al. Pronounced haemodynamic changes during and after robotic-assisted laparoscopic prostatectomy: A prospective observational study. BMJ Open. 2020;**10**:e038045

[75] Haas S, Haese A, Goetz AE, Kubitz JC. Haemodynamics and cardiac function during robotic-assisted

laparoscopic prostatectomy in steep Trendelenburg position. International Journal of Medical Robotics and Computer Assisted Surgery. 2011;**7**:408-413. DOI: 10.1002/rcs.410

[76] Kılınç E, Yildirim SA, Ulugöl H, Büyüköner EE, Güçyetmez B, Toraman F. The evaluation of cardiac functions in deep Trendelenburg position during robotic-assisted laparoscopic prostatectomy. Frontiers in Medicine. 2023;**10**:1273180. DOI: 10.3389/fmed.2023.1273180

[77] Kim NY, Kim KJ, Kim TL, Shin HJ, Oh C, Lee MH, et al. Prediction of hypotension after postural change in robot-assisted laparoscopic prostatectomy using esophageal Doppler monitoring: A prospective observational trial. Scientific Reports. 2021;**11**:14589. DOI: 10.1038/s41598-021-93990-3

[78] Wesselink EM, Wagemakers SH, van Waes JAR, Wanderer JP, van Klei WA, Kappen TH. Associations between intraoperative hypotension, duration of surgery and postoperative myocardial injury after noncardiac surgery: A retrospective single-centre cohort study. British Journal of Anaesthesia. 2022;**129**:487-496. DOI: 10.1016/j.bja.2022.06.034

[79] Endo Y, Akatsuka J, Kuwahara K, Takasaki S, Takeda H, Yanagi M, et al. A case of well leg compartment syndrome after robot-assisted laparoscopic prostatectomy: With review. The Journal of Medical Investigation. 2022;**69**(1.2):145-147. DOI: 10.2152/jmi.69.145

[80] Tantry TP, Muralishankar BG, Karanth H, Shetty PK, Shenoy SP, Kadam D, et al. Prophylactic measures to prevent cerebral oxygen desaturation events in elective beach-chair position shoulder surgeries: A systematic review and meta-analysis. Korean Journal of Anesthesiology. 2021;**74**:422-438. DOI: 10.4097/kja.21069

[81] Li X, Eichinger JK, Hartshorn T, Zhou H, Matzkin EG, Warner JP. A comparison of the lateral decubitus and beach-chair positions for shoulder surgery: Advantages and complications. The Journal of the American Academy of Orthopaedic Surgeons. 2015;**23**:18-28. DOI: 10.5435/JAAOS-23-01-18

[82] Thanaboriboon C, Vanichvithya P, Jinaworn P. What is the risk of intraoperative cerebral oxygen desaturation in patients undergoing shoulder surgery in the beach chair position? Clinical Orthopaedics and Related Research. 2021;**479**(12):2677-2687. DOI: 10.1097/CORR.0000000000001864

[83] Dippmann C, Winge S, Nielsen HB. Severe cerebral desaturation during shoulder arthroscopy in the beach-chair position. Arthroscopy. 2010;**26**(9 Suppl):S148-S150. DOI: 10.1016/j.arthro.2010.03.012

[84] De Rojas JO, Syre P, Welch WC. Regional anesthesia versus general anesthesia for surgery on the lumbar spine: A review of the modern literature. Clinical Neurology and Neurosurgery. 2014;**119**:39-43. DOI: 10.1016/j.clineuro.2014.01.016

[85] Ono M, Joshi B, Brady K, Easley RB, Zheng Y, Brown C, et al. Risks for impaired cerebral autoregulation during cardiopulmonary bypass and postoperative stroke. British Journal of Anaesthesia. 2012;**109**:391-398. DOI: 10.1093/bja/aes148

[86] Fried LP, Tangen CM, Walston J, Newman AB, Hirsch C, Gottdiener J, et al. Frailty in older adults: Evidence for a phenotype. The Journals of

Gerontology. Series A, Biological Sciences and Medical Sciences. 2001;**56**(3):M146-M156. DOI: 10.1093/gerona/56.3.m146

[87] Sabaté S, Gomar C, Huguet J, Castillo J, Canet J, Villalonga A. Anesthesia for urological surgery in a European region with 6.7 million inhabitants (Catalonia, Spain). Journal of Clinical Anesthesia. 2009;**21**(1):30-37. DOI: 10.1016/j.jclinane.2008.06.017

[88] Suskind AM, Jin C, Cooperberg MR, Finlayson E, Boscardin WJ, Sen S, et al. Preoperative frailty is associated with discharge to skilled or assisted living facilities after urologic procedures of varying complexity. Urology. 2016;**97**:25-32. DOI: 10.1016/j.urology.2016.03.073

[89] Scheipner L, Zurl H, Altziebler JV, Pichler GP, Schöpfer-Schwab S, Jasarevic S, et al. Charlson-Deyo comorbidity index as a novel predictor for recurrence in non-muscle-invasive bladder cancer. Cancers (Basel). 2023;**15**:5770. DOI: 10.3390/cancers15245770

[90] Sanada F, Taniyama Y, Muratsu J, Otsu R, Shimizu H, Rakugi H, et al. Source of chronic inflammation in aging. Frontiers in Cardiovascular Medicine. 2018;**5**:12. DOI: 10.3389/fcvm.2018.00012

[91] Henein MY, Vancheri S, Longo G, Vancheri F. The role of inflammation in cardiovascular disease. International Journal of Molecular Sciences. 2022;**23**:12906. DOI: 10.3390/ijms232112906

[92] Lee A, Kim SH, Hong JY, Hwang JH. Effect of anesthetic methods on cerebral oxygen saturation in elderly surgical patients: Prospective, randomized, observational study. World Journal of Surgery. 2012;**36**:2328-2334. DOI: 10.1007/s00268-012-1676-z

[93] Dutton RP. Controlled hypotension for spinal surgery. European Spine Journal. 2004;**3 Suppl 1**(Suppl 1):S66-S71. DOI: 10.1007/s00586-004-0756-7

[94] Choi H, Huh J, Koo J, Lee J, Hwang W, Schaller B. Effects of milrinone on cerebral perfusion and postoperative cognitive function in spine surgery: Secondary analysis of a CONSORT-compliant randomized controlled trial. Medicine. 2020;**99**(46):e21717. DOI: 10.1097/MD.0000000000021717

[95] Nissen P, Pacino H, Frederiksen HJ, Novovic S, Secher NH. Near-infrared spectroscopy for evaluation of cerebral autoregulation during orthotopic liver transplantation. Neurocritical Care. 2009;**11**(2):235-241. DOI: 10.1007/s12028-009-9226-8

[96] Baltrūnas T, Mosenko V, Mackevičius A, Dambrauskas V, Ašakienė I, Ručinskas K, et al. The use of near-infrared spectroscopy in the diagnosis of peripheral artery disease: A systematic review. Vascular. 2022;**30**:715-727. DOI: 10.1177/17085381211025174

[97] Taudorf M, Nielsen MB, Schroeder TV, Lönn L, Nielsen HB. Endovascular aortic repair reduces gluteal oxygenation. Acta Radiologica Open. 2019;**8**:2058460119850115. DOI: 10.1177/2058460119850115

[98] Newton E, Butskiy O, Shadgan B, Prisman E, Anderson DW. Outcomes of free flap reconstructions with near-infrared spectroscopy (NIRS) monitoring: A systematic review. Microsurgery. 2020;**40**(2):268-275. DOI: 10.1002/micr.30526

[99] Futier E, Christophe S, Robin E, Petit A, Pereira B, Desbordes J, et al. Use of near-infrared spectroscopy during a vascular occlusion test to assess the

microcirculatory response during fluid challenge. Critical Care. 2011;**15**(5):R214. DOI: 10.1186/cc10449

[100] Svendsen LB, Flink P, Wøjdemann M, Riber C, Mogensen T, Secher NH. Muscle oxygen saturation during surgery in the lithotomy position. Clinical Physiology. 1997;7(5):433-438. DOI: 10.1046/j.1365-2281.1997.04747.x

[101] Nissen P, Bjørnholdt K, Secher NH. Crural compartment syndrome following surgery in the lithotomy position. Ugeskrift for Laeger. 2008;**170**(33):2467

[102] Shuler MS, Roskosky M, Kinsey T, Glaser D, Reisman W, Ogburn C, et al. Continual near-infrared spectroscopy monitoring in the injured lower limb and acute compartment syndrome: An FDA-IDE trial. The Bone & Joint Journal. 2018;**100-B**(6):787-797. DOI: 10.1302/0301-620X.100B6.BJJ-2017-0736.R3

[103] Holmgaard F, Vedel AG, Langkilde A, Nilsson JC, Ravn HB. Does depth of the frontal sinus affect near-infrared spectroscopy measurement? Perfusion. 2016;**31**(8):659-661. DOI: 10.1177/0267659116649425

[104] Vedamurthy M. Beware what you inject: Complications of injectables-dermal fillers. Journal of Cutaneous and Aesthetic Surgery. 2018;**11**(2):60-66. DOI: 10.4103/JCAS.JCAS_68_18

[105] Madsen PL, Skak C, Rasmussen A, Secher NH. Interference of cerebral near-infrared oximetry in patients with icterus. Anesthesia and Analgesia. 2000;**90**:489-493. DOI: 10.1097/00000539-200002000-00046

[106] Nielsen HB, Larsen FS. Cerebral oximetry and hyperbilirubinemia. Anesthesia and Analgesia. 2001;**93**(1):245-246. DOI:10.1097/00000539-200107000-00060

[107] Egesborg AH, Sørensen H, Olesen ND, Secher NH. Phenylephrine increases near-infrared spectroscopy determined muscle oxygenation during head-up tilt in men. Scandinavian Journal of Clinical and Laboratory Investigation. 2018;**78**:601-605. DOI: 10.1080/00365513.2018.1528505

[108] Sørensen H, Secher NH, Siebenmann C, Nielsen HB, Kohl-Bareis M, Lundby C, et al. Cutaneous vasoconstriction affects near-infrared spectroscopy determined cerebral oxygen saturation during administration of norepinephrine. Anesthesiology. 2012;**117**(2):263-270. DOI: 10.1097/ALN.0b013e3182605afe

[109] Foss VT, Christensen R, Rokamp KZ, Nissen P, Secher NH, Nielsen HB. Effect of phenylephrine vs. ephedrine on frontal lobe oxygenation during caesarean section with spinal anesthesia: An open label randomized controlled trial. Frontiers in Physiology. 2014;**5**:81. DOI: 10.3389/fphys.2014.00081

[110] Rokamp KZ, Staalsoe JM, Gartmann M, Sletgaard A, Nordsborg NB, Secher NH, et al. G16R single nucleotide polymorphism but not haplotypes of the β2-adrenergic receptor gene alters cardiac output in humans. Clinical Science. 2013;**8**:661. DOI: 10.3389/fphys.2017.00661

[111] Staalsø JM, Rokamp KZ, Olesen ND, Lonn L, Secher NH, Olsen NV, et al. ADRB2 gly16gly genotype, cardiac output, and cerebral oxygenation in patients undergoing anesthesia for abdominal aortic aneurysm surgery. Anesthesia and Analgesia. 2016;**123**:1408-1415. DOI: 10.1213/ANE.0000000000001563

[112] Kitchen CC, Nissen P, Secher NH, Nielsen HB. Preserved frontal lobe oxygenation following calcium chloride for treatment of anesthesia-induced hypotension. Frontiers in Physiology. 2014;**5**:407. DOI: 10.3389/fphys.2014.00407

[113] Nissen P, van Lieshout JJ, Nielsen HB, Secher NH. Frontal lobe oxygenation is maintained during hypotension following propofol-fentanyl anesthesia. American Association of Nurse Anesthesiology. 2009;**77**:271-276

[114] Davie SN, Grocott HP. Impact of extracranial contamination on regional cerebral oxygen saturation: A comparison of three cerebral oximetry technologies. Anesthesiology. 2012;**116**:834-840. DOI: 10.1097/ALN.0b013e31824c00d7

Chapter 6

Methodological Issues and Safety Considerations in Enhancing Exercise Performance through Ischemic Preconditioning

Yilin Zhang and Yun Xie

Abstract

Ischemic preconditioning (IPC), a technique involving short, intermittent bouts of limb ischemia followed by reperfusion, has gained significant attention in sports science as an intervention to enhance exercise performance. Although empirical studies have reported beneficial effects on endurance, strength, and recovery, methodological inconsistencies and safety concerns remain unresolved. This chapter systematically reviews key methodological variables of IPC, including intervention devices, pressure protocols, target limbs and cycles, timing intervals, experimental designs, and participant characteristics, highlighting their potential moderating effects on IPC outcomes. Furthermore, the chapter evaluates existing safety issues in IPC applications and proposes practical strategies—such as individualized pressure control, rating of perceived exertion (RPE) monitoring, and standardized warm-up procedures—to improve the feasibility and applicability of IPC interventions. Results suggest that IPC is a low-risk and highly adaptable method with potential to enhance physical performance. However, its underlying mechanisms are yet to be unified, and its applicability remains limited. There is an urgent need for future studies with higher ecological validity across variables such as gender, age, and athletic level. This review aims to provide methodological guidance and safety references for the scientific use and further development of IPC interventions.

Keywords: ischemia, pressure, blood flow restriction, perceived exertion, method, safety

1. Introduction

Ischemic preconditioning (IPC) refers to a process in which the body is exposed to several brief, non-lethal episodes of ischemia followed by reperfusion, thereby enhancing tissue tolerance to subsequent prolonged and severe ischemic insults, ultimately providing protective effects to target organs [1]. This mechanism was initially discovered for its cardioprotective effects and gained widespread attention through clinical and experimental studies in the 1980s and 1990s [2, 3]. Subsequent research has demonstrated that IPC also confers protective benefits to the liver [4], kidneys [5], brain [6], intestines [7], and skeletal muscle [8].

In the field of sports science, IPC is defined as the repeated application of localized limb ischemia and reperfusion prior to exercise or testing, with the aim of enhancing physical performance within a specific time window [9, 10]. The primary mechanism is thought to involve an increased tolerance to subsequent ischemia induced by IPC [11], along with a reduction in the energy metabolism rate during exercise without affecting adenosine triphosphate (ATP) levels [3]. This line of research gained traction in the early twenty-first century, with a pivotal 2005 study showing that IPC provided both early and late protection against endothelial ischemia-reperfusion injury in humans [12]. In 2010, it was further demonstrated that performing IPC before an incremental cycling test could improve maximal oxygen uptake (VO_2max) by 3% and power output by 1.6% [13]. Over the past two decades, research in this area has grown exponentially, with over 200 original studies on IPC and exercise performance currently available in both domestic and international databases.

Despite the extensive body of research on IPC, the field remains characterized by substantial methodological heterogeneity [14]. A recent study found that although IPC significantly improves exercise performance, the underlying mechanism may stem more from placebo effects—such as low-pressure ischemia (e.g., 20 mmHg)—than from IPC's direct physiological efficacy [15]. Their results indicated a significant placebo effect compared to control conditions (e.g., effect size for resistance exercise repetitions = 0.45; p = 0.03) [15]. However, Zhang Yilin et al. identified considerable methodological inconsistencies across 79 studies [15, 16]: (1) 61 studies included a warm-up between IPC and performance testing, meaning the reported interval actually reflected the time between IPC and the warm-up, not the test itself; (2) only 13 studies employed a direct IPC-to-test protocol without a warm-up; (3) 3 studies used a warm-up–IPC–test sequence. This methodological heterogeneity extends beyond placebo effects and experimental sequencing. Variables such as time interval between IPC and testing [17], ischemia-reperfusion protocol [18], pressure standards [18], and participant characteristics (e.g., sex, age, and training background) [17] may all directly or indirectly influence the effectiveness of IPC on performance outcomes [19]. For instance, regarding time interval, Seeley et al. found that a 45-minute delay between IPC and warm-up enhanced muscle oxygen saturation during recovery from sprinting, outperforming a 5-minute delay [17]. In terms of sex differences, IPC significantly enhanced sympathetic functional sympatholysis in men (Δ-3% ± 9% vs. baseline Δ-8% ± 7%, p = 0.02), but not in women (Δ-5% ± 10% vs. baseline Δ-8% ± 9%, p = 0.13) [20]. Age-related physiological changes, such as reduced vascular elasticity and metabolic efficiency, may also diminish IPC's effectiveness in older adults. Furthermore, because IPC involves acute limb occlusion, it can induce blood pressure fluctuations in the treated or adjacent regions [19, 21]. Therefore, uncertainty in IPC parameter protocols and improper implementation may raise safety concerns.

In light of these issues, the present study focuses on original research combining ischemic preconditioning with exercise interventions, with an emphasis on synthesizing methodological findings in existing literature. Given that many methodological factors are closely related to safety, this review also addresses safety concerns associated with IPC. The aim is to provide a scientific basis for the informed and safe application of IPC in both fitness and elite sports contexts.

2. Methodological issues in optimizing exercise performance through ischemic preconditioning

Ischemic preconditioning IPC involves short-duration, high-frequency cycles of limb blood flow occlusion and reperfusion, eliciting physiological responses that are highly time-dependent and subject to individual variability [19, 22]. Although its potential to enhance exercise performance has been supported by systematic reviews [23, 24], significant methodological heterogeneity continues to hinder the standardization of IPC protocols and the comparability of results. IPC is primarily applied prior to exercise, testing, or competition, aiming to improve subsequent performance through repeated ischemia-reperfusion cycles. As such, factors such as the type of occlusion device, protocol design, applied pressure, site of occlusion, time interval before performance, and participant characteristics may all potentially influence the effectiveness of IPC interventions [19].

2.1 Types of ischemic preconditioning devices

In studies examining the acute effects of ischemic preconditioning IPC on exercise performance, the type of occlusion device used plays a crucial role in ensuring standardized protocol implementation, reproducibility of outcomes, and control of safety margins. Current mainstream IPC devices can be broadly categorized into three types based on their method of pressure application: traditional manually inflatable cuffs, elastic compression bands, and automated closed-loop systems. Each device type exhibits varying degrees of efficacy advantages, and practical limitations in both research and applied settings [22, 25, 26].

First, traditional manually inflatable cuffs remain the most widely used basic tool in IPC research. These devices typically employ standard medical sphygmomanometer cuffs, which are manually inflated to a pressure above the limb's arterial systolic pressure (typically 220–250 mmHg) to induce brief cycles of ischemia and reperfusion [25, 27]. Their primary advantages lie in their wide availability, low cost, and operational simplicity, making them highly practical in early exploratory studies. For example, Ferreira et al. used specially designed dual-chamber inflatable cuffs and monitored posterior tibial artery blood flow with Doppler ultrasound to confirm complete vascular occlusion, thereby ensuring consistent pressure across intervention groups [28]. However, such devices rely heavily on operator experience, making them vulnerable to human error in pressure magnitude, duration, and release timing. These factors can introduce systematic bias and inconsistencies in intervention delivery, ultimately compromising the internal validity and reproducibility of studies [16, 22].

Among elastic compression devices, blood flow restriction (BFR) training bands offer a lightweight, training-integrated alternative. These bands wrap around the limb using elastic materials to partially restrict venous return, creating a state of "limited ischemia" while still allowing some arterial inflow [29]. BFR bands are widely used in resistance training, rehabilitation, and IPC-related research. Their advantages include ease of wear, compact size, low cost, and suitability for everyday training environments or home-based interventions [30]. However, studies have pointed out that due to the inherent elasticity of the material and variability in how well the bands conform to individual limb shapes, these devices often lack precise pressure regulation, resulting in substantial inter-individual variability [31, 32]. Citherlet et al. found that elastic BFR bands produced considerable pressure fluctuations during use when comparing subjective discomfort scores with objective pressure monitoring data. In more severe cases, such fluctuations may affect participants' tolerance and muscle perfusion efficiency, thereby weakening the overall effectiveness of the intervention [32].

To enhance intervention precision and minimize human error, automated IPC devices have recently become the mainstream tools for ischemic interventions. These systems are based on microprocessor-controlled closed-loop circuits that allow precise setting and monitoring of pressure and duration, while also responding in real-time to the physiological feedback of the participant. Their advantages include standardized intervention processes, fine-tuned pressure regulation, and the ability to record data. Currently, automated IPC devices can be broadly divided into three categories. The first category includes laboratory-grade high-precision equipment, such as the Hokanson Rapid Cuff Inflation System and the Delfi Personalized Tourniquet System. The Hokanson Rapid Cuff Inflator (D.E. Hokanson Inc., USA) is widely used in physiological experiments due to its ultra-fast inflation speed (completed within 0.3 seconds) and its ability to maintain consistent pressure [33]. In a study utilizing this device, Bouffard et al. found that it effectively improved 30-second Wingate anaerobic performance in endurance athletes [34]. In contrast, the Delfi system offers more advanced individualized closed-loop control by measuring each participant's limb occlusion pressure (LOP) in real time and applying a pressure percentage based on that value (e.g., 80% LOP). This significantly enhances the individualization and safety margin of pressure application [35–37]. Scott et al. reported that the Delfi system outperformed traditional cuff methods in repeated sprint performance and muscle reoxygenation. Loenneke et al. also noted that the Delfi system supports comprehensive pressure history tracking and data export, making it one of the most data-integrated platforms currently available in BFR and IPC research [38]. The second category includes smart devices designed for athletic training, such as SmartCuff, Kaatsu Master, and BStrong. These devices are typically equipped with microprocessors, Bluetooth modules, and mobile app control systems, enabling rapid parameter configuration, real-time monitoring, and training log recording—particularly suitable for coach-led interventions in athletic settings [26, 39].

The third category comprises compact, personalized devices such as the Occlude Pro, which are smaller, more affordable, and suitable for beginners or recreational users performing low-intensity, self-administered IPC (https://occlusioncuff.com). While these devices offer portability and accessibility advantages, they still face technical limitations in pressure control, feedback mechanisms, and safety assurance, and are currently more appropriate for low-risk intervention contexts.

Although automated smart IPC devices offer significant advantages in intervention efficiency and standardization, the suitability of different device types for various populations and research purposes still requires clear delineation. Medical-grade devices such as the Delfi and Hokanson systems are well-suited for high-standard physiological research and elite athletic interventions due to their high precision, parameter stability, and comprehensive safety mechanisms. However, their high cost and bulky size limit their applicability in practical training environments. Smart training devices excel in functional convenience and adaptability to various settings, making them ideal for use by coaching teams and non-elite populations. Nevertheless, some models still require improvements in pressure resolution and over-limit warning systems. Handheld portable devices, while offering a degree of flexibility, generally lack precise pressure control and physiological feedback features, resulting in limited risk management capabilities. These are more appropriate for low-intensity exercise or early-stage rehabilitation training.

In summary, for experimental research and high-performance athletes, the use of high-precision devices such as Delfi and Hokanson is recommended to ensure standardized intervention protocols and reproducible outcomes. For the general population, smart and portable devices like SmartCuff may be selected based on the training context, but it is advisable to complement their use with assessments of limb circumference or blood pressure parameters [40]. Moreover, it is essential to enhance users' understanding of device operation procedures, pressure-related risk identification, and emergency response protocols to minimize adverse events caused by improper use.

2.2 Pressure standards and intensity levels

In IPC applications, the setting of pressure parameters is a critical factor affecting both safety and efficacy. The lack of standardized pressure guidelines has become a major point of contention in current methodologies. Traditional protocols often employ a fixed high pressure (e.g., 220 mmHg), overlooking substantial individual differences in arterial pressure, limb circumference, and vascular characteristics [18, 21, 41]. This one-size-fits-all approach poses dual risks: insufficient pressure may lead to incomplete blood flow occlusion, thereby diminishing physiological effects [25]; whereas excessive pressure can cause severe pain (average VAS score of 6.5/10) and even tissue damage [42, 43]. As such, determining the minimum effective pressure based on individualized total occlusion pressure (TOP) has become a key direction for optimizing IPC. However, TOP measurement presents technical challenges—while medical ultrasound is the gold standard, it is expensive [44, 45], and pulse oximetry is susceptible to environmental interference [46]. Incorporating systolic blood pressure (SBP) into a predictive formula (e.g., TOP = 0.7 × SBP + 0.3 × thigh circumference – 15.2) can increase estimation success rates to 90%, offering a viable solution for field applications [47]. Notably, cuff width is significantly and negatively correlated with occlusion pressure ($r = -0.81$); a 13 cm wide cuff requires only 161.2 mmHg on average to achieve complete occlusion [48, 49]—125 mmHg less than narrower 5 cm cuffs—while also reducing the risk of subcutaneous nerve compression [48].

After establishing the importance and methodological approach for determining individualized pressure settings, understanding the differential effects of varying pressure magnitudes—namely high pressure (HP) versus low pressure (LP)—on exercise performance becomes essential. At the efficacy level, HP (220 mmHg) and LP (20 mmHg) IPC protocols exhibit paradoxical outcomes. Although neither condition significantly impacts isometric strength or fatigue index, both result in increased total work during repeated knee extensions (HP: ES = 0.29; LP: ES = 0.34 vs. Con: ES = 0.17), suggesting potentially distinct underlying mechanisms [50]. A study monitoring autonomic nervous system responses indicated that LP significantly elevated sympathetic-vagal balance (LF/HF%) and suppressed parasympathetic activity (RMSSD%) [51, 52], whereas HP elicited a weaker neural response, implying that LP may exert physiological effects *via* neural reflex pathways mediated by group III/IV afferent fibers [53]. Further research has revealed a more complex dose-response relationship between pressure magnitude and recovery outcomes: moderate pressure (MP: 100 mmHg) improved maximal voluntary contraction recovery rate, whereas HP (220 mmHg) and LP (20 mmHg) were ineffective. This effect appeared to be independent of muscle oxygenation, as no significant differences in SmO_2 were observed between groups [54].

Current debates primarily center on the fundamental mechanisms underlying the effects of IPC. The performance enhancement observed in the low-pressure (LP) group may be attributed to placebo effects or centrally mediated expectation mechanisms—specifically, the presence of a cuff may enhance motor cortex excitability through perceptual cues [55]. However, the stronger pain stimulus reported in the high-pressure (HP) group (VAS 6.2 vs. 1.8) did not translate into differences in subjective fatigue (RPE) [42, 43], suggesting that nociceptive afferent signals originating from peripheral tissues (i.e., pain) may be modulated or suppressed by higher-order central expectations or regulatory processes. Another critical point of contention involves the temporal nature of metabolic adaptations: IPC appears ineffective—or even detrimental—for maximal efforts lasting ≤10 seconds (e.g., 30-meter sprints) [56], yet improves performance in submaximal efforts exceeding 10 seconds [57]. This discrepancy may relate to the differential regulation of ATP utilization efficiency—IPC has been shown to help preserve phosphocreatine levels [58], but may simultaneously suppress glycolytic flux during maximal power output [59].

From a practical standpoint, three major limitations must be addressed. First, measurements of total occlusion pressure (TOP) are predominantly conducted in the supine position [60], neglecting the impact of posture-induced arterial pressure changes during real-world applications in seated or standing positions. Second, the vast majority of studies have focused on male participants, overlooking the influence of sex-based physiological differences—such as the faster accumulation of fatigue observed in females—on IPC responsiveness [61]. Third, anatomical factors such as limb circumference and adipose tissue distribution have not been adequately integrated into pressure determination models [49, 62]. Future research should develop posture-adjusted TOP algorithms, expand validation in sex-specific contexts, and explore adaptable IPC protocols for diverse exercise scenarios in order to facilitate the translation of IPC from controlled laboratory settings to practical training environments.

2.3 Implementation sites and protocol duration

In terms of implementation site selection, current research generally suggests that the application of ischemic preconditioning IPC should correspond to the primary working limbs involved in the target exercise. That is, the choice of IPC site often depends on the specific nature of the activity, such as whether it predominantly engages upper- or lower-limb muscle groups. For example, in upper-limb–dominant sports such as rowing [63], bench press [51], and climbing [64], IPC is typically applied to the upper limbs. Conversely, in activities like running [65], cycling [66], jumping [36], and various forms of lower-limb resistance training [67], IPC is more frequently administered to the lower limbs. In contrast, Lisbôa et al. implemented IPC simultaneously on both upper and lower limbs and found additional benefits for swimmers' 50-meter performance (+1.0%–1.2%). Similarly, a recent study by Urbanski et al. demonstrated that combined upper- and lower-limb IPC enhanced relative peak power output during rowing (6.5–6.8 W/kg) [63]. Moreover, some studies have investigated the effects of IPC applied to non-exercising limbs, indicating that even when the intervention site does not align with the primary working musculature, IPC can still extend time to exhaustion in male participants during fatiguing resistance tests (+5 min, P = 0.01) [68]. Although no studies to date have directly compared the intervention effects between upper- and lower-limb IPC, the current literature has not reported any adverse outcomes associated with site selection, suggesting that IPC exhibits high safety and adaptability across different limb regions.

The IPC implementation cycle refers to the selection of ischemia and reperfusion durations, as well as the number of repeated cycles. The most widely adopted IPC protocol consists of 3 to 4 cycles of 5-minute ischemia followed by 5-minute reperfusion—a classical regimen originally derived from clinical studies [2, 3, 11, 58] and subsequently validated across numerous sports performance studies [27, 67, 69, 70]. For example, in a systematic review, Marocolo et al. [8, 22] reported that nearly all IPC research has employed this standard protocol, confirming its effectiveness and broad applicability in enhancing athletic performance. Nevertheless, an increasing number of studies have begun to explore alternative cycle durations and frequencies in an effort to further optimize IPC efficacy. Recent investigations have tested both shorter and longer ischemia/reperfusion durations to assess their impact on performance outcomes. Urbanski et al. [63] found that although a single 5-minute IPC cycle (1 × 5 min) did not significantly affect test duration, power output, heart rate, or blood lactate (BLa) concentration, it significantly reduced the time required to reach peak power during a 500-meter rowing ergometer trial ($p = 0.017$). Furthermore, this protocol was associated with a notably lower rating of perceived exertion (RPE), showing nearly a 2-point reduction compared to the control group (IPC: 5.2 ± 0.5 vs. Con: 6.9 ± 0.5, $p < 0.001$; effect size = 1.19), suggesting that IPC may enhance performance while simultaneously reducing perceived fatigue, thereby improving the performance–perception relationship [71]. In another study aimed at determining the optimal IPC dosage for improving cycling time trial performance, Cocking et al. [72] compared the effects of four-cycle and eight-cycle IPC protocols, concluding that while the four-cycle protocol effectively shortened time trial completion time, the eight-cycle protocol provided no additional benefit to performance.

Although the classical IPC protocol of 3–4 × 5 minutes is widely effective for acute enhancement of exercise performance, recent studies have begun to investigate IPC as a "chronic" intervention strategy within training cycles, exploring its adaptive effects when applied over multiple consecutive days or even weeks—such as for 7 days [73], 10 days [74], 2 weeks [75], or 8 weeks [76]. Lindsay et al. [77] reported that applying a 4 × 5 min bilateral leg IPC protocol daily for 7 days led to a 3.4% increase in average power output during a simulated Keirin sprint, an 18.5% improvement in maximal aerobic power, and a significant 12.8% enhancement in VO_2peak, with additional benefits in ventilatory capacity when combined with hypoxic exposure [73]. In contrast, Tanaka et al. found that a two-week IPC intervention (6 sessions per week) did not improve systemic or localized performance outcomes. Specifically, there were no significant changes in VO_2peak pre- and post-intervention ($P = 0.147$, 95% CI: −0.67 to 1.09), nor in time to exhaustion ($P = 0.923$, 95% CI: −0.86 to 0.89) [75]. Moreover, no significant differences were observed in repeated moderate-intensity cycling tests, knee extensor strength, or quadriceps muscle volume [75]. Similarly, Slysz and Burr [76] conducted an 8-week unilateral leg IPC intervention (three sessions per week) in well-trained middle- and long-distance runners and reported no significant improvements in 1-km run time or maximal oxygen uptake (VO_2max), with only a marginal trend toward improved running economy during low-intensity efforts ($P = 0.057$).

In summary, IPC site selection should ideally align with the primary working limbs; however, both combined and non-matching applications have shown to be potentially effective and safe. Regarding protocol duration, the classical 3–4 × 5-minute regimen remains a reliable strategy for acutely enhancing performance. Nevertheless, tailoring the duration and number of cycles (e.g., shorter protocols or four-cycle schemes) to specific sporting contexts may confer additional benefits, such as faster attainment of peak power and reduced perceived exertion. In contrast, the use of IPC as a chronic intervention strategy—applied over multiple weeks as a training aid—yields inconsistent findings, and current evidence remains insufficient to support its generalized efficacy as a routine training adjunct.

2.4 Timing intervals and experimental design IPC

The interval between IPC application and subsequent exercise testing is a critical variable influencing its physiological effects. Early IPC studies in animal models clearly identified a biphasic effect, characterized by an initial early protection window and a delayed second window of protection [2, 78, 79]. The early window typically lasts 1–2 hours, while the delayed second window appears 12–24 hours post-intervention and persists longer. Its mechanisms involve angiogenic activation, myofibrillar structural preservation, and enhanced mitochondrial activity [8, 9, 80, 81]. However, within the field of exercise science, most studies have focused on the early effect window, typically around 45 minutes after IPC intervention [15, 16]. Empirical findings have demonstrated that, compared to a 5-minute interval, a 45-minute delay prior to high-intensity sprint cycling elicits a greater rebound in skeletal muscle metabolism and facilitates better muscle reoxygenation during active recovery at lower intensities [17]. These results suggest that implementing an appropriately delayed interval after IPC may help optimize muscle deoxygenation efficiency and mitochondrial oxidative function, thereby creating a more favorable physiological state for subsequent exercise performance.

It is worth noting that the structure of the warm-up routine during experimental procedures is also a critical factor influencing the effectiveness of IPC. Currently, more than 70% of experimental designs follow the sequence of "IPC → warm-up → performance test," whereas relatively few adopt a direct "IPC → performance test" approach [16]. Although meta-analyses have synthesized the overall effects of IPC interventions on exercise performance [15, 16], they did not distinguish between studies with or without warm-up protocols, thereby introducing potential confounding in the interpretation of results. As warm-up routines are well known to independently enhance athletic performance, the effect sizes reported in these meta-analyses may not accurately reflect the isolated contribution of IPC. Furthermore, previous studies have suggested that placebo effects significantly influence IPC outcomes [15], and warm-up routines themselves may elicit psychological expectancy effects. Therefore, whether the combined or synergistic effects of "warm-up + IPC" amplify the performance-enhancing mechanisms of IPC warrants further investigation. Our research team has previously highlighted that the lack of precise reporting on the interval between IPC and performance testing is a major barrier to standardizing IPC protocols [16]. For example, although Kaur et al. [82] reported a 15-minute interval following IPC, this actually included 3 minutes of warm-up and 2 minutes of measurement, making the true interval closer to 20 minutes. In another study, Lisbôa et al. [83] found no significant improvement in 50-m sprint swimming performance when tested 1 hour post-IPC, but observed significant enhancements at 2 and 8 hours post-intervention—both of which included approximately 20 minutes of warm-up. Similarly, Richard et al. [84] reported a 1-hour interval, but this also incorporated 20–40 minutes of warm-up activities. These findings suggest that warm-up routines are often embedded within the stated pre-test interval, potentially obscuring accurate interpretation of IPC's temporal effect window.

Over the past two decades, the lack of standardized warm-up protocols and inconsistent reporting of interval durations have hindered the standardization of IPC procedures in the field of exercise science. Therefore, scientific rigor in experimental design and control over the implementation process have become critical factors for improving research quality. Current research efforts have primarily focused on controlling placebo effects and clarifying underlying physiological mechanisms. Standardized study designs often adopt a three-arm trial structure—including IPC, sham (placebo) intervention, and a no-intervention control group—combined with randomized controlled or crossover trial formats to effectively minimize placebo-related confounding. This approach has emerged in response to growing evidence that significant placebo effects may be present in IPC interventions, potentially driven by mechanisms involving brain–somatic sensory integration and vagal nerve regulation [21]. More specifically, the tactile sensations experienced during ischemic procedures can elicit a cascade of psychophysiological responses, which may subtly influence participants' behavioral performance through complex interactions among perceptual, motor, and cognitive systems [85]. As a result, recent studies have begun incorporating psychophysiological indicators—such as emotional valence and subjective experience—into IPC protocols that gradually increase cuff pressure from sham (low pressure) to true IPC (high pressure), aiming to systematically explore the role of perceived placebo-induced enhancements in performance [51, 54, 86–89]. Subtle yet often overlooked elements of sham IPC—such as heightened sensitivity of tactile receptors, increased experimenter attention, and resulting psychological priming—may also exert significant influence on motor behavior [90–92]. Although the existence of placebo effects is widely acknowledged, some studies still fall short in interpreting these outcomes. For instance, several trials have shown that sham IPC significantly outperforms control conditions, yet fail to strictly control for variables such as warm-up routines and interventional timing [16]. In the context of performance research, warm-up is already recognized as an essential prerequisite, while the interval between intervention and testing has been confirmed as a critical modulatory factor [9].

In summary, effective control of placebo effects is a critical component of IPC experimental design. If the objective is to elucidate the physiological mechanisms of IPC itself, it is recommended that intervention studies be conducted under no-warm-up conditions to minimize potential confounding variables. However, in athletic training and competitive settings, IPC interventions are more appropriately administered prior to warm-up. This approach not only reduces the risk of injury associated with high-intensity exercise but may also allow low-intensity activity to synergistically potentiate the latent effects of IPC. For example, Telles et al. [51] demonstrated that both low- and high-pressure IPC protocols can enhance maximal strength performance through favorable psychophysiological responses, such as the activation of group III and IV afferent nerve fibers. Moreover, combining IPC with different exercise intensities—such as 50% MVC handgrip training [93], 5-km time trials [94], or exhaustive tests at 70% VO_2max [95, 96]—has consistently shown positive effects on both athletic performance and physiological indicators.

2.5 Participant characteristics

Among the various factors influencing the efficacy of ischemic preconditioning IPC in enhancing exercise performance, individual participant characteristics—such as age, sex, and training experience—are widely recognized as important moderating variables that may substantially affect both the effectiveness and applicability of the intervention. Existing studies have shown that individuals at different ages exhibit marked differences in cardiovascular regulation, metabolic responses to exercise, and tissue tolerance. Sex-related differences may also mediate heterogeneity in IPC outcomes through mechanisms involving hormonal profiles, muscular strength, and blood flow regulation. Furthermore, an individual's training status and competitive level directly influence the magnitude of physiological response and the capacity for adaptation to exogenous interventions. Currently, the participant pool in most IPC research is heavily concentrated among young, recreationally active males, limiting the generalizability of findings and constraining the interpretation of IPC responsiveness across diverse populations. Therefore, it is essential to systematically consider the moderating and confounding effects of participant characteristics in both study design and practical application. Tailoring IPC protocols to account for population-specific physiological traits and athletic backgrounds will be key to improving the ecological validity and practical relevance of IPC research.

2.5.1 Age and sex

In recent years, although the number of original studies combining IPC with exercise has increased significantly, research subjects remain predominantly young or middle-aged males, while empirical data on females and older adults remain limited [8]. In one study focusing on elderly populations, researchers compared the effects of different interventions on blood pressure and found that handgrip training and high-intensity interval training (HIIT) were more effective than IPC. However, it is important to note that the IPC group in this study did not incorporate any form of exercise [97]. In contrast, recent findings suggest that IPC combined with aerobic exercise can significantly improve general health indicators, quality of life, and endurance performance in older adults aged 70 years, demonstrating promising intervention potential [98]. Specifically, a 6-week IPC intervention significantly increased the six-minute walk distance (from 489 m to 540 m), along with notable improvements in several functional fitness parameters, including balance score (from 3.73 to 3.80), Timed Up and Go (TUG) test score (from 3.20 to 4.13), and lower-limb maximal strength (from 114 N to 149 N) [98]. In comparison, Telles et al. [99] analyzed the acute effects of IPC in physically active older women and found that the IPC group exhibited a significantly shorter TUG time than the sham group (a 7.2% reduction), although no significant difference was observed in the six-minute walk test (IPC group improved by 2.1% compared to sham). This finding contrasts with the 17.13% improvement reported by Muñoz-Gómez et al. [98], which may be attributed to differences in intervention protocol design. Nevertheless, the results indirectly suggest that longer-term (e.g., 6-week) IPC interventions combined with aerobic activities such as walking may offer more pronounced benefits than acute applications. Supporting this, another study employing a similar 6-week IPC protocol also reported positive effects on functional indicators in older adults [100].

In sports science research, it is widely acknowledged that males and females exhibit distinct cardiovascular regulatory mechanisms both at rest and during exercise [101, 102]. Gibson et al. [56] reported that ischemic preconditioning IPC did not significantly affect performance in male and female team sport athletes completing five sets of 6-second repeated sprint cycling. However, more recent studies suggest that the ergogenic effects of IPC may exhibit sex-specific differences, potentially related to disparities in metabolic responses and functional sympathetic inhibition during exercise between males and females [20, 63]. For instance, Paradis-Deschênes et al. [103], in a study involving five sets of five maximal voluntary knee extensions, found that males experienced greater improvements in total work following IPC.

Further evidence from time-to-exhaustion protocols [68] and handgrip training trials [20] showed that IPC significantly increased endurance duration and grip strength only in male participants. A key mechanism underlying this sex-specific response may lie in the tighter coupling between muscle blood flow and absolute muscle strength in males [20]. Supporting this, previous studies have shown that when absolute muscle contraction intensity is controlled between sexes, the exercise-induced blood pressure response differences largely disappear [104–106], further reinforcing the physiological basis for sex-specific IPC effects.

2.5.2 Experience level

The training experience and athletic level of participants—such as elite athletes versus recreationally active individuals—may significantly influence the actual effectiveness of IPC interventions. Existing findings indicate that individuals with lower training status or without systematic training tend to exhibit more pronounced improvements in rating of perceived exertion (RPE) following IPC, whereas highly trained or elite athletes often experience limited benefits [15]. This disparity suggests that baseline training status or physiological adaptation capacity may serve as important modulators of IPC efficacy.

However, the vast majority of empirical studies on IPC and performance enhancement have focused on recreational or amateur populations, limiting the generalizability of findings to higher-level athletic cohorts. In elite sports environments, the marginal gains from exogenous or physiological modulation strategies are often already saturated, and whether IPC still offers meaningful performance improvements in such settings remains unclear. Furthermore, most studies employ open-ended laboratory testing protocols, in which participants are unaware of the test endpoint. This design contrasts significantly with the demands of competitive sport, where pacing strategies and self-regulated effort allocation are critical. Conversely, field-based assessments or pacing-controlled tests in simulated competitive environments are more ecologically valid, yet remain underrepresented in the literature, with limited empirical evidence available. Therefore, a key priority for advancing this field is to increase research on IPC applications in real-world or sport-specific contexts, particularly focusing on performance outcomes among elite-level athletes.

Currently, the evaluation of IPC intervention effects is primarily based on statistical significance testing (e.g., p-values) or the estimation of effect sizes (ES). However, there remains considerable debate within the academic community regarding the appropriateness and interpretation of such statistical indicators in exercise performance research [107, 108]. While this chapter does not aim to elaborate on the broader controversies surrounding statistical methodologies, it is important to emphasize that statistical outcomes—whether derived from t-tests, analysis of variance, or effect size calculations—must be interpreted cautiously in the context of the specific research setting. For elite athletes, even a small observed effect may translate into meaningful advantages in competitive scenarios; conversely, among recreational athletes, moderate or even large effect sizes may lack practical relevance or generalizability [109].

A review of nearly 50 experimental studies investigating the effects of IPC on exercise performance in healthy individuals reveals that only two have specifically targeted elite competitive athletes: one study involved national-level speed skaters [84], and the other focused on professional road cyclists [110]. The remaining literature predominantly features recreationally trained individuals, casual participants, and even sedentary or healthy control subjects. Although some studies describe their participants as "highly trained," they often fail to meet the standards of elite athletic performance. Notably, a field-based study conducted by Foster et al. evaluated the impact of IPC on a 12.8-km time trial in a hypoxic environment. While the intervention group showed a slight improvement in performance, the difference was not statistically significant, and the effect size was minimal [111]. Another study examining IPC's impact on swimming performance reported modest improvements; however, the 100-meter freestyle times in the intervention group were close to 60 seconds—substantially slower than elite competitive swimmers, who typically complete the event in under 50 seconds—thus disqualifying the sample as truly elite [112].

In summary, current evidence does not yet support the conclusion that IPC produces consistent and significant performance-enhancing effects in self-paced events or field-based competitive settings. As a performance-enhancement strategy, IPC still presents considerable uncertainty. Future research should aim to overcome limitations related to participant sampling and the artificiality of testing conditions. In particular, it is essential to conduct ecologically valid intervention studies involving professional athletes under authentic competitive scenarios to comprehensively evaluate the practical utility of IPC in high-performance sport.

3. Safety considerations of ischemic preconditioning for performance enhancement

When evaluating the impact of ischemic preconditioning IPC on exercise performance, safety remains one of the most critical considerations in both research and practice. This is particularly relevant when applying IPC to healthy individuals or clinically vulnerable populations, where balancing intervention efficacy with the avoidance of potential discomfort or risk is essential for assessing feasibility. To date, no study has reported adverse safety outcomes associated with IPC. However, because IPC involves the intermittent occlusion of limb blood flow, it inherently introduces a degree of invasiveness and nociceptive stimulation. Therefore, the ability to continuously assess participants' subjective experience and anticipate potential risks is key to ensuring the safe and effective delivery of the intervention. In this context, the rating of perceived exertion (RPE) scale—a simple and sensitive self-perception tool—has gained increasing attention as a means of monitoring subjective responses during IPC procedures.

During IPC procedures, RPE is commonly used to monitor intervention tolerability and to evaluate the presence of pain or discomfort responses in participants [113]. Clinical studies often record both RPE and subjective discomfort scores to assess the tolerability and safety of IPC. RPE is considered a key indicator reflecting participants' real-time subjective load and pain perception. An abnormally elevated RPE often suggests that ischemia-induced discomfort may be exceeding the individual's tolerance threshold. To ensure safety, some studies have recommended the immediate cessation of IPC stimulation when participants report intolerable discomfort, indicated by excessively high RPE or pain scores [114]. Therefore, continuous monitoring of RPE during IPC application is essential for identifying adverse subjective responses in a timely manner, positioning RPE as a potential early warning marker of pain or intolerance.

Existing research has shown that performing IPC prior to exercise interventions may help reduce RPE scores during subsequent physical activity [115]. For instance, ter Beek et al. reported that, in healthy males, IPC significantly reduced RPE during cycling at high power outputs compared to a placebo group—specifically, at workloads of 210 W and 245 W, RPE scores were significantly lower in the IPC group ($p < 0.01$) [37]. Similarly, a study by Montoye et al. involving 115 female athletes found that, although IPC did not improve overall performance during a 2.4-km run, RPE scores in the IPC group were approximately 0.8 units lower than those in the placebo group (based on the 6–20 scale) [115]. Additionally, a systematic review by Caru et al. [23] noted that IPC may delay the rate of RPE increase during exercise, potentially reducing the body's sensitivity to fatigue-related signals and thereby alleviating the perceived exertion associated with high-intensity effort. This reduction in RPE suggests that IPC may improve subjective exercise experience [116]. However, it is important to note that not all studies have observed changes in RPE. In certain clinical populations—such as heart failure patients undergoing six-minute walk tests—IPC failed to improve performance or significantly affect exercise RPE [117]. Overall, most studies involving healthy individuals and athletes support the notion that IPC can attenuate perceived exertion without compromising exercise safety.

When IPC leads to a significant increase in RPE, it is often accompanied by intense pain and heightened sympathetic nervous system activity. Ischemic stimulation activates group III/IV muscle afferent fibers, which trigger a central sympathetic reflex, resulting in elevated heart rate and blood pressure [118]. Excessively high RPE may indicate excessive sympathetic activation, which could pose risks—such as large fluctuations in blood pressure or arrhythmias—particularly for individuals with cardiovascular dysfunction or other vulnerable populations. Albuquerque et al. [119] reported that discomfort or pain induced by excessively high cuff pressures not only elevates RPE but may also alter the expected physiological response pattern of IPC. Meanwhile, a study by Incognito et al. [118] found that a single bout of IPC did not significantly reduce blood pressure or muscle sympathetic nerve activity during static exercise, suggesting that IPC might not suppress exercise-induced sympathetic excitation. However, in practical settings, when high RPE arises due to intense pain, excessive sympathetic activation remains a potential concern. Therefore, the safe implementation of IPC requires avoiding extreme elevations in RPE. If participants report perceived exertion levels classified as "very hard" or approaching their tolerance limit (e.g., scores above 18 on the Borg 6–20 scale), this is typically regarded as a warning sign [120]. In such cases, pressure should be reduced or the intervention paused to prevent adverse physiological responses caused by nociceptive stress. Fortunately, no serious adverse events directly linked to IPC have been reported in current human studies. On the contrary, multiple clinical trials have indicated that IPC is generally well-tolerated across different populations—for example, no serious adverse reactions were observed following a single RIPC session in individuals with multiple sclerosis [113], and no negative hemodynamic events were reported in patients with chronic heart failure undergoing RIPC [117].

In summary, IPC is considered safe when applied under standardized conditions; however, monitoring indicators such as RPE remains essential to prevent excessive sympathetic activation or other adverse responses in individual cases.

4. Conclusion and future perspectives

As a low-cost and non-pharmacological physiological intervention, ischemic preconditioning IPC has demonstrated potential in enhancing exercise performance.

However, current literature indicates that the efficacy of IPC remains highly influenced by numerous methodological variables. These include the type of equipment used, pressure settings, site and duration of occlusion, timing intervals, warm-up protocols, and individual participant characteristics—all of which may modulate IPC outcomes through complex physiological mechanisms. Furthermore, some studies suggest that the performance-enhancing effects of IPC may be partly attributable to placebo or expectancy-related mechanisms, thereby adding further complexity to its research and practical application.

In terms of safety, although most studies have not reported serious adverse events, notable inter-individual variability in subjective tolerability remains. This is particularly relevant under high-pressure IPC conditions, where the risks of pain and heightened sympathetic nervous responses cannot be overlooked. Therefore, developing individualized pressure assessment models, enhancing device feedback mechanisms, and optimizing intervention protocols represent critical directions for improving the safety boundaries of IPC in future applications.

In conclusion, the mechanisms underlying IPC interventions remain inconclusive, and their efficacy is constrained by multiple interacting factors. As such, the practical implementation of IPC in both elite sports and health promotion should proceed with caution. Future research should prioritize the following areas: first, clarifying the causal pathways between various methodological variables and IPC effects within a standardized experimental framework; second, expanding the diversity of study samples, particularly by including female participants, older adults, and elite athletes; third, advancing ecologically valid IPC research in real-world training environments, with long-term monitoring of training adaptations and performance outcomes; and fourth, strengthening the integration of psychophysiological assessments to better delineate the boundaries of placebo effects in IPC interventions. Only through a clearer understanding of both theoretical mechanisms and practical application logic can IPC truly transition from controlled laboratory settings to applied contexts, thereby serving broader goals in performance enhancement and health promotion.

Author details

Yilin Zhang and Yun Xie*
School of Sports Training, Tianjin University of Sport, China

*Address all correspondence to: xieyun@tjus.edu.cn

References

[1] Yao X, Feng D. Advances in the application of ischemic preconditioning in acute kidney injury. Journal of Practical Medicine. 2017;**33**(21):3507-3510

[2] Ce M, Rb J, Ka R. Preconditioning with ischemia: A delay of lethal cell injury in ischemic myocardium. Circulation. 1986;**74**(5):1124-1136. DOI: 10.1161/01.cir.74.5.1124

[3] Ce M, Vj R, Ka R, Rb J. Ischemic preconditioning slows energy metabolism and delays ultrastructural damage during a sustained ischemic episode. Circulation Research. 1990;**66**(4):913-931. DOI: 10.1161/01.res.66.4.913

[4] Feng Z, Yang W, Junwei S, Nie Lei W, Dongde YT. Effect of ischemic preconditioning on the activity of the IL-6-STAT3 signaling pathway during hepatic ischemia-reperfusion. Journal of Huazhong University of Science and Technology (Medical Sciences). 2019;**48**(6):667-670

[5] Wei Wei F, Ping ZY. Research progress on remote ischemic preconditioning in acute kidney injury. Journal of Nephropathy, Dialysis & Kidney Transplantation. 2025;**34**(2):174-179

[6] Fangfang L, Wei W. Research progress on the neuroprotective mechanisms of remote ischemic preconditioning. Journal of Clinical Pediatrics. 2016;**34**(8):634-636

[7] Zhongzhi J. Mechanisms, prevention, and treatment of intestinal ischemia-reperfusion injury. Journal of Interventional Radiology. 2018;**27**(7):700-703

[8] Marocolo M, Souza HLR, Surke P, Ferrauti A. Potential short- and long-term physiological effects of ischemic preconditioning as an ergogenic aid: Revisiting foundational mechanisms and applications. Sports Medicine. 2025;**55**(7):1547-1557. DOI: 10.1007/s40279-025-02232-3

[9] Yuying S, Wei L. Research progress on the effects of remote ischemic preconditioning on exercise performance and its physiological mechanisms. China Sport Science and Technology. 2024;**60**(10):31-39. DOI: 10.16470/j.csst.2024096

[10] Jun W, Qijiang Z, Shuangyu L, Lei Z, Honggang W. Research progress on the application of remote ischemic conditioning and its endogenous protective mechanisms. Chinese Journal of Pathophysiology. 2021;**37**(8):1511-1518

[11] Reimer KA, Murry CE, Jennings RB. Cardiac adaptation to ischemia. Ischemic preconditioning increases myocardial tolerance to subsequent ischemic episodes. Circulation. 1990;**82**(6):2266-2268. DOI: 10.1161/01.cir.82.6.2266

[12] Loukogeorgakis SP, Panagiotidou AT, Broadhead MW, Donald A, Deanfield JE, MacAllister RJ. Remote ischemic preconditioning provides early and late protection against endothelial ischemia-reperfusion injury in humans: Role of the autonomic nervous system. Journal of the American College of Cardiology. 2005;**46**(3):450-456. DOI: 10.1016/j.jacc.2005.04.044

[13] De Groot PCE, Thijssen DHJ, Sanchez M, Ellenkamp R, Hopman MTE. Ischemic preconditioning improves maximal performance in humans. European Journal of Applied Physiology. 2010;**108**(1):141-146. DOI: 10.1007/s00421-009-1195-2

[14] Wang Zhou W, Ying. Ischemic preconditioning enhances exercise performance: Methods, applications, and mechanisms. Chinese Journal of Tissue Engineering Research. 2023;**27**(30):4869-4875

[15] LRS H, TO G, Anderson M. Does ischemic preconditioning enhance sports performance more than placebo or no intervention? A systematic review with meta-analysis. Journal of Sport and Health Science. 2024;**14**:101010. DOI: 10.1016/j.jshs.2024.101010

[16] Zhang Y, Kong H, Xu K, Yin M, Xie Y. Comment on "does ischemic preconditioning enhance sports performance more than placebo or no intervention? A systematic review with meta-analysis.". Journal of Sport and Health Science. 2025;**14**:101056. DOI: 10.1016/j.jshs.2025.101056

[17] Seeley AD, Jacobs KA. IPC recovery length of 45 minutes improves muscle oxygen saturation during active sprint recovery. European Journal of Sport Science. 2022;**22**(9):1383-1390. DOI: 10.1080/17461391.2021.1939429

[18] Souza HLR, Oliveira GT, Meireles A, et al. Response to the comment on "does ischemic preconditioning enhance sports performance more than placebo or no intervention? A systematic review with meta-analysis.". Journal of Sport and Health Science. 2025;**14**:101057. DOI: 10.1016/j.jshs.2025.101057

[19] Incognito AV, Burr JF, Millar PJ. The effects of ischemic preconditioning on human exercise performance. Sports Medicine. 2016;**46**(4):531-544. DOI: 10.1007/s40279-015-0433-5

[20] Teixeira AL, Gangat A, Bommarito JC, Burr JF, Millar PJ. Ischemic preconditioning acutely improves functional sympatholysis during handgrip exercise in healthy males but not females. Medicine and Science in Sports and Exercise. 2023;**55**(7):1250-1257. DOI: 10.1249/MSS.0000000000003148

[21] Marocolo M, Hohl R, Arriel RA, Mota GR. Ischemic preconditioning and exercise performance: Are the psychophysiological responses underestimated? European Journal of Applied Physiology. 2023;**123**(4):683-693. DOI: 10.1007/s00421-022-05109-9

[22] Marocolo M, Billaut F, da Mota GR. Ischemic preconditioning and exercise performance: An ergogenic aid for whom? Frontiers in Physiology. 2018;**9**:1874. DOI: 10.3389/fphys.2018.01874

[23] Caru M, Levesque A, Lalonde F, Curnier D. An overview of ischemic preconditioning in exercise performance: A systematic review. Journal of Sport and Health Science. 2019;**8**(4):355-369. DOI: 10.1016/j.jshs.2019.01.008

[24] Chen Z, Wu W, Qiang L, Wang C, He Z, Wang Y. The effect of ischemic preconditioning on physical fitness and performance: A meta-analysis in healthy adults. European Journal of Applied Physiology. 2024;**125**(3):823. DOI: 10.1007/s00421-024-05633-w

[25] Salvador AF, De Aguiar RA, Lisbôa FD, Pereira KL, Cruz RS, Caputo F. Ischemic preconditioning and exercise performance: A systematic review and meta-analysis. International Journal of Sports Physiology and Performance. 2016;**11**(1):4-14. DOI: 10.1123/ijspp.2015-0204

[26] Patterson SD, Hughes L, Warmington S, et al. Blood flow restriction exercise: Considerations of methodology, application, and safety. Frontiers in Physiology. 2019;**10**:533. DOI: 10.3389/fphys.2019.00533

[27] Jessee MB, Buckner SL, Mouser JG, et al. Muscle adaptations to high-load training and very low-load training with and without blood flow restriction. Frontiers in Physiology. 2018;**9**:1448. DOI: 10.3389/fphys.2018.01448

[28] Ferreira TN, Sabino-Carvalho JLC, Lopes TR, et al. Ischemic preconditioning and repeated sprint swimming: A placebo and nocebo study. Medicine and Science in Sports and Exercise. 2016;**48**(10):1967-1975. DOI: 10.1249/MSS.0000000000000977

[29] Yue W, Yameng Y, Le C, Kanglai T, Dianwei L, Li Z. Effects of two different blood flow restriction training methods on the immediate response of upper limb muscles in military academy cadets. Journal of Army Medical University. 2023;**45**(22):2343-2351. DOI: 10.16016/j.2097-0927.202303123

[30] Gao X, Wang A, Fan J, et al. The effect of ischemic preconditioning on repeated sprint cycling performance: A randomized crossover study. The Journal of Sports Medicine and Physical Fitness. 2024;**64**(11):1147-1156. DOI: 10.23736/S0022-4707.24.16015-X

[31] Hughes L, Jeffries O, Waldron M, et al. Influence and reliability of lower-limb arterial occlusion pressure at different body positions. PeerJ. 2018;**6**:e4697. DOI: 10.7717/peerj.4697

[32] Citherlet T, Willis SJ, Chaperon A, Millet GP. Differences in the limb blood flow between two types of blood flow restriction cuffs: A pilot study. Frontiers in Physiology. 2022;**13**:931270. DOI: 10.3389/fphys.2022.931270

[33] Jeffries O, Waldron M, Pattison JR, Patterson SD. Enhanced local skeletal muscle oxidative capacity and microvascular blood flow following 7-day ischemic preconditioning in healthy humans. Frontiers in Physiology. 2018;**9**:e463. DOI: 10.3389/fphys.2018.00463

[34] Bouffard S, Paradis-Deschênes P, Billaut F. Neuromuscular adjustments following sprint training with ischemic preconditioning in endurance athletes: Preliminary data. Sports. 2021;**9**(9):124. DOI: 10.3390/sports9090124

[35] Pandorf Z, Erickson S, Scholten SD. Ischemic preconditioning on swimming performance: An exploration into practical application. Medicine and Science in Sports and Exercise. 2023;**55**(9):377-377

[36] Lindner TD, Scholten SD, Halverson JM, Baumgarten KM, Birger CB, Nowotny BG. The acute effects of ischemic preconditioning on power and sprint performance. South Dakota Medicine. 2021;**74**(5):210-219

[37] Ter Beek F, Jokumsen PS, Sloth BN, Stevenson AJT, Larsen RG. Ischemic preconditioning attenuates rating of perceived exertion but does not improve maximal oxygen consumption or maximal power output. Journal of Strength and Conditioning Research. 2022;**36**(9):2479-2485. DOI: 10.1519/JSC.0000000000003625

[38] Loenneke JP, Kim D, Mouser JG, et al. Are there perceptual differences to varying levels of blood flow restriction? Physiology & Behavior. 2016;**157**:277-280. DOI: 10.1016/j.physbeh.2016.02.022

[39] Wilk M, Trybulski R, Krzysztofik M, et al. Acute effects of different blood flow restriction protocols on bar velocity during the squat exercise. Frontiers in Physiology. 2021;**12**:652896. DOI: 10.3389/fphys.2021.652896

[40] Mouser JG, Dankel SJ, Mattocks KT, et al. Blood flow restriction and cuff

width: Effect on blood flow in the legs. Clinical Physiology and Functional Imaging. 2018;**38**(6):944-948. DOI: 10.1111/cpf.12504

[41] Hughes L, Paton B, Rosenblatt B, Gissane C, Patterson SD. Blood flow restriction training in clinical musculoskeletal rehabilitation: A systematic review and meta-analysis. British Journal of Sports Medicine. 2017;**51**(13):1003-1011. DOI: 10.1136/bjsports-2016-097071

[42] Sharma V, Marsh R, Cunniffe B, Cardinale M, Yellon DM, Davidson SM. From protecting the heart to improving athletic performance - the benefits of local and remote ischaemic preconditioning. Cardiovascular Drugs and Therapy. 2015;**29**(6):573-588. DOI: 10.1007/s10557-015-6621-6

[43] Sharma V, Cunniffe B, Verma AP, Cardinale M, Yellon D. Characterization of acute ischemia-related physiological responses associated with remote ischemic preconditioning: A randomized controlled, crossover human study. Physiological Reports. 2014;**2**(11):e12200. DOI: 10.14814/phy2.12200

[44] Vehrs PR, Richards S, Blazzard C, et al. Use of a handheld Doppler to measure brachial and femoral artery occlusion pressure. Frontiers in Physiology. 2023;**14**:1239582. DOI: 10.3389/fphys.2023.1239582

[45] Vehrs PR, Richards S, Allen J, et al. Measurements of arterial occlusion pressure using hand-held devices. Journal of Strength and Conditioning Research. 2024;**38**(5):873-880. DOI: 10.1519/JSC.0000000000004716

[46] Zeng Z, Centner C, Gollhofer A, König D. Blood-flow-restriction training: Validity of pulse oximetry to assess arterial occlusion pressure. International Journal of Sports Physiology and Performance. 2019;**14**(10):1408-1414. DOI: 10.1123/ijspp.2019-0043

[47] Brekke AF, Sørensen AN, Buhr C, Johannesdottír ÍO, Jakobsen TL. The validity and reliability of the handheld oximeter to determine limb occlusion pressure for blood flow restriction exercise in the lower extremity. International Journal of Sports Physical Therapy. 2020;**15**(5):783-791. DOI: 10.26603/ijspt20200783

[48] Loenneke JP, Allen KM, Mouser JG, et al. Blood flow restriction in the upper and lower limbs is predicted by limb circumference and systolic blood pressure. European Journal of Applied Physiology. 2015;**115**(2):397-405. DOI: 10.1007/s00421-014-3030-7

[49] Loenneke JP, Fahs CA, Rossow LM, et al. Effects of cuff width on arterial occlusion: Implications for blood flow restricted exercise. European Journal of Applied Physiology. 2012;**112**(8):2903-2912. DOI: 10.1007/s00421-011-2266-8

[50] de Souza HLR, Arriel RA, Hohl R, da Mota GR, Marocolo M. Is ischemic preconditioning intervention occlusion-dependent to enhance resistance exercise performance? Journal of Strength and Conditioning Research. 2021;**35**(10):2706-2712. DOI: 10.1519/JSC.0000000000003224

[51] Telles LG, Billaut F, de Souza RA, et al. Ischemic preconditioning with high and low pressure enhances maximum strength and modulates heart rate variability. International Journal of Environmental Research and Public Health. 2022;**19**(13):7655. DOI: 10.3390/ijerph19137655

[52] Lopes KG, Farinatti P, Bottino DA, et al. Does resistance training with blood flow restriction affect blood pressure and

cardiac autonomic modulation in older adults? International Journal of Exercise Science. 2021;**14**(3):410-422

[53] RSO d C, Pereira KL, Lisbôa FD, Caputo F. Could small-diameter muscle afferents be responsible for the ergogenic effect of limb ischemic preconditioning? Journal of Applied Physiology 1985. 2017;**122**(3):718-720. DOI: 10.1152/japplphysiol.00662.2016

[54] Meireles A, Souza HLR, Arriel RA, et al. Attenuation of neuromuscular fatigue by ischemic preconditioning with moderate cuff pressure is not related to muscle oxygen saturation in men. International Journal of Exercise Science. 2023;**16**(2):1025-1037

[55] Moerman DE, Jonas WB. Deconstructing the placebo effect and finding the meaning response. Annals of Internal Medicine. 2002;**136**(6):471-476. DOI: 10.7326/0003-4819-136-6-200203190-00011

[56] Gibson N, Mahony B, Tracey C, Fawkner S, Murray A. Effect of ischemic preconditioning on repeated sprint ability in team sport athletes. Journal of Sports Sciences. 2015;**33**(11):1182-1188. DOI: 10.1080/02640414.2014.988741

[57] Slysz JT, Petrick HL, Marrow JP, Burr JF. An examination of individual responses to ischemic preconditioning and the effect of repeated ischemic preconditioning on cycling performance. European Journal of Sport Science. 2020;**20**(5):633-640. DOI: 10.1080/17461391.2019.1651401

[58] Reimer KA, Murry CE, Yamasawa I, Hill ML, Jennings RB. Four brief periods of myocardial ischemia cause no cumulative ATP loss or necrosis. American Journal of Physiology-Heart and Circulatory Physiology. 1986;**251**(6 Pt 2):H1306-15. DOI: 10.1152/ajpheart.1986.251.6.H1306

[59] Paixão RC, da Mota GR, Marocolo M. Acute effect of ischemic preconditioning is detrimental to anaerobic performance in cyclists. International Journal of Sports Medicine. 2014;**35**(11):912-915. DOI: 10.1055/s-0034-1372628

[60] Crisafulli A, Tangianu F, Tocco F, et al. Ischemic preconditioning of the muscle improves maximal exercise performance but not maximal oxygen uptake in humans. Journal of Applied Physiology. 2011;**111**(2):530-536. DOI: 10.1152/japplphysiol.00266.2011

[61] Lalonde F, Curnier DY. Can anaerobic performance be improved by remote ischemic preconditioning? The Journal of Strength & Conditioning Research. 2015;**29**(1):80. DOI: 10.1519/JSC.0000000000000609

[62] Loenneke JP, Wilson JM, Marín PJ, Zourdos MC, Bemben MG. Low intensity blood flow restriction training: A meta-analysis. European Journal of Applied Physiology. 2012;**112**(5):1849-1859. DOI: 10.1007/s00421-011-2167-x

[63] Urbanski R, Aschenbrenner P, Zmijewski P, Ewertowska P, Switala K, Krzysztofik M. Effect of simultaneous lower- and upper-body ischemic preconditioning on lactate, heart rate, and rowing performance in healthy males and females. Applied Sciences-Basel. 2024;**14**(9):3539. DOI: 10.3390/app14093539

[64] MacDougall KB, McClean ZJ, MacIntosh BR, Fletcher JR, Aboodarda SJ. Ischemic preconditioning, but not priming exercise, improves exercise performance in trained rock climbers. Journal of Strength and Conditioning Research. 2023;**37**(11):2149-2157. DOI: 10.1519/JSC.0000000000004565

[65] Paull EJ, Van Guilder GP. Remote ischemic preconditioning increases

accumulated oxygen deficit in middle-distance runners. Journal of Applied Physiology. 2019;**126**(5):1193-1203. DOI: 10.1152/japplphysiol.00585.2018

[66] Christiansen D, Olsen CBL, Kehler F, et al. Active relative to passive ischemic preconditioning enhances intense endurance performance in well-trained men. International Journal of Sports Physiology and Performance. 2022;**17**(6):979-990. DOI: 10.1123/ijspp.2021-0397

[67] Cruz R, Tramontin AF, Oliveira AS, Caputo F, Denadai BS, Greco CC. Ischemic preconditioning increases spinal excitability and voluntary activation during maximal plantar flexion contractions in men. Scandinavian Journal of Medicine & Science in Sports. 2024;**34**(3):e14591. DOI: 10.1111/sms.14591

[68] Pereira HM, de Lima FF, Silva BM, Kohn AF. Sex differences in fatigability after ischemic preconditioning of non-exercising limbs. Biology of Sex Differences. 2020;**11**(1):59. DOI: 10.1186/s13293-020-00338-z

[69] Lopes TR, Sabino-Carvalho JL, Ferreira THN, Succi JE, Silva AC, Silva BM. Effect of ischemic preconditioning on the recovery of cardiac autonomic control from repeated Sprint exercise. Frontiers in Physiology. 2018;**9**:1465. DOI: 10.3389/fphys.2018.01465

[70] Zihan F, Ying W. Application of ischemic conditioning in sports training: Effects, mechanisms, and challenges. Chinese Journal of Sports Medicine. 2024;**43**(9):753-766. DOI: 10.16038/j.1000-6710.2024.09.001

[71] Salagas A, Tsoukos A, Terzis G, et al. Effectiveness of either short-duration ischemic pre-conditioning, single-set high-resistance exercise, or their combination in potentiating bench press exercise performance. Frontiers in Physiology. 2022;**13**:1083299. DOI: 10.3389/fphys.2022.1083299

[72] Cocking S, Wilson MG, Nichols D, ct al. Is there an optimal ischemic-preconditioning dose to improve cycling performance? International Journal of Sports Physiology and Performance. 2018;**13**(3):274-282. DOI: 10.1123/ijspp.2017-0114

[73] Seeley AD, Caldwell AR, Cahalin LP, et al. Seven days of ischemic preconditioning augments hypoxic exercise ventilation and muscle oxygenation in recreationally trained males. American Journal of Physiology. Regulatory, Integrative and Comparative Physiology. 2022;**323**(4):R457-R466. DOI: 10.1152/ajpregu.00335.2021

[74] Niespodzinski B, Mieszkowski J, Kochanowicz M, Kochanowicz A, Antosiewicz D. Effect of 10 consecutive days of remote ischemic preconditioning on local neuromuscular performance. Journal of Electromyography and Kinesiology. 2021;**60**:102584. DOI: 10.1016/j.jelekin.2021.102584

[75] Tanaka D, Suga T, Shimoho K, Isaka T. Effect of 2-weeks ischemic preconditioning on exercise performance: A pilot study. Front Sports Act Living. 2021;**3**:646369. DOI: 10.3389/fspor.2021.646369

[76] Slysz JT, Burr JF. Impact of 8 weeks of repeated ischemic preconditioning on running performance. European Journal of Applied Physiology. 2019;**119**(6):1431-1437. DOI: 10.1007/s00421-019-04133-6

[77] Lindsay A, Petersen C, Blackwell G, et al. The effect of 1 week of repeated ischaemic leg preconditioning on simulated Keirin cycling performance:

A randomised trial. BMJ Open Sport & Exercise Medicine. 2017;**3**(1):e000229. DOI: 10.1136/bmjsem-2017-000229

[78] Nukada A. Muscular performance in reactive hyperemia of muscles. Internationale Zeitschrift für Angewandte Physiologie. 1955;**16**(1):81-82

[79] Muller EA. Muscular work and muscular blood circulation in reactive hyperemia. Pflügers Archiv für die Gesamte Physiologie des Menschen und der Tiere. 1958;**265**(5):29-39. DOI: 10.1007/BF00369771

[80] Dirnagl U, Becker K, Meisel A. Preconditioning and tolerance against cerebral ischaemia: From experimental strategies to clinical use. Lancet Neurology. 2009;**8**(4):398-412. DOI: 10.1016/S1474-4422(09)70054-7

[81] Heusch G. Molecular basis of cardioprotection: Signal transduction in ischemic pre-, post-, and remote conditioning. Circulation Research. 2015;**116**(4):674-699. DOI: 10.1161/CIRCRESAHA.116.305348

[82] Kaur G, Binger M, Evans C, Trachte T, Van Guilder GP. No influence of ischemic preconditioning on running economy. European Journal of Applied Physiology. 2017;**117**(2):225-235. DOI: 10.1007/s00421-016-3522-8

[83] Lisbôa FD, Turnes T, Cruz RSO, Raimundo JAG, Pereira GS, Caputo F. The time dependence of the effect of ischemic preconditioning on successive sprint swimming performance. Journal of Science and Medicine in Sport. 2017;**20**(5):507-511. DOI: 10.1016/j.jsams.2016.09.008

[84] Richard P, Billaut F. Time-trial performance in elite speed skaters after remote ischemic preconditioning. International Journal of Sports Physiology and Performance. 2018;**13**(10):1308-1316. DOI: 10.1123/ijspp.2018-0111

[85] Behrens M, Gube M, Chaabene H, et al. Fatigue and human performance: An updated framework. Sports Medicine. 2023;**53**(1):7-31. DOI: 10.1007/s40279-022-01748-2

[86] de Oliveira GT, Souza HLR, Prazeres EO, et al. A practical approach for ischemic preconditioning intervention in sports: A pilot study for cuff thigh occlusion pressure estimation based on systolic blood pressure. Journal of Human Kinetics. 2024;**91**(Spec Issue):157-164. DOI: 10.5114/jhk/186064

[87] Dantas PAM, Da Silva NJ, Paz CR, et al. Acute effect of ischemic preconditioning in different blood flow restriction compressions on the anaerobic performance of trained individuals. Retos. 2024;**54**:721-727

[88] Hammert WB, Kataoka R, Yamada Y, et al. Are the effects of ischemic preconditioning on fatigue performance testing influenced by the applied pressure? Medicine and Science in Sports and Exercise. 2023;**55**(9):211-212

[89] Pizzo Junior E, de Souza Cavina AP, Lemos LK, Biral TM, Pastre CM, Vanderlei FM. Effects of different ischemic preconditioning occlusion pressures on muscle damage induced by eccentric exercise: A study protocol for a randomized controlled placebo clinical trial. Trials. 2021;**22**(1):326. DOI: 10.1186/s13063-021-05285-7

[90] Cromwell HC, Panksepp J. Rethinking the cognitive revolution from a neural perspective: How overuse/misuse of the term "cognition" and the

neglect of affective controls in behavioral neuroscience could be delaying progress in understanding the BrainMind. Neuroscience and Biobehavioral Reviews. 2011;**35**(9):2026-2035. DOI: 10.1016/j.neubiorev.2011.02.008

[91] Ellingson JM, Verges A, Littlefield AK, Martin NG, Slutske WS. Are bottom-up and top-down traits in dual-systems models of risky behavior genetically distinct? Behavior Genetics. 2013;**43**(6):480-490. DOI: 10.1007/s10519-013-9615-9

[92] Hohl R, Deslandes AC, Mármora CHC. The effect of single-dose massage session on autonomic activity, mood, and affective responses in major depressive disorder. Journal of Holistic Nursing. 2019;**37**(4):312-321. DOI: 10.1177/0898010119832493

[93] Daniel JB, Montrezol FT, Maxwell JD, et al. Impact of handgrip exercise and ischemic preconditioning on local and remote protection against endothelial reperfusion injury in young men. American Journal of Physiology. Regulatory, Integrative and Comparative Physiology. 2023;**324**(3):R329-R335. DOI: 10.1152/ajpregu.00061.2022

[94] Bailey TG, Birk GK, Cable NT, et al. Remote ischemic preconditioning prevents reduction in brachial artery flow-mediated dilation after strenuous exercise. American Journal of Physiology-Heart and Circulatory Physiology. 2012;**303**(5):H533-H538. DOI: 10.1152/ajpheart.00272.2012

[95] Kido K, Suga T, Tanaka D, et al. Ischemic preconditioning accelerates muscle deoxygenation dynamics and enhances exercise endurance during the work-to-work test. Physiological Reports. 2015;**3**(5):e12395. DOI: 10.14814/phy2.12395

[96] Kido K, Suga T, Tanaka D, et al. Remote ischemic preconditioning accelerates systemic O_2 dynamics and enhances endurance during work-to-work cycling exercise. Translational Sports Medicine. 2018;**1**(5):204-211. DOI: 10.1002/tsm2.36

[97] Herrod PJJ, Lund JN, Phillips BE. Time-efficient physical activity interventions to reduce blood pressure in older adults: A randomised controlled trial. Age and Ageing. 2021;**50**(3):980-984. DOI: 10.1093/ageing/afaa211

[98] Muñoz-Gómez E, Mollà-Casanova S, Sempere-Rubio N, et al. Effectiveness of an endurance exercise programme preceded by ischaemic preconditioning in older people. Geriatric Nursing. 2025;**63**:442-449. DOI: 10.1016/j.gerinurse.2025.03.043

[99] da Silva Telles LG, Billaut F, Cunha G, et al. Ischemic preconditioning improves handgrip strength and functional capacity in active elderly women. International Journal of Environmental Research and Public Health. 2022;**19**(11):6628. DOI: 10.3390/ijerph19116628

[100] Clarkson MJ, Conway L, Warmington SA. Blood flow restriction walking and physical function in older adults: A randomized control trial. Journal of Science and Medicine in Sport. 2017;**20**(12):1041-1046. DOI: 10.1016/j.jsams.2017.04.012

[101] Hart EC, Charkoudian N, Wallin BG, Curry TB, Eisenach JH, Joyner MJ. Sex differences in sympathetic neural-hemodynamic balance: Implications for human blood pressure regulation. Hypertension. 2009;**53**(3):571-576. DOI: 10.1161/HYPERTENSIONAHA.108.126391

[102] Teixeira AL, Ritti-Dias R, Antonino D, Bottaro M, Millar PJ,

Vianna LC. Sex differences in cardiac Baroreflex sensitivity after isometric handgrip exercise. Medicine and Science in Sports and Exercise. 2018;**50**(4):770-777. DOI: 10.1249/MSS.0000000000001487

[103] Paradis-Deschênes P, Joanisse DR, Billaut F. Sex-specific impact of ischemic preconditioning on tissue oxygenation and maximal concentric force. Frontiers in Physiology. 2016;**7**:674. DOI: 10.3389/fphys.2016.00674

[104] Notay K, Lee JB, Incognito AV, Seed JD, Arthurs AA, Millar PJ. Muscle strength influences pressor responses to static handgrip in men and women. Medicine and Science in Sports and Exercise. 2018;**50**(4):778-784. DOI: 10.1249/MSS.0000000000001485

[105] Lee JB, Lutz W, Omazic LJ, et al. Blood pressure responses to static and dynamic knee extensor exercise between sexes: Role of absolute contraction intensity. Medicine and Science in Sports and Exercise. 2021;**53**(9):1958-1968. DOI: 10.1249/MSS.0000000000002648

[106] Lee JB, Notay K, Seed JD, Nardone M, Omazic LJ, Millar PJ. Sex differences in muscle metaboreflex activation after static handgrip exercise. Medicine and Science in Sports and Exercise. 2021;**53**(12):2596-2604. DOI: 10.1249/MSS.0000000000002747

[107] Batterham AM, Hopkins WG. The case for magnitude-based inference. Medicine and Science in Sports and Exercise. 2015;**47**(4):885. DOI: 10.1249/MSS.0000000000000551

[108] Welsh AH, Knight EJ. "Magnitude-based inference": A statistical review. Medicine and Science in Sports and Exercise. 2015;**47**(4):874-884. DOI: 10.1249/MSS.0000000000000451

[109] Marocolo M, Simim MAM, Bernardino A, Monteiro IR, Patterson SD, da Mota GR. Ischemic preconditioning and exercise performance: Shedding light through smallest worthwhile change. European Journal of Applied Physiology. 2019;**119**(10):2123-2149. DOI: 10.1007/s00421-019-04214-6

[110] Paradis-Deschênes P, Joanisse DR, Billaut F. Ischemic preconditioning improves time trial performance at moderate altitude. Medicine & Science in Sports & Exercise. 2018;**50**(3):533-541. DOI: 10.1249/MSS.0000000000001473

[111] Foster GP, Giri PC, Rogers DM, Larson SR, Anholm JD. Ischemic preconditioning improves oxygen saturation and attenuates hypoxic pulmonary vasoconstriction at high altitude. High Altitude Medicine & Biology. 2014;**15**(2):155-161. DOI: 10.1089/ham.2013.1137

[112] Jean-St-Michel E, Manlhiot C, Li J, et al. Remote preconditioning improves maximal performance in highly trained athletes. Medicine and Science in Sports and Exercise. 2011;**43**(7):1280-1286. DOI: 10.1249/MSS.0b013e318206845d

[113] Chotiyarnwong C, Nair K, Angelini L, et al. Effect of remote ischaemic preconditioning on walking in people with multiple sclerosis: Double-blind randomised controlled trial. BMJ Neurology Open. 2020;**2**(1):e000022. DOI: 10.1136/bmjno-2019-000022

[114] Wang Z, Li X, Li N, et al. Safety and tolerability of both arm ischemic conditioning in patients with major depression: A proof of concept study. Frontiers in Psychiatry. 2020;**11**:570. DOI: 10.3389/fpsyt.2020.00570

[115] AHK M, Mitchinson CJ, Townsend OR, Nemmers CH, Serkaian CN, Rider BC. Ischemic preconditioning does not improve time trial performance in

recreational runners. International Journal of Exercise Science. 2020;**13**(6):1402-1417. DOI: 10.70252/ZXRT9304

[116] Kataoka R, Song JS, Yamada Y, et al. The impact of different ischemic preconditioning pressures on pain sensitivity and resistance exercise performance. Journal of Strength and Conditioning Research. 2024;**38**(5):864-872. DOI: 10.1519/JSC.0000000000004718

[117] Martin SM, Lalonde F, Legault É, Ribeiro P, Comtois AS, Tournoux F. Remote ischemic preconditioning does not improve the six minutes walk test performance in chronic heart failure patients: A randomised pilot trial. International Journal of Exercise Science. 2021;**14**(2):1354-1362. DOI: 10.70252/KBNF6433

[118] Incognito AV, Doherty CJ, Lee JB, Burns MJ, Millar PJ. Ischemic preconditioning does not alter muscle sympathetic responses to static handgrip and metaboreflex activation in young healthy men. Physiological Reports. 2017;**5**(14):e13342. DOI: 10.14814/phy2.13342

[119] Albuquerque MR, Flôr CAG, Ribeiro AIS, Mesquita PHC, Franchini E, Laurentino GC. Effects of ischemic preconditioning on sport-specific performance in highly trained taekwondo athletes. Sports (Basel). 2024;**12**(7):179. DOI: 10.3390/sports12070179

[120] Hansen D, Abreu A, Ambrosetti M, et al. Exercise intensity assessment and prescription in cardiovascular rehabilitation and beyond: Why and how: A position statement from the secondary prevention and rehabilitation section of the European Association of Preventive Cardiology. European Journal of Preventive Cardiology. 2022;**29**(1):230-245. DOI: 10.1093/eurjpc/zwab007

Chapter 7

Hemodynamic Stability during Spinal Anesthesia

Maliha Khalid and Muhammad Khalid

Abstract

Spinal anesthesia, also known as subarachnoid block, is a regional anesthesia technique often preferred over general anesthesia for surgeries involving the lower abdomen, perineum, and lower limbs. This approach helps avoid serious complications associated with general anesthesia, such as intubation difficulties, aspiration, and opioid-related issues. For lower limb surgeries, various anesthetic options are available, including general anesthesia, central neuraxial blocks, peripheral nerve blocks, and local anesthesia. Compared to general anesthesia, spinal anesthesia provides more stable vital signs, less postoperative pain, reduced blood loss, and a lower risk of deep vein thrombosis and delirium. However, spinal anesthesia can cause hypotension, bradycardia, and other cardiovascular effects due to sympathetic blockage, with hypotension being the most common complication. This is primarily due to decreased systemic vascular resistance and vasodilation, leading to reduced cardiac output. Despite these potential drawbacks, spinal anesthesia remains a widely used and effective technique for lower limb surgeries globally.

Keywords: spinal anesthesia, hyperbaric bupivacaine, mean arterial pressure, hemodynamic stability, neuraxial block

1. Introduction

Spinal anesthesia has become a crucial component of modern anesthetic practice, particularly for surgeries involving the lower abdomen, limbs, and obstetrics [1]. This technique offers a safer alternative to general anesthesia, with benefits including reduced risk of intubation difficulties, aspiration, and cardiodepressant effects [2]. It provides effective anesthesia with muscle relaxation, is cost-effective, and has been shown to lower blood loss and mortality rates, especially in obstetric cases [3]. Bupivacaine is a commonly used medication for spinal anesthesia, and studies have reported varying frequencies of hypotension with different concentrations of hyperbaric bupivacaine. For instance, a study conducted by Goyal and colleagues found that the frequency of hypotension was 66.67% when 0.5% hyperbaric bupivacaine was used in a lower segment cesarean operation [4]. The study observed a notable difference in systolic blood pressure (SBP) between the 0.75 and 0.5% hyperbaric bupivacaine groups, with SBP after 5 minutes of spinal anesthesia being 109.20 ± 21.65 and 113.23 ± 20.27 mmHg, respectively. Another study led by Ali et al. discovered that the frequency of hypotension was 30.8% with 0.75% hyperbaric bupivacaine in lower segment cesarean section [5]. In contrast, a study by Rani et al. found that a high intrathecal dose of 15 mg of hyperbaric 0.5% and 15 mg of hyperbaric 0.75% bupivacaine had no significant effect on mean arterial pressure in patients undergoing elective surgery under conventional spinal anesthesia [6]. However, a study conducted by Rai et al. found that pregnant females undergoing elective cesarean section and receiving conventional dose (15 mg) of spinal anesthesia with 0.5 versus 0.75% hyperbaric bupivacaine had a statistically significant difference hemodynamically, with the group of patients receiving 0.75% hyperbaric bupivacaine experiencing more hypotension [7].

Unilateral spinal anesthesia is a subset of spinal anesthesia that offers benefits like stable hemodynamics, reduced urine retention, increased patient satisfaction, and faster recovery but it limits the anesthetic effects to the operative side only [8]. This study aims to investigate the effects of low-dose hyperbaric bupivacaine (7.5 mg) in different concentrations (0.5 and 0.75%) on hemodynamic stability in patients undergoing unilateral spinal anesthesia, building upon the existing research on spinal anesthesia and its applications.

2. Anatomy

Understanding the anatomy and physiology of the spinal column and its contents is essential for effective spinal anesthesia.

2.1 Spinal column

The spinal column comprises 33 vertebrae, divided into cervical, thoracic, lumbar, sacrum, and coccyx regions, with four distinct curves [1]. Each vertebra consists of a weight-bearing body, pedicles, and laminae that form transverse and spinous processes. Five key ligaments support the vertebral bodies, with the ligamentum flavum playing a significant role in spinal procedures due to its thickness and elasticity [1].

2.2 Contents of spinal column

The vertebral canal houses key structures, including the meninges, cerebrospinal fluid (CSF), spinal cord, nerve roots, and vessels.

2.2.1 Meninges

The spinal meninges consist of three protective layers: dura mater, arachnoid mater, and pia mater [2]. These layers protect the spinal cord and facilitate substance movement within the spinal canal.

2.2.2 Cerebrospinal fluid

CSF is a complex solution produced through plasma ultrafiltration and glucose oxidation, with specific characteristics, including a specific gravity of 1.003–1.009 and a volume of approximately 20 mL in the spinal subarachnoid space.

2.2.3 Spinal cord

The spinal cord originates from the medulla oblongata and gives rise to 31 pairs of spinal nerves, each corresponding to specific dermatomes [2]. Specific dermatomes correspond to specific areas of the body.

2.2.4 Vessels

The spinal cord's blood supply comes from three main arteries: one anterior spinal artery and two posterior spinal arteries, which supply the anterior and posterior spinal cord, respectively [9]. Venous drainage occurs through a network of anterior and posterior veins.

3. Structures pierced during subarachnoid block

When administering spinal anesthesia, a needle must traverse several structures to reach the subarachnoid space. The sequence of structures is as follows [10]: the needle first passes through the skin and subcutaneous tissue, followed by the supraspinous ligament and interspinous ligament. Next, it encounters the ligamentum flavum, a thick and elastic ligament. After penetrating the ligamentum flavum, the needle enters the epidural space, which contains areolar tissue. Finally, the needle passes through the dura mater to reach the subarachnoid space, where the anesthetic is administered.

4. Physiology of neuraxial blockade

Neuraxial block can have various physiological effects on the body [11]:

4.1 Cardiovascular effects

Spinal anesthesia can cause decreased heart rate and arterial blood pressure due to sympathectomy-induced vasodilation, with the extent of these effects depending on the block height. Venodilation has a more significant impact due to the large volume of blood in the venous system. High neuraxial blockade can slow heart rate by blocking cardiac accelerator fibers (T1-T4).

4.2 Respiratory effects

In healthy patients, neuraxial block typically has minimal effects on pulmonary function, with tidal volume remaining stable and vital capacity decreasing slightly due to reduced expiratory reserve volume (4.05 –3.73 L). However, patients with severe respiratory compromise may be at risk due to respiratory muscle paralysis.

4.3 Gastrointestinal effects

Nausea and vomiting occur in up to 20% of patients undergoing neuraxial anesthesia, primarily due to unopposed parasympathetic activation leading to gastrointestinal hyperperistalsis. This can create favorable surgical conditions due to the contracted state of the intestines.

4.4 Effect on renal function

Neuraxial blockade can lead to decreased renal blood flow, but this typically has minimal physiological impact. Urine retention is a notable effect, which can delay discharge and require catheterization. Lower doses of local anesthetics can impair bladder function.

4.5 Endocrine effects

Spinal anesthesia can effectively block many endocrine and metabolic changes associated with the stress response by limiting sensory signals to the central nervous system in order to mitigate the body's stress reaction to surgery.

5. Factors affecting block height

Several factors influence the block height in spinal anesthesia. These include patient characteristics, technique of injection, and characteristics of the local anesthetic solution.

5.1 Patient characteristics

Patient-specific factors that influence block height include cerebrospinal fluid (CSF) volume, age, weight, and body mass index (BMI). While patient height and age do not directly correlate with block features, BMI significantly predicts total sensory block development. Other factors like intra-abdominal pressure and spinal column anatomy also play a role [12, 13].

5.2 Technique of injection

The injection technique is crucial in determining block height, with factors like bevel direction and injection rate impacting anesthetic spread. These variables can significantly influence the effectiveness of spinal anesthesia.

5.3 Characteristics of local anesthetic solution

The effectiveness of local anesthetics depends on baricity, dose, volume, and concentration [14]. Baricity affects anesthetic spread, with isobaric, hyperbaric, and hypobaric solutions behaving differently. Dose and concentration also impact block height, with controllable factors including dose, site of injection, baricity, and patient posture. Understanding these factors enables tailored spinal anesthesia for specific surgical needs and patient conditions. The concentration of local anesthetics affects the type of block achieved, with varying concentrations providing different levels of motor block.

6. Pharmacokinetics of local anesthetics in spinal anesthesia

After injecting a local anesthetic into the subarachnoid space, its concentration rapidly declines due to several factors. Initially, cerebrospinal fluid (CSF) dilution and mixing occur within 2–3 minutes, driven by the force and volume of the injection. The anesthetic then undergoes diffusion, distribution, and binding to neural tissues. Ultimately, vascular absorption and elimination via the arachnoid villi and parenchymal capillary bed contribute to the decrease in anesthetic concentration over time.

7. Sequence of nerve modality block

The sequence of sensory and motor blockade typically follows a specific order. It begins with vasomotor block, leading to vasodilation, followed by a loss of temperature sensation, pain perception, and tactile sensation. As the block progresses, motor function is impaired, resulting in muscle weakness or paralysis. Finally, deep sensations such as pressure, position sense, and vibration are lost, marking the progression of the blockade. Understanding this sequence is essential for effective spinal anesthesia management.

8. Hemodynamic instability during neuraxial blockade

8.1 Managing hypotension in spinal anesthesia

Hypotension is a common consequence of spinal anesthesia, particularly with higher dermatomal levels, due to sympathetic chain suppression [15]. This can lead to nausea, vomiting, and potential spinal cord ischemia. Research has identified various strategies to prevent and manage hypotension, including positioning patients in the Trendelenburg position, fluid loading with lactated Ringer's solution or 6% hydroxyethyl starch solution, and vasopressor therapy. Co-hydration has been found to be more effective than pre-hydration, and colloid loading is better at sustaining cardiac output and blood pressure. According to Shin et al., crystalloid pre-treatment may delay the cranial distribution of the block and stimulate cerebrospinal fluid production [16].

8.2 Preventing hypotension in obstetric patients

In obstetric patients undergoing spinal anesthesia, factors contributing to hypotension include increased venodilation due to hormonal changes, hypertension, advanced age, higher BMI, higher birth weight, and higher block level [17, 18]. Common measures to prevent and manage hypotension include fluid loading, lateral tilt or wedge under the right buttock, and vasopressor therapy [19, 20]. Phenylephrine is often preferred over ephedrine due to its effectiveness in maintaining hemodynamic stability without increasing fetal acidity [21]. A variable infusion of phenylephrine (25–50 μg/min) is more effective than constant infusion [22]. However, phenylephrine infusion can cause bradycardia due to a baroreflex-mediated mechanism.

8.3 Special consideration

For patients with severe heart disease, non-invasive cardiac output monitoring may be beneficial [23]. In patients with conditions like pre-eclampsia, sympathetic inhibition affecting arterial vasculature plays a major role in reducing arterial pressure, supporting the use of vasopressor therapy [20].

8.4 Understanding spinal hypotension and bradycardia

Spinal hypotension and bradycardia are primarily caused by the blockade of spinal sympathetic nerve fibers [24]. As the block extends to higher thoracic levels, the body's ability to compensate for these changes is impaired. The blockade of T5-L1 spinal nerve fibers reduces efferent input to the adrenal glands, limiting the release of catecholamines that help counteract hypotension and bradycardia.

8.5 Mechanisms and risk factors

Systemic blood pressure is determined by cardiac output and systemic vascular resistance (SVR), with the latter being the primary cause of spinal hypotension [25]. Factors like aortocaval compression in pregnant women can exacerbate the condition, and high thoracic blocks can further worsen hypotension by reducing myocardial contractility [26]. A T4 sensory block can cause a significant drop in mean arterial pressure, resulting from a reduction in SVR and cardiac output.

8.6 Predictors and incidence

According to Carpenter et al., the strongest predictor of hypotension during spinal anesthesia is a peak sensory block height at or above T5, with an odds ratio of 3.8 [27]. Other significant risk factors for hypotension include being over 40 years old and having a baseline systolic blood pressure below 120 mmHg [28, 29]. Studies have shown that hypotension requiring treatment occurs in around 33–38% of patients, while bradycardia occurs in 13% of patients [30–32].

8.7 Prevention and treatment

Prophylactic crystalloid injection only temporarily increases blood pressure and cardiac indices, with short-lived effects [33, 34]. Volume preloading with colloid solutions results in greater and longer-lasting volume expansion, but still fails to avoid hypotension in all patients [35]. Due to the lack of consistent evidence, prophylactic volume preloading is not recommended for euvolemic patients receiving spinal anesthesia [36]. Vasopressor therapy depends on the patient's hemodynamic profile, with ephedrine being the preferred choice for postpartum spinal hypotension [37]. Phenylephrine is suitable for hypotensive and tachycardic patients, while low-dose epinephrine can increase cardiac output and arterial pressure [38, 39]. For severe bradycardia or asystole, 5–20 µg of epinephrine should be administered intravenously, with the dose gradually increasing every minute [39]. In cases of asystole, 1 mg of epinephrine should be injected immediately. Atropine treats mild to severe bradycardia while epinephrine provides strong alpha- and beta-adrenergic stimulation [39].

9. Unilateral spinal anesthesia: A better option for lower limb procedures

Unilateral spinal anesthesia (ULSA) may be a better option than traditional spinal anesthesia for procedures involving one lower leg, reducing hypotension risk, facilitating faster recovery, and increasing patient satisfaction [40]. Techniques such as lateral decubitus position, low anesthetic doses, specific needle orientation, and slow injection rates can achieve ULSA using hypobaric, isobaric, or hyperbaric solutions.

9.1 Effective doses and solutions

Studies have found that low doses of bupivacaine can be effective in ULSA. Nair et al. found that an intrathecal dose of 4–5 mg hyperbaric bupivacaine was sufficient for arthroscopic knee surgery [41]. Minville et al. demonstrated the effectiveness of low intrathecal doses (mean dose of 5 mg) in elderly patients undergoing hip fracture surgery, providing stable operating conditions and improved hemodynamic stability [42]. Atef et al. found that 7.5 mg of 0.5% hyperbaric bupivacaine resulted in less hypotension compared to 10 mg in elderly patients undergoing arthroscopy under ULSA [43].

9.2 Comparison of hyperbaric and hypobaric solutions

Kaya et al.'s study compared hyperbaric and hypobaric bupivacaine (7.5 mg) in 50 patients undergoing lower limb orthopedic surgery, finding both effective with intraoperative hemodynamic stability and rapid recovery [44]. However, bilateralization was more likely with hypobaric bupivacaine. Imbelloni et al. investigated 5 mg of bupivacaine in ULSA in 150 patients, finding all three approaches (hypobaric, isobaric, or hyperbaric) successful [45, 46].

9.3 Minimizing hemodynamic instability

Perioperative hemodynamic instability can be minimized by reducing cardiovascular effects of neuraxial blockade, and techniques like one-sided sympathetic block and dose restriction are effective [47]. ULSA with low doses (7.5 mg) significantly reduces the risk of hypotension compared to traditional spinal anesthesia (15 mg) which ranges from 25 to 69% [48–50].

9.4 Clinical trial on unilateral spinal anesthesia

Our study involved 100 patients aged 20–70 years who underwent lower limb surgery and were divided into two groups: Group A received 0.5% hyperbaric bupivacaine, while Group B received 0.75% hyperbaric bupivacaine. To achieve unilateral anesthesia, patients were placed in a lateral position tilted 30 degrees toward the surgical side immediately after intrathecal injection. The results showed significant differences in mean arterial pressure (MAP) between the groups, with more pronounced hemodynamic changes in patients receiving 0.75% hyperbaric bupivacaine (p-value <0.05). The study's limitations included limited outcomes, but the use of sequential sampling reduced bias. A multicenter study is needed for future therapeutic implications due to our single-center design.

10. Conclusion

Our study indicates that 7.5 mg of 0.5% hyperbaric bupivacaine maintains more stable mean arterial pressure compared to 7.5 mg of 0.75% hyperbaric bupivacaine in patients undergoing lower limb surgery under unilateral spinal anesthesia. We suggest that 7.5 mg of 0.5% hyperbaric bupivacaine is a suitable dose for minimizing hypotensive effects in these patients. This dose may be considered for routine use in similar surgical procedures.

Acknowledgements

Parts of the chapter were previously published in this work (Maliha Khalid. Comparison of hemodynamic effect caused by intrathecal low dose administration of 0.5% against 0.75% hyperbaric bupivacaine in patients undergoing lower limb surgery under unilateral spinal anesthesia. Vol. 35 No. 4 (2023): Journal of Ayub Medical College Abbottabad/Original Article. Available from https://demo.ayubmed.edu.pk/jamc/index.php/jamc/article/download/12270/3615/49495).

Conflict of interest

Nil.

Nomenclature

ULSA	unilateral spinal anesthesia
CSF	cerebrosspinal fluid
MAP	mean arterial pressure

Appendix

See **Tables 1** and **2** and **Figure 1.**

Mean Arterial Pressure MAP	Mean ± SD Group A n = 50	Mean ± SD Group B n = 50	P value
Baseline MAP	88.72 ± 1.71	88.94 ± 1.95	0.551
MAP at 15 minutes post unilateral spinal anesthesia	86.22 ± 2.55	81.78 ± 1.52	0.000
MAP at 30 minutes post unilateral spinal anesthesia	83.72 ± 3.36	75.84 ± 1.34	0.000
MAP at 45 minutes post unilateral spinal anesthesia	80.02 ± 3.40	70.90 ± 0.97	0.000
MAP at 60 minutes post unilateral spinal anesthesia	77.14 ± 4.24	66.06 ± 1.62	0.000

Source: Khan et al. [51].

Table 1.
Mean arterial pressure measured at different time intervals in both groups of patients.

Complications	Group A n = 50 (%)	Group B n = 50 (%)	P Value
Nausea and vomiting	1 (2%)	2 (4%)	
Bradycardia	1 (2%)	1 (2%)	0.842
Hypotension	0	0	
No complications	48	47	

Source: Khan et al. [51].

Table 2.
Comparison of complications in both groups of patients.

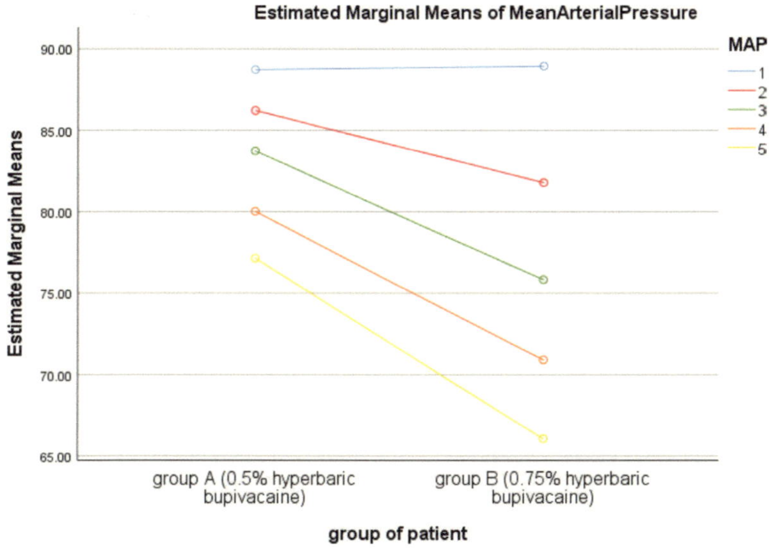

Figure 1.
Mean arterial pressure (MAP) was measured at various time points after administering unilateral spinal anesthesia in two patient groups. The measurements were taken at baseline (MAP1), 15 minutes post-anesthesia (MAP2), 30 minutes post-anesthesia (MAP3), 45 minutes post-anesthesia (MAP4), and 60 minutes post-anesthesia (MAP5). By tracking MAP at these different intervals, the study allowed for a comparison of hemodynamic changes between the two groups over time, providing insight into the effects of unilateral spinal anesthesia on blood pressure. Source: Khan et al. [51].

Author details

Maliha Khalid* and Muhammad Khalid
PAF Hospital Mushaf, Sargodha, Pakistan

*Address all correspondence to: dowite18malyha@yahoo.com

References

[1] Brown DL. Spinal, epidural and caudal anesthesia. In: Miller RD, editor. Miller's Anesthesia. 7th ed. Philadelphia: Elsevier Churchill Livingstone; 2010. pp. 1611-1638

[2] Bernards CM. Epidural and spinal anesthesia. In: Clinical Anaesthesia. 6th ed. New York: Wolters Kluwer Lippioncott Williams and Wilkins; 2009. pp. 927-950

[3] Bano N, Firdous R. Effects of intrathecal hyperbaric versus isobaric bupivacaine in elective caesarean section. Journal of Univeristy Medical and Dental College. 2015;**6**(2):1-6. Available from: https://www.jumdc.com/index.php/jumdc/article/view/224

[4] Goyal A, Shankaranarayan P, Ganapathi P. A randomized clinical study comparing spinal anesthesia with isobaric levobupivacaine with fentanyl and hyperbaric bupivacaine with fentanyl in elective cesarean sections. Anesthesia, Essays and Researches. 2015;**9**(1):57-62. DOI: 10.4103/0259-1162.150169

[5] Ali M, Iqbal A. A comparative study of two different doses of 0.75% hyperbaric bupivacaine for spinal anaesthesia in elective caesarean section a. Pakistan Armed Forces Medical Journal. 2019;**69**(1):154-159. Available from: https://www.pafmj.org/PAFMJ/article/view/2514

[6] Rani Z, Mehmood T, Ishrat Z. Comparison of efficacy and hemodynamic effects of two different concentrations of hyperbaric bupivacain 0.5 and 0.75% during spinal anesthesia. The Pakistan Journal of Medical and Health Sciences. 2019;**13**(3):659-664

[7] Rai SA, Malak AM, Ali CA. Comparison between 0.5% and 0.75% hyperbaric bupivacaine given intrathecally in elective caesarean section. Journal of Postgraduate Medical Institute. 2018;**32**(1):87-90

[8] Cindea I, Balcan A, Gherghina V, Nicolae G. Unilateral spinal anesthesia versus conventional spinal anesthesia in ambulatory lower abdominal surgery. European Journal of Anaesthesiology (EJA). 2007;**24**:10

[9] Ganong WF. Review of Medical Physiology. 23rd ed. Chapter 34, Circulation through Special Regions. New York: McGraw-Hill Company; 2010. p. 571

[10] Boon JM, Abrahams PH, Meiring JH, Welch T. Lumbar puncture: Anatomical review of a clinical skill. Clinical Anatomy. 2004;**17**(7):544-553. DOI: 10.1002/ca.10250

[11] William and Wilkins. Physiology of Spinal Anesthesia. Baltimore: Williams and Wilkins; 2001. pp. 78-108

[12] Karim MA, Banik D, Hye A, Huda Q, Laskar MMH, Banik D, et al. Effect of site of injection on spread of spinal anaesthesia with hyperbaric bupivacaine. Journal of the Bangladesh Society of Anaesthesiologists. 2007;**20**(2):51-55

[13] Veering BT, Immink-Speet TT, Burm AG, Stienstra R, van Kleef JW. Spinal anaesthesia with 0.5% hyperbaric bupivacaine in elderly patients: Effects of duration spent in the sitting position. British Journal of Anaesthesia. 2001;**87**(5):738-742. DOI: 10.1093/bja/87.5.738

[14] Gupta R, Bogra J, Singh PK, Saxena S, Chandra G, Kushwaha JK. Comparative study of intrathecal

hyperbaric versus isobaric ropivacaine: A randomized control trial. Saudi Journal of Anaesthesia. 2013;**7**(3):249-253. DOI: 10.4103/1658-354X.115326

[15] Amjad QUA, Sharif A, Khan A. Comparison of 0.5% and 0.75% hyperbaric bupivacaine given intrathecally in elective lower segment caesarean section. Khyber Medical University Journal. 2016;**8**(2):78-81

[16] Shin BS, Kim CS, Sim WS, Lee CJ, Kim ST, Kim GH, et al. A comparison of the effects of preanesthetic administration of crystalloid versus colloid on intrathecal spread of isobaric spinal anesthetics and cerebrospinal fluid movement. Anesthesia and Analgesia. 2011;**112**(4):924-930. DOI: 10.1213/ANE.0b013e31820d93d8. Epub 2011 Feb 2

[17] Hwang JW, Oh AY, Song IA, Na HS, Ryu JH, Park HP, et al. Influence of a prolonged lateral position on induction of spinal anesthesia for cesarean delivery: A randomized controlled trial. Minerva Anestesiologica. 2012 Jun;**78**(6):646-652. Epub 2012 Mar 13

[18] Zhang N, He L, Ni JX. Level of sensory block after spinal anesthesia as a predictor of hypotension in parturient. Medicine (Baltimore). 2017;**96**(25):e7184. DOI: 10.1097/MD.0000000000007184

[19] Sharwood-Smith G, Drummond GB. Hypotension in obstetric spinal anaesthesia: A lesson from pre-eclampsia. British Journal of Anaesthesia. 2009;**102**(3):291-294. DOI: 10.1093/bja/aep003

[20] Langesæter E, Dyer RA. Maternal haemodynamic changes during spinal anaesthesia for caesarean section. Current Opinion in Anaesthesiology. 2011;**24**(3):242-248. DOI: 10.1097/ACO.0b013e32834588c5

[21] Ngan Kee WD, Khaw KS, Lau TK, Ng FF, Chui K, Ng KL. Randomised double-blinded comparison of phenylephrine vs ephedrine for maintaining blood pressure during spinal anaesthesia for non-elective caesarean section. Anaesthesia. 2008;**63**(12):1319-1326. DOI: 10.1111/j.1365-2044.2008.05635.x

[22] Ngan Kee WD, Khaw KS, Ng FF, Lee BB. Prophylactic phenylephrine infusion for preventing hypotension during spinal anesthesia for cesarean delivery. Anesthesia and Analgesia. 2004;**98**(3):815-821, table of contents. DOI: 10.1213/01.ane.0000099782.78002.30

[23] Moschovaki N, Saranteas T, Spiliotaki E, Giannoulis D, Anagnostopoulos D, Talliou C, et al. Point of care transthoracic echocardiography for the prediction of post – Spinal anesthesia hypotension in elderly patients with cardiac diseases and left ventricular dysfunction: Inferior vena cava and post-spinal anesthesia hypotension in elderly patients. Journal of Clinical Monitoring and Computing. 2023;**37**(5):1207-1218. DOI: 10.1007/s10877-023-00981-y. Epub 2023 Feb 21

[24] Hofhuizen C, Lemson J, Snoeck M, Scheffer GJ. Spinal anesthesia-induced hypotension is caused by a decrease in stroke volume in elderly patients. Local and Regional Anesthesia. 2019;**12**:19-26. DOI: 10.2147/LRA.S193925

[25] DeMers D, Wachs D. Physiology, mean arterial pressure. In: StatPearls. Treasure Island (FL): StatPearls Publishing; 2023. p. 2025

[26] Šklebar I, Bujas T, Habek D. Spinal anaesthesia-induced hypotension In obstetrics: Prevention and therapy. Acta Clinica Croatica. 2019;**58**(Suppl 1):90-95. DOI: 10.20471/acc.2019.58.s1.13

[27] Carpenter RL, Caplan RA, Brown DL, Stephenson C, Wu R. Incidence and risk factors for side effects of spinal anesthesia. Anesthesiology. 1992;**76**(6):906-916. DOI: 10.1097/00000542-199206000-00006

[28] Hartmann B, Junger A, Klasen J, Benson M, Jost A, Banzhaf A, et al. The incidence and risk factors for hypotension after spinal anesthesia induction: An analysis with automated data collection. Anesthesia and Analgesia. 2002;**94**(6):1521-1529, table of contents. DOI: 10.1097/00000539-200206000-00027

[29] Buggy D, Higgins P, Moran C, O'Brien D, O'Donovan F, McCarroll M. Prevention of spinal anesthesia-induced hypotension in the elderly: Comparison between preanesthetic administration of crystalloids, colloids, and no prehydration. Anesthesia and Analgesia. 1997;**84**(1):106-110. DOI: 10.1097/00000539-199701000-00020

[30] Caplan RA, Ward RJ, Posner K, Cheney FW. Unexpected cardiac arrest during spinal anesthesia: A closed claims analysis of predisposing factors. Anesthesiology. 1988;**68**(1):5-11. DOI: 10.1097/00000542-198801000-00003

[31] Kaimar P, Sanji N, Upadya M, Mohammed KR. A comparison of hypotension and bradycardia following spinal anesthesia in patients on calcium channel blockers and β-blockers. Indian Journal Of Pharmacology. 2012;**44**(2):193-196. DOI: 10.4103/0253-7613.93847

[32] Chooi C, Cox JJ, Lumb RS, Middleton P, Chemali M, Emmett RS, et al. Techniques for preventing hypotension during spinal anaesthesia for caesarean section. Cochrane Database of Systematic Reviews. 2017;**8**(8):CD002251. DOI: 10.1002/14651858.CD002251.pub3. Update in: Cochrane Database Syst Rev. 2020 Jul 1;7:CD002251. Doi: 10.1002/14651858.CD002251.pub4

[33] Gousheh MR, Akhondzade R, Asl Aghahoseini H, Olapour A, Rashidi M. The effects of pre-spinal anesthesia administration of crystalloid and colloid solutions on hypotension in elective cesarean section. Anesthesia and Pain Medicine. 2018;**8**(4):e69446. DOI: 10.5812/aapm.69446

[34] Rout CC, Rocke DA, Levin J, Gouws E, Reddy D. A reevaluation of the role of crystalloid preload in the prevention of hypotension associated with spinal anesthesia for elective cesarean section. Anesthesiology. 1993;**79**(2):262-269. DOI: 10.1097/00000542-199308000-00011. Erratum in: Anesthesiology 1994;81(2):529.

[35] Tawfik MM, Hayes SM, Jacoub FY, Badran BA, Gohar FM, Shabana AM, et al. Comparison between colloid preload and crystalloid co-load in cesarean section under spinal anesthesia: A randomized controlled trial. International Journal of Obstetric Anesthesia. 2014;**23**(4):317-323. DOI: 10.1016/j.ijoa.2014.06.006 Epub 2014 Jun 30

[36] Jackson R, Reid JA, Thorburn J. Volume preloading is not essential to prevent spinal-induced hypotension at caesarean section. British Journal of Anaesthesia. 1995;**75**(3):262-265. DOI: 10.1093/bja/75.3.262

[37] Biricik E, Ünlügenç H. Vasopressors for the treatment and prophylaxis of spinal induced hypotension during caesarean section. The Turkish Journal

of Anaesthesiology and Reanimation. 2021;**49**(1):3-10. DOI: 10.5152/TJAR.2020.70. Epub 2020 May 5

[38] Richards E, Lopez MJ, Maani CV. Phenylephrine. In: StatPearls. Treasure Island (FL): StatPearls Publishing; 2023. p. 2025

[39] Dalal R, Grujic D. Epinephrine. In: StatPearls. Treasure Island (FL): StatPearls Publishing; 2024. p. 2025

[40] Khatouf M, Loughnane F, Boini S, Heck M, Meuret P, Macalou D, et al. Rachianesthésie hypobare unilatérale chez le sujet âgé pour la chirurgie traumatique de la hanche: étude pilote [Unilateral spinal anaesthesia in elderly patient for hip trauma: a pilot study]. Annales Françaises d'Anesthèsie et de Rèanimation. 2005;**24**(3):249-254. French. DOI: 10.1016/j.annfar.2004.12.027

[41] Nair GS, Abrishami A, Lermitte J, Chung F. Systematic review of spinal anaesthesia using bupivacaine for ambulatory knee arthroscopy. British Journal of Anaesthesia. 2009;**102**(3):307-315. DOI: 10.1093/bja/aen389. Epub 2009 Feb 3

[42] Minville V, Fourcade O, Grousset D, Chassery C, Nguyen L, Asehnoune K, et al. Spinal anesthesia using single injection small-dose bupivacaine versus continuous catheter injection techniques for surgical repair of hip fracture in elderly patients. Anesthesia and Analgesia. 2006;**102**(5):1559-1563. DOI: 10.1213/01.ane.0000218421.18723.cf

[43] Atef H, El-Kasaby A, Omera M, Badr M. Optimal dose of hyperbaric bupivacaine 0.5% for unilateral spinal anesthesia during diagnostic knee arthroscopy. Local and Regional Anesthesia. 2010;**3**:85-91. DOI: 10.2147/LRA.S11815. Epub 2010 Aug 26

[44] Kaya M, Oğuz S, Aslan K, Kadioğullari N. A low-dose bupivacaine: A comparison of hyperbaric and hypobaric solutions for unilateral spinal anesthesia. Regional Anesthesia and Pain Medicine. 2004;**29**(1):17-22. DOI: 10.1016/j.rapm.2003.09.006

[45] Imbelloni LE, Beato L, Gouveia MA, Cordeiro JA. Baixa dose de bupivacaína isobárica, hiperbárica ou hipobárica para raquianestesia unilateral [Low dose isobaric, hyperbaric, or hypobaric bupivacaine for unilateral spinal anesthesia.]. Revista Brasileira de Anestesiologia. 2007;**57**(3):261-270. Portuguese

[46] Esmaoğlu A, Boyaci A, Ersoy O, Güler G, Talo R, Tercan E. Unilateral spinal anaesthesia with hyperbaric bupivacaine. Acta Anaesthesiologica Scandinavica. 1998;**42**(9):1083-1087. DOI: 10.1111/j.1399-6576.1998.tb05380.x

[47] Fanelli G, Borghi B, Casati A, Bertini L, Montebugnoli M, Torri G. Unilateral bupivacaine spinal anesthesia for outpatient knee arthroscopy. Italian study group on unilateral spinal anesthesia. Canadian Journal of Anaesthesia. 2000;**47**(8):746-751. DOI: 10.1007/BF03019476

[48] Kahloul M, Nakhli MS, Chouchene A, Chebbi N, Mhamdi S, Naija W. Comparison of two doses of hypobaric bupivacaine in unilateral spinal anesthesia for hip fracture surgery: 5 mg versus 7.5 mg. The Pan African Medical Journal. 2017;**28**:108. DOI: 10.11604/pamj.2017.28.108.11421

[49] Moosavi Tekye SM, Alipour M. Comparison of the effects and complications of unilateral spinal anesthesia versus standard spinal anesthesia in lower-limb orthopedic surgery. Brazilian Journal of Anesthesiology. 2014;**64**(3):173-176.

DOI: 10.1016/j.bjane.2013.06.014. Epub 2013 Oct 25

[50] Gong C, Ye X, Liao Y, Ye P, Zheng T, Zheng X. Hypotension after unilateral versus bilateral spinal anaesthesia: A systematic review with meta-analysis. European Journal of Anaesthesiology. 2025;**42**(3):203-223. DOI: 10.1097/EJA.0000000000002098. Epub 2024 Nov 21

[51] Khan MK, Hafiz A, Feroze F, Tahir AA, Farooq S, Faheem SB, et al. Comparison of hemodynamic effect caused by intrathecal low dose administration of 0.5% against 0.75% hyperbaric bupivacaine In patients undergoing lower limb surgery under unilateral spinal anaesthesia. Journal of Ayub Medical College, Abbottabad. 2023;**35**(4):549-552. DOI: 10.55519/JAMC-04-12270

Chapter 8

Minimally Invasive Cardiac Output Monitoring Devices: Principles, Applications, and Limitations

Bhavya Naithani Dube, Mallikarjun Dube and Neeraj Kumar

Abstract

Minimally invasive cardiac output monitoring (MICOM) devices have revolutionized hemodynamic monitoring in critically ill patients. This chapter reviews the principles and applications of various MICOM devices, including pulse contour analysis (e.g., LiDCO and PiCCO), esophageal Doppler, and bioimpedance cardiography. LiDCO and PiCCO devices use pulse contour analysis to estimate cardiac output, providing valuable insights into hemodynamic function. Their clinical utility spans diverse patient populations, such as those undergoing surgery or experiencing shock. Evidence supporting their use in goal-directed therapy protocols is also examined. However, MICOM devices have limitations, including issues related to accuracy, precision, and clinical interpretation. Understanding these limitations is crucial to harnessing their potential. By providing a comprehensive overview of MICOM devices, this chapter empowers clinicians to make informed decisions about hemodynamic management in critical care settings, ultimately enhancing patient outcomes and driving progress in critical care medicine.

Keywords: MICOM, LiDCO, PiCCO, hemodynamic monitoring, cardiac output

1. Introduction

The quantification of cardiac output, a crucial macrohemodynamic variable, is essential in evaluating hemodynamically unstable, critically ill patients. This key metric, which measures the blood flow produced by the heart, plays a vital role that is closely tied to the nuanced interpretation of associated hemodynamic and metabolic parameters. As therapeutic interventions progress, the interaction between cardiac output values and their fluctuations often guides treatment decisions, highlighting the necessity for accurate measurement and contextual comprehension.

Managing circulatory shock in intensive care unit (ICU) patients requires precise hemodynamic monitoring to assess cardiac function, vascular filling, and tone. Monitoring cardiac output has become an essential part of anesthesia and critical care, acting as a key indicator of oxygen delivery to tissues and identifying patients at increased risk of significant morbidity and mortality. This parameter informs treatment decisions, particularly in fluid resuscitation and the use of vasoactive and

IntechOpen

inotropic medications. Basic monitoring tools such as heart rate and blood pressure are necessary, but they are often insufficient for assessing volume status and predicting cardiac output. Advanced hemodynamic monitoring offers valuable insights, aiding clinicians in diagnosing and treating shock more effectively [1].

The Swan-Ganz catheter, introduced in 1970, has been fundamental in measuring cardiac output and providing insights into patients' hemodynamic status. Although its use has declined due to studies questioning its impact on clinical outcomes, it remains the benchmark against which newer monitoring technologies are evaluated. The invasive nature of the Swan-Ganz catheter presents certain challenges and risks, including infection, pulmonary artery rupture, arrhythmias, thrombosis, and embolism [2].

Researchers have developed minimally invasive cardiac output monitors to address the limitations of the Swan-Ganz catheter. These devices, such as transpulmonary thermodilution and non-invasive technologies, use different techniques to calculate cardiac output, each with its own potential errors and invasiveness levels [1]. Understanding these devices' principles and the clinical contexts that affect their accuracy is crucial for evaluating their reliability in ICU patients. This chapter provides a comprehensive review of cardiac output calculation principles, potential errors, and the clinical scenarios where monitor accuracy may be compromised, helping clinicians make informed decisions and optimize patient care.

2. Overview of cardiac output monitoring devices

Table 1 provides a comparative overview of cardiac output monitoring devices, highlighting their principles, advantages, and limitations.

3. Rationale for excluding the pulmonary artery catheter

In this chapter, we focus exclusively on the minimally invasive and non-invasive methods of cardiac output monitoring. While the pulmonary artery catheter (PAC)—commonly referred to as the Swan-Ganz catheter—was revolutionary in providing direct hemodynamic assessment, its current use in clinical practice is notably restricted due to significant limitations.

The PAC is highly invasive. Placement and use are associated with considerable risks, including infection, pulmonary artery rupture, arrhythmias, thrombosis, and embolism. Over the past two decades, substantial research has questioned whether these risks are justified by clinical benefit. Multiple large clinical trials and systematic reviews have failed to demonstrate an improvement in patient outcomes when PACs are routinely used in critically ill or high-risk surgical populations [3].

For instance, a landmark randomized controlled trial published in 2003 in The New England Journal of Medicine found no advantage of catheter-guided therapy over standard care for high-risk elderly surgery patients admitted to the intensive care unit [4]. Additionally, the 2013 Cochrane review by Rajaram and colleagues concluded that PAC use does not improve outcomes in adult intensive care unit patients [5]. These data suggest that routine use of the pulmonary artery catheter is unwarranted and may actually increase morbidity and mortality in certain patients.

Device/method	Principle of measurement	Advantages	Disadvantages
Pulmonary artery catheter (PAC)	Thermodilution via pulmonary artery catheter	Reference standard; direct measurement; full hemodynamics	Highly invasive; risks of infection, rupture, arrhythmia, thrombosis, embolism
Transpulmonary thermodilution (TPTD)	Cold saline bolus and arterial thermistor analysis	Less invasive than PAC; measures extra parameters	Requires both central venous and arterial access
Pulse contour analysis (e.g. PiCCO and LiDCO)	Analysis of arterial pressure waveform	Minimally invasive; continuous, real-time monitoring	Accuracy affected by arrhythmias, vascular tone, algorithm/ calibration limits
Lithium dilution cardiac output (LiDCO)	Lithium chloride bolus; arterial lithium detection	Minimally invasive; repeated measurements possible	Special equipment/lithium required; contraindicated in patients on lithium
FloTrac/Vigileo	Proprietary arterial waveform statistical analysis	Minimally invasive; easy continuous use	Decreased accuracy in low-flow/high-resistance/ vasoconstriction states
Esophageal Doppler	Doppler ultrasound in distal esophagus	Minimally invasive; tracks fluid responsiveness	Requires probe placement; operator and patient dependent; unreliable in aortic disease
Bioimpedance/ bioreactance cardiac output monitors	Electrical impedance/phase shift across thorax	Non-invasive; simple, rapid application	Less accurate in obesity, pulmonary edema, severe arrhythmias
Ultrasonic cardiac output monitor (USCOM)	Doppler ultrasound across heart valves	Non-invasive; portable; rapid assessment	Operator dependent; less reliable in complex cardiac anatomy

CO = cardiac output; PAC = pulmonary artery catheter; TPTD = transpulmonary thermodilution; PiCCO = pulse contour cardiac output.

Table 1.
Cardiac output monitoring devices: principles, advantages, and disadvantages.

In light of these findings, the prevalence of PAC use has significantly declined. Many contemporary guidelines and expert recommendations suggest restricting or discontinuing the routine application of PAC monitoring for most modern critical care and perioperative scenarios, given its limited efficacy and potential for patient harm.

Given these concerns, the need for accurate yet safer alternatives has driven advances in both minimally invasive and non-invasive cardiac output monitoring methods. The remainder of this chapter is devoted to the principles, devices, and clinical applications of these newer technologies, which aim to provide actionable hemodynamic data while minimizing procedural risks [6]. **Figure 1** demonstrates the properties of an ideal haemodynamic monitoring system.

4. Precision, accuracy, and the evolving role of volumetric indices

To replace the gold standard in cardiac output measurement, a new technique must demonstrate both high precision and accuracy. While accuracy ensures that measured values reflect the true cardiac output, precision—the ability to reliably detect consistent changes—may be even more critical for monitoring dynamic patient responses and evaluating therapeutic interventions.

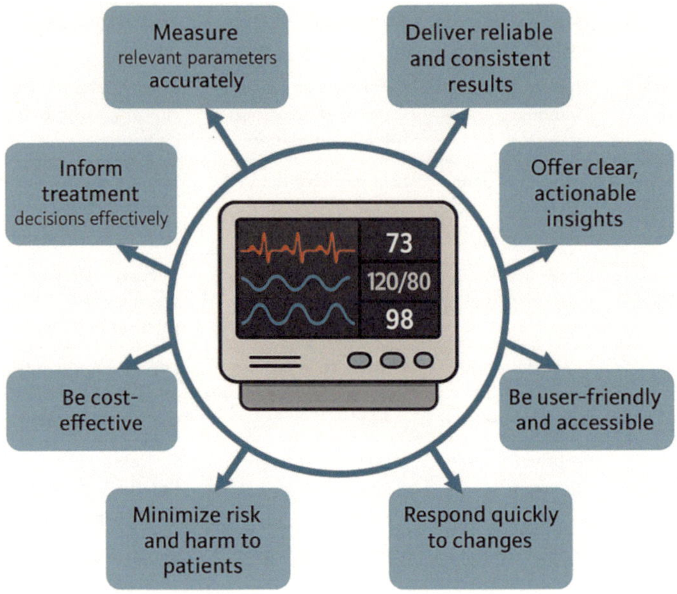

Figure 1.
An ideal heamodynamic monitoring system.

The complexities of cardiac function are aptly described by the Frank-Starling mechanism, which highlights the relationship between left ventricular preload and the fiber length of myocardial muscles at the end of diastole [7]. This interplay is best expressed in terms of the left ventricular end-diastolic volume, a direct volumetric measure. Unfortunately, accurate bedside measurement of left ventricular end-diastolic volume is not readily feasible in clinical practice [7].

Historically, clinicians have relied on pressure-based surrogate markers such as central venous pressure (CVP) and pulmonary artery occlusion pressure (PAOP) to estimate preload. These indices are based on the assumption of a stable relationship between pressure and volume within the heart. However, in critically ill patients, this assumption often fails due to significant alterations in ventricular compliance, fluctuating intrathoracic pressures, and changes in cardiac geometry. As a result, pressure-based parameters can be misleading and poorly reflect true intravascular volume status [8].

Low values of CVP and PAOP may sometimes indicate low preload, but crucially, these parameters do not predict fluid responsiveness and should not guide resuscitation toward arbitrary thresholds. Attempting to optimize hemodynamics based only on absolute CVP or PAOP values risks both under- and over-resuscitation, especially in patients experiencing increased intrathoracic pressure—a condition reported in more than 30% of patients receiving critical care. Consequently, modern resuscitation algorithms emphasize the limitations of pressure-based monitoring and increasingly promote volumetric assessment as a more faithful representation of true cardiac filling status [9].

This clinical recognition has fueled the development and routine clinical adoption of volumetric preload indices, which directly measure the volume status of the heart and central circulation, providing actionable data for fluid management—particularly in patients with altered chest and cardiac compliance [9].

Parameter	Definition/description	Unit
Cardiac output (CO)	Total volume of blood pumped by the heart per minute	L/min
Stroke volume (SV)	Amount of blood ejected from the ventricle with each heartbeat	mL
Stroke volume index (SVI)	Stroke volume standardized for body surface area	mL/m^2
Cardiac index (CI)	Cardiac output normalized for body surface area	$L/min/m^2$
End-diastolic volume (EDV)	Volume of blood in the ventricle at end of diastole (preload)	mL
End-systolic volume (ESV)	Volume of blood remaining in the ventricle at end of systole	mL
Ejection fraction (EF)	Percentage of end-diastolic volume ejected with each contraction (indicator of systolic function)	%
Global end-diastolic volume index (GEDVI)	Cumulative volume of blood in all four cardiac chambers at end-diastole, normalized for body surface area	mL/m^2
Intrathoracic blood volume index (ITBVI)	Total blood volume within the thoracic compartment (all cardiac chambers and pulmonary vasculature), per body surface area	mL/m^2
Extravascular lung water index (EVLWI)	Amount of fluid in pulmonary interstitium and alveolar space, normalized for body weight (indicator of pulmonary edema risk)	mL/kg

Table 2.
Hemodynamic parameters and their definitions.

4.1 Key hemodynamic and volumetric indices

The following volumetric and functional indices now guide advanced hemodynamic management in critically ill and surgical patients and are summarized in **Table** 2.

Table 2 summarizes key volumetric and flow-based parameters used in advanced hemodynamic monitoring. Units are standardized to facilitate comparison across individuals of varying body size. Parameters such as GEDVI, ITBVI, and EVLWI are particularly relevant in critical care settings for assessing preload, thoracic blood volume, and pulmonary fluid status [10].

Collectively, these volumetric parameters provide comprehensive insights into cardiac function, true preload (volume status), and the patient's overall fluid balance. Their use allows clinicians to tailor fluid therapy and optimize hemodynamic management more precisely, markedly improving decision-making in patients—particularly those with increased intrathoracic pressure, altered cardiac compliance, or complex critical illness [11].

5. Principles of physics behind cardiac output monitoring

Cardiac output (CO)—the volume of blood pumped by the heart per minute—is a fundamental parameter in evaluating cardiac function, perfusion, and overall circulatory status. Its measurement relies on several distinct physical principles and methods, each with unique strengths and limitations. The main approaches include the following [12]:

1. Fick method
2. Dilution techniques (thermodilution, dye densitometry, and lithium dilution) [13]
3. Arterial pulse analysis [14, 15]
4. Electrical impedance methods (transthoracic impedance and bioreactance) [15, 16]
5. Doppler ultrasound [17]

Each of these approaches offers a distinct way to assess cardiac function, with its own strengths and weaknesses.

5.1 The Fick Principle

The Fick Principle, developed by Adolf Eugen Fick in 1870, is a fundamental concept in cardiovascular physiology that enables the calculation of cardiac output based on the relationship between oxygen consumption and blood flow. At its core, it posits that the amount of oxygen extracted by the body's tissues is directly proportional to the difference in oxygen content between the arterial blood supplying the tissues and the venous blood returning to the lungs, which implies that CO—the volume of blood pumped by the heart per unit time—can be determined by measuring the difference in oxygen content between arterial and venous blood and dividing the oxygen consumption by this difference.

Mathematically, this relationship can be expressed as follows:

$$\mathbf{CO} = \frac{VO_2}{(CaO_2 - CvO_2)} \tag{1}$$

Where:
CO = Cardiac output (L/min)
VO_2 = Oxygen consumption (ml O_2/min, typically 125 × BSA for indirect method)
CaO_2 = Arterial oxygen content (ml O_2/L)
CvO_2 = Mixed venous oxygen content (ml O_2/L)

The Fick principle's application extends to various substances beyond oxygen, including carbon dioxide and specific markers, enabling assessment of blood flow and metabolic activity in specific organs and tissues, in addition to whole-body measurements (**Figure 2**).

The Fick principle relies on two fundamental assumptions. Firstly, it assumes a steady state condition where oxygen consumption and delivery are balanced, meaning the rate at which tissues uptake oxygen equals the rate at which oxygen is delivered to them. Secondly, it assumes that cardiac output is equal in both ventricles, implying that blood volume pumped by the right ventricle into the lungs is matched by that pumped by the left ventricle into the systemic circulation. These assumptions are necessary for accurately applying the Fick Principle to calculate cardiac output [18].

$$\text{Cardiac Output (CO)}\ \frac{\text{Oxygen Consumption } (VO_2)}{\text{Arterial Oxygen Content } (CaO_2) - \text{Venous Oxygen Content } (CvO_2)}$$

Figure 2.
Fick Principle equation illustrating the relationship between cardiac output, oxygen consumption, and arterial-venous oxygen content difference.

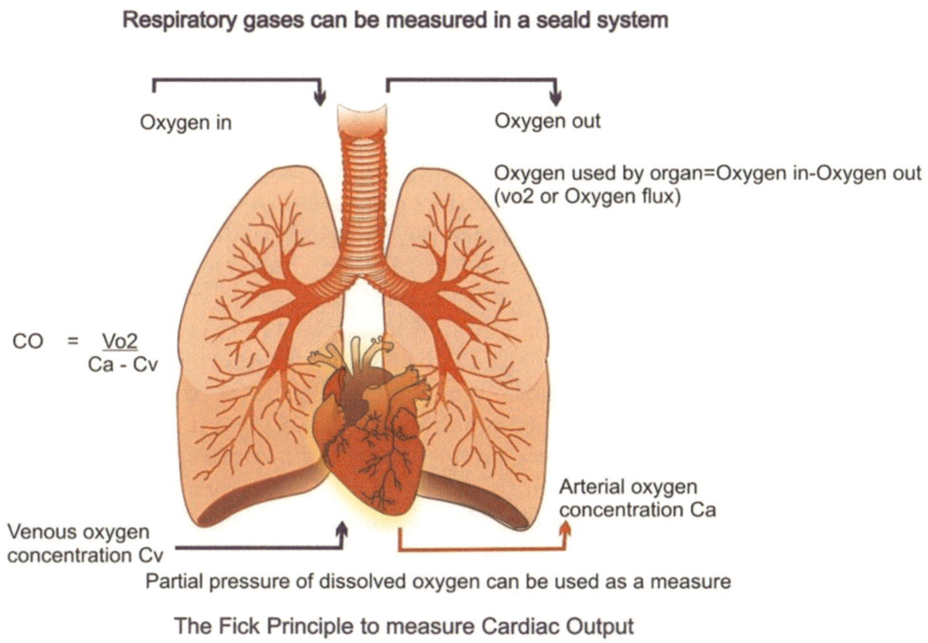

Figure 3.
The Fick's Principle to measure cardiac output.

The Direct Fick method is considered the benchmark for measuring cardiac output. It involves directly measuring the difference in oxygen levels between inspired and expired air to determine oxygen consumption (VO_2). Additionally, arterial and mixed venous blood gases are analyzed to calculate oxygen content in arterial (CaO_2) and venous (CvO_2) blood, with the latter requiring a pulmonary artery sample. This method provides a precise calculation of cardiac output (**Figure 3**) [19].

5.2 Indirect Fick methods

In contrast, Indirect Fick methods estimate one or more variables, introducing potential errors. They include estimation of oxygen consumption (VO_2) using nomograms, which are charts that predict normal values based on factors like age, sex, and weight; carbon dioxide content ($CaCO_2$) based on end-tidal CO_2 measurements, which measure CO_2 levels in exhaled breath; venous CO_2 content ($CvCO_2$) during rebreathing, where a patient rebreathes CO_2 to alter CO_2 levels in the blood; and finally estimation of arterial oxygen content (CaO_2) using pulse oximetry. Arterial oxygen saturation can be non-invasively monitored using pulse oximetry, a technique that measures SpO_2 levels [19].

Needless to say, indirect methods may be less precise than the Direct Fick method due to the potential for estimation errors. As mentioned earlier, a modified indirect version of the Fick principle uses carbon dioxide (CO_2) to measure cardiac output in mechanically ventilated patients. This technique involves a specialized device that includes a rebreathing loop, CO_2 sensor, and airflow sensor, and by analyzing changes in CO_2 elimination during normal and partial rebreathing states, the device estimates cardiac output.

Nevertheless, this approach has drawbacks, such as necessitating intubation and mechanical ventilation with consistent settings. Its suitability is also limited for patients with substantial respiratory diseases, making it mainly applicable to those who are mechanically ventilated and hemodynamically stable.

5.3 Limitations of the Fick method and indirect approaches

The Fick method for calculating cardiac output is subject to several limitations that can compromise its accuracy. Notably, indirect estimates can introduce significant errors, particularly in patients with complex physiological conditions, such as morbid obesity, hypothermia, or sepsis. Even the direct Fick method is not entirely infallible, exhibiting an inherent margin of error of approximately ±8%. Certain pulmonary conditions, such as severe pneumonia, can lead to augmented oxygen consumption, thereby resulting in an overestimation of cardiac output. Furthermore, the method's presumption of a condition of equilibrium may not be correct as oxygen consumption may not precisely reflect tissue oxygen requirements. Moreover, in high-output states characterized by narrow arteriovenous oxygen content differences, even miniscule errors in measurement can be substantially magnified. Lastly, intracardiac shunts can confound the measurement by inducing changes in oxygen content that are unrelated to alterations in cardiac output, thereby underscoring the need for cautious interpretation of Fick's method to results (**Figure 4**) [20].

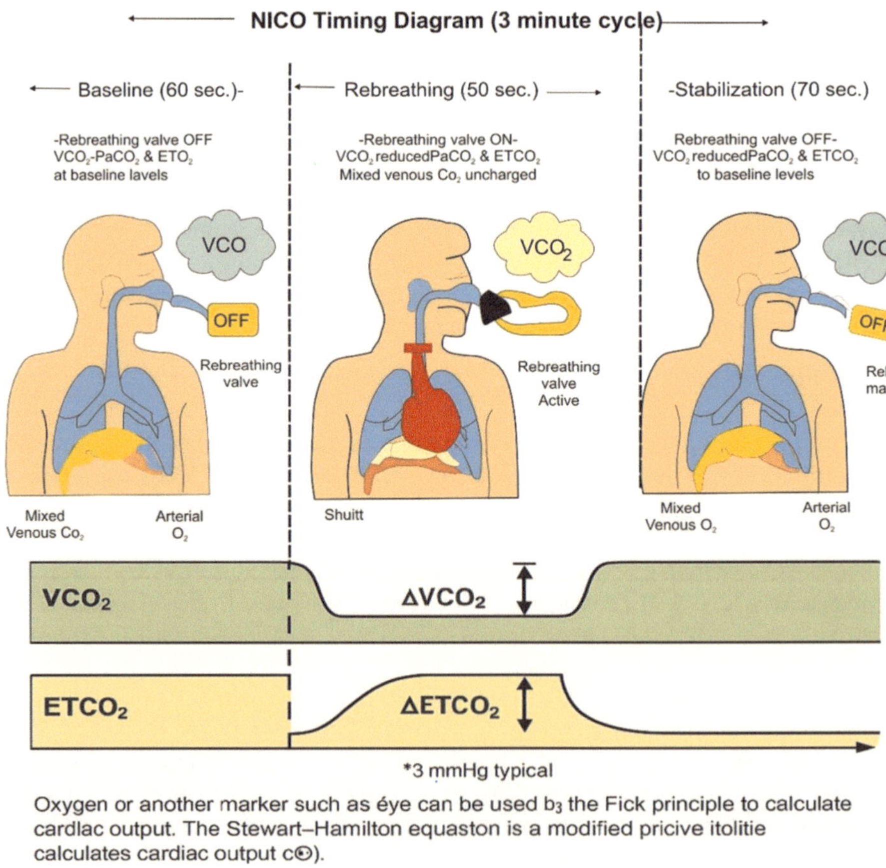

Figure 4.
Rebreathing circuit and sequence of breathing using the NICO system. Partial rebreathing is initiated every 3 minutes by opening the valve and pulmonary blood flow is calculated by difference between normal and rebreathing ratio.

5.4 Thermodilution techniques

In a recent advancement, transpulmonary thermodilution, the principle of which was obtained from the Stewart Hamilton Equation, has emerged as a promising technique, endeavoring to replicate the accuracy of the venerable pulmonary artery catheter (PAC) thermodilution method while mitigating its attendant complications. The Stewart-Hamilton equation has its origins in the concept of thermal dilution, where a cold saline bolus is injected into the bloodstream, causing a temporary drop in blood temperature. As the cold saline mixes with the blood, the temperature change is measured over time, creating a thermodilution curve. The area under this curve is inversely proportional to cardiac output: a larger area indicates slower blood flow (lower cardiac output), while a smaller area indicates faster blood flow (higher cardiac output). By analyzing this curve, the equation calculates cardiac output, providing a quantitative measure of the heart's pumping efficiency [21].

Innovative devices such as the PiCCOplus and EV1000/VolumeView have harnessed this technology to facilitate intermittent calibration of their sophisticated pulse pressure analysis-based cardiac output monitors. It involves the judicious injection of cold saline into the superior vena cava via a central venous catheter, while an arterial cannula, strategically placed in a major artery, incorporates a thermistor to meticulously measure the subtle changes in blood temperature. Advanced computer software then generates a thermodilution curve, elegantly plotting the temperature fluctuations over time [22].

Notably, cannulation via the femoral vein is generally eschewed, as it may precipitate an overestimation of intrathoracic blood volume. Furthermore, if femoral venous access is deemed necessary, the catheter should be positioned contralateral to the femoral arterial catheter to preclude crosstalk phenomena [23].

These cutting-edge monitors also provide a wealth of additional hemodynamic parameters, including global end-diastolic volume, intrathoracic blood volume, extravascular lung water, and a pulmonary vascular permeability index, all derived from the transpulmonary thermodilution technique. This comprehensive suite of metrics offers clinicians a nuanced understanding of cardiovascular dynamics, thereby informing therapeutic decision-making [21].

A myriad of potential sources of error has been discerned in the transpulmonary thermodilution technique as it exhibits a heightened susceptibility to errors precipitated by drift and indicator recirculation, yet paradoxically demonstrates a reduced vulnerability to errors stemming from respiratory variation [24]. The fundamental difference in measurement sites, wherein PAC thermodilution assesses right heart cardiac output and transpulmonary thermodilution evaluates left heart cardiac output, can lead to disparate measurements in the presence of intracardiac or intrapulmonary shunts.

Furthermore, the magnitude of error induced by valvular regurgitation is inherently unpredictable, being contingent upon the site and severity of the regurgitation. Notwithstanding these potential pitfalls, a robust correlation between PAC and transpulmonary thermodilution has been established in diverse experimental and clinical contexts, including cardiac surgery and intensive care settings involving septic and burn patients. Intriguingly, underestimation of cardiac output has been reported due to indicator recirculation, despite the fact that a substantial proportion (approximately 96–97%) of the indicator is recovered in the aorta. Indicator recirculation refers to the phenomenon wherein the cold injectate diffuses into tissues and subsequently reenters the bloodstream, potentially leading to measurement inaccuracies.

Moreover, indicator loss into the lungs, particularly in patients with pulmonary edema, has been posited as a contributing factor to poor correlation in some studies. The interplay between indicator loss and recirculation appears to be complex, with the effects of these two parameters tending to counterbalance each other; however, the relative significance of each remains to be fully elucidated [25].

5.5 Pulse dye densitometry

Pulse dye densitometry (PDD) employs the DDG-2001 analyzer to estimate arterial indocyanine green (ICG) concentration following intravenous injection. This non-invasive technique utilizes a fingertip sensor emitting specific wavelengths to detect ICG levels after pulmonary circulation. The relative ICG concentration ratio is then used to calculate cardiac output [26]. Notably, ICG is a safe and non-toxic dye, rarely associated with allergic reactions, and is exclusively cleared by the liver. Furthermore, the magnitude of error induced by valvular regurgitation is inherently unpredictable, being contingent upon the site and severity of the regurgitation. Notwithstanding these potential pitfalls, a robust correlation between pulmonary artery catheter (PAC) and transpulmonary thermodilution has been established in diverse experimental and clinical contexts, including cardiac surgery and intensive care settings involving septic and burn patients [27].

Intriguingly, underestimation of cardiac output has been reported due to indicator recirculation, despite the fact that a substantial proportion (approximately 96–97%) of the indicator is recovered in the aorta. Indicator recirculation refers to the phenomenon wherein the cold injectate diffuses into tissues and subsequently reenters the bloodstream, potentially leading to measurement inaccuracies [28]. Moreover, indicator loss into the lungs, particularly in patients with pulmonary edema, has been posited as a contributing factor to poor correlation in some studies. The interplay between indicator loss and recirculation appears to be complex, with the effects of these two parameters tending to counterbalance each other; however, the relative significance of each remains to be fully elucidated.

5.6 Pulse dye densitometry

Pulse dye densitometry (PDD) uses the DDG-2001 analyzer to measure arterial indocyanine green (ICG) concentration after intravenous injection. This non-invasive method employs a fingertip sensor to detect ICG levels post-pulmonary circulation and calculates cardiac output based on the ICG concentration ratio. ICG is a safe, non-toxic dye cleared exclusively by the liver. The PDD technique enables repeated measurements every 20 minutes once ICG levels drop to 1%. However, study results on PDD accuracy are inconsistent, necessitating further research (**Figure** 5) [26].

5.7 The lithium dilution method

The LiDCOplus system offers real-time cardiac output monitoring through pulse power analysis via the PulseCO algorithm, complemented by lithium dilution for intermittent calibration. The LiDCOplus system is an amalgamation of two proprietary algorithms: the LiDCO system, which meticulously measures cardiac output through indicator dilution, and the PulseCO system, which provides a continuous, nuanced analysis of the arterial waveform. The harmonious union of these two systems is calibrated to perfection, yielding a precise and reliable measurement of cardiac function [23].

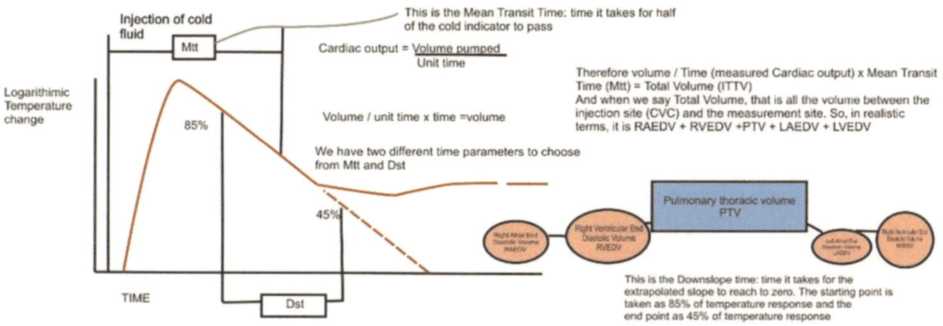

Figure 5.
Diagram explaining the principle of thermodilution and how the mean transit time and downslope time are used to calculate intrathoracic blood volumes.

A delicate lithium sensor, attached to the arterial line, senses the lithium ions as they flow through the circulation, generating a concentration-time curve that holds the secrets of cardiac output. This subtle yet powerful technique requires only an arterial line and a peripheral intravenous line, a testament to its minimally invasive nature. The PulseCO system is a marvel of mathematical wizardry, employing an autocorrelation algorithm to distill the arterial pressure waveform into a precise calculation of stroke volume [24]. The root mean square method, a clever mathematical trick, determines the volume of the arterial tree, while patient-specific factors are carefully woven into the calculation to yield an accurate measurement of cardiac function. This method involves injecting small boluses of lithium chloride, which are then measured by a sensor attached to an arterial cannula, generating a concentration-time curve that facilitates calculation of plasma flow using the Stewart-Hamilton equation [13, 24].

Lithium's unique properties render it an ideal indicator, but certain limitations apply. Patients on long-term lithium therapy may experience reduced accuracy. Moreover, the presence of non-depolarizing neuromuscular blocking agents, particularly atracurium and rocuronium, can lead to overestimation of cardiac output due to sensor cross-reactivity. Additionally, contraindications include patients weighing under 40 kg and those in the first trimester of pregnancy [24].

Despite these limitations, studies have demonstrated excellent correlation between lithium dilution cardiac output measurement and the pulmonary artery catheter thermodilution technique in various clinical settings. Research has shown minimal bias between the LiDCO device and thermodilution, with some variability in specific patient populations, such as those undergoing coronary artery bypass grafting or aortic clamping/unclamping. Nonetheless, current evidence suggests that LiDCOplus technology is a trustworthy alternative to the more invasive thermodilution method that uses a pulmonary artery catheter [13, 24].

There are various publications about the LiDCOplus system in multiple clinical settings, yielding promising results. Studies have supported the use of LiDCOplus with thermodilution in post-coronary artery bypass graft (CABG) patients [13], satisfactory correlation in post-liver transplant patients [28], and good correlation in post-cardiac surgery patients [29]. Moreover, LiDCOplus-based goal-directed therapy has been shown to significantly reduce complications and hospital stay [30]. However, its accuracy may be limited in certain situations, such as off-pump CABG, where a poor correlation was observed [31]. In contrast, LiDCOplus has proven sensitive in assessing intravascular volume in off-pump coronary artery bypass (OPCAB) surgery patients [32]. Furthermore, comparative studies have found LiDCO to be the least erroneous among other devices like PiCCO, FloTrac, and PAC [33]. These findings reiterate its benefits and limitations in different clinical contexts.

5.8 Arterial waveform analysis method

The arterial waveform method for cardiac output monitoring uses the blood pressure waveform to estimate stroke volume and cardiac output. This technique, first introduced by Otto Frank in 1899, utilizes a "Windkessel" model to describe the circulation. The Windkessel effect is a physiological phenomenon that describes how the left ventricle's contraction generates a systolic pressure wave that is then converted into a constant pressure in the systemic vasculature, maintaining a stable blood pressure and ensuring continuous blood flow to the tissues, even during diastole [21].

When the left ventricle contracts, it ejects blood into the aorta, causing the aortic walls to expand and stretch. This expansion stores potential energy, which is then converted to kinetic energy as the walls recoil, propelling blood forward into the systemic vasculature during diastole. This process, likened by Otto Frank to the 'Windkessel' air chamber used in fire engines, enables the conversion of the sinusoidal pressure wave generated by the heart into a positive and constant pressure at the tissue (**Figure 6**) [34].

The pulse pressure conceptual principle has been studied in clinical practice for a long time, initially through assessing the character and volume of the pulse. With advancements in technology, arterial cannulation and pulse pressure waveform analysis have become ubiquitous techniques for monitoring cardiac output. Pulse pressure analysis involves calculating stroke volume from the arterial waveform, considering factors like systolic and diastolic portions, aortic impedance, compliance, and peripheral vascular resistance. The pressure-recording analytical method (PRAM) is a technique that calculates cardiac output using physical parameters, including left ventricular ejection force, arterial impedance, compliance, and peripheral resistance [35].

The pulse pressure analysis technique utilizes the arterial waveform, obtained from an arterial catheter or finger probe, to calculate stroke volume and systemic vascular resistance. However, this method is complicated by the nonlinear and age-related compliance of the aortic wall, which precludes a direct correlation between pressure and volume. To address this limitation, in 1983, Wesseling et al. [36] introduced an algorithm that accounts for the nonlinear compliance of the aortic wall, allowing stroke volume to be calculated by analyzing the area under the systolic portion of the arterial waveform.

A distinct approach to estimating stroke volume involves analyzing pulse contour characteristics using models of systemic circulation. Conversely, pulse power analysis adopts a different strategy, focusing on the power changes within each heartbeat. This method posits that the net power change results from the balance between incoming blood volume and peripheral blood loss. By leveraging autocorrelation over time and sidestepping frequency-based methods, pulse power analysis reduces the impact of arterial damping and waveform irregularities. Although it can monitor stroke volume changes, calibration against a reference method, such as lithium dilution, is necessary to obtain precise absolute values.

The arterial waveform method has various benefits, including its less invasive nature, attenuating complications associated with traditional methods. It provides continuous, real-time monitoring of cardiac output, allowing for prompt interventions. Some systems, like the Nexfin monitor, are completely non-invasive, making them extremely useful for patients where invasive monitoring is not feasible.

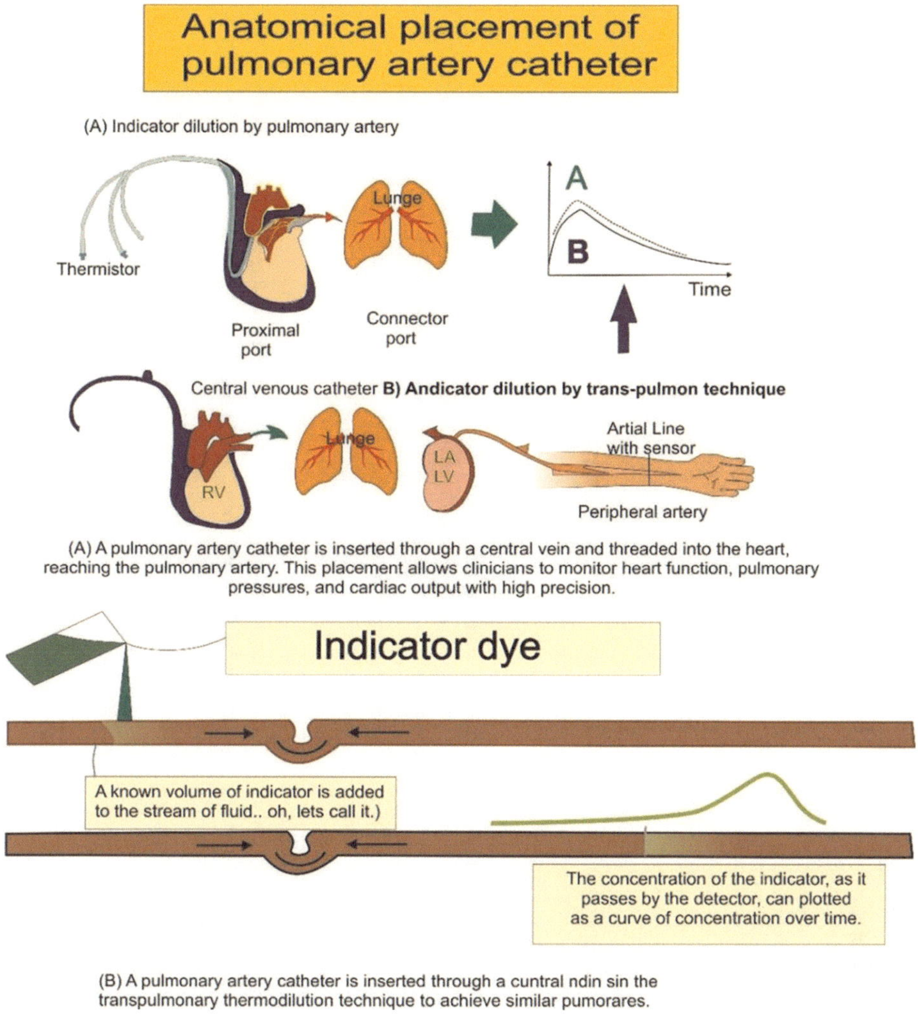

Figure 6.
The Windkesel model translating into a normal and abnormal pulse pressure waveform. (A) Pulmonary artery catheter inserted through central vein measures cardiac output via indicator dilution. Known volume of indicator (dye) added to bloodstream; its concentration as it passes detector plotted as curve over time. (B) Transpulmonary thermodilution technique achieves similar parameters.

However, the arterial waveform method also has several disadvantages. It requires an ideal arterial pressure tracing, which can be affected by under- or over-damped waveforms. Moreover, its accuracy may be limited when patients are on significant inotropic or vasopressor support, off-pump coronary artery bypass surgery, and open aortic abdominal aneurysm repair [34, 35].

Various commercial systems utilizing arterial waveform analysis have been developed, including auto/non-calibrated and externally calibrated devices (**Table 3**). Auto/non-calibrated devices include the FloTrac sensor, ProAQT sensor, LiDCO rapid system, Nexfin monitor, and esCCO. Calibrated devices include the LiDCOplus, PiCCOplus monitor, and EV1000/VolumeView monitor. These systems employ various techniques to determine cardiac output, including analysis of pulse contour, pulse power, or pulse wave transit time.

Device/manufacturer	Method/principle	Description	Advantages	Disadvantages
LiDCOplus (LiDCO Ltd., UK)	Lithium dilution calibration + pulse power analysis	Uses two proprietary algorithms: the LiDCO system for intermittent cardiac output via lithium dilution, and the PulseCO system for continuous arterial waveform analysis.	Useful in post-coronary artery bypass graft (CABG) patients; shown to be least erroneous among devices.	May overestimate cardiac output with non-depolarizing muscle relaxants; contraindicated in pregnancy and morbid obesity.
PiCCOplus (Pulsion Medical Systems, Germany)	Transpulmonary thermodilution calibration + pulse pressure analysis	Intermittent calibration via cold saline bolus and continuous real-time cardiac output calculation via pulse pressure analysis with arterial thermistor-tipped catheter.	Reliable in pediatric patients, one-lung ventilation, and during renal replacement therapy.	Requires regular calibration (every 8 hours in stable patients; every 15 minutes if hemodynamically unstable).
EV1000/ VolumeView (Edwards Lifesciences, USA)	Transpulmonary thermodilution + pulse contour analysis	Uses both thermodilution and continuous pulse wave analysis; measures global end-diastolic volume (GEDV) and extravascular lung water (EVLW) for fluid/preload management.	Provides additional volumetric parameters to guide fluid therapy and assess cardiac preload.	Accuracy may be affected by incorrect catheter placement or issues with the thermodilution curve.
FloTrac sensor/ ProAQT sensor	Uncalibrated pulse contour analysis	Algorithm derives stroke volume and cardiac output directly from the arterial waveform (standard arterial line).	Less invasive; algorithm-based calculation, no external calibration required.	Accuracy may decrease in extreme hemodynamic conditions, arrhythmias, or vasopressor use.
LiDCO rapid system	Uncalibrated pulse power analysis	Uses arterial line waveform and pulse power algorithms to track stroke volume changes; estimates cardiac output using nomograms.	Simple setup; continuous trend monitoring.	Provides trends but may be less accurate for absolute values.
Nexfin monitor	Non-invasive finger cuff arterial pressure waveform reconstruction	Inflatable finger cuff derives the arterial pressure waveform, reconstructs brachial waveform; measures continuous blood pressure, heart rate, and cardiac output.	Completely non-invasive; suitable for patients where arterial cannulation is not feasible.	Operator and patient dependent; peripheral vasoconstriction can affect accuracy; less robust in shock states.
esCCO	Pulse Wave Transit Time (PWTT) analysis	Non-invasive; uses the time delay between electrocardiogram (ECG) R-wave and pulse wave rise (PWTT) to estimate stroke volume and cardiac output.	Non-invasive; allows continuous cardiac output measurement without an arterial line.	Estimation can be affected by arrhythmias and poor ECG/pulse signal; less validated in rapidly changing conditions.

PWTT, pulse wave transit time; ECG, electrocardiogram; SV, stroke volume; CO, cardiac output; CABG, coronary artery bypass grafting; GEDV, global end-diastolic volume; EVLW, extravascular lung water.

Table 3.
Pulse contour and pulse wave transit time cardiac output monitoring devices: principles, advantages, and disadvantages [10].

5.9 Non-calibrated and uncalibrated devices

Non-calibrated (uncalibrated) cardiac output monitoring devices estimate cardiac output and stroke volume using proprietary algorithms, without depending on external reference calibration. The most widely used systems include the following:

1. *FloTrac sensor*: This device uses advanced algorithms to calculate stroke volume (SV) from the arterial waveform obtained from a standard arterial catheter. The ProAQT sensor in the Pulsioflex monitor uses a similar approach.

2. *LiDCO rapid system*: This monitor uses pulse power analysis to track changes in stroke volume and calculates cardiac output (CO) using nomograms.

3. *Nexfin monitor*: This non-invasive device uses an inflatable finger cuff to derive the finger arterial pressure waveform, which is then reconstructed into a brachial arterial pressure waveform. It measures various hemodynamic parameters, including continuous blood pressure, heart rate, and cardiac output.

4. *esCCO*: This non-invasive monitor uses pulse wave transit time (PWTT) analysis technology to calculate cardiac output. PWTT is the time delay between the electrocardiogram (ECG) R-wave peak and the pulse wave rise point, which is used to estimate stroke volume and cardiac output (**Figure** 7) [37].

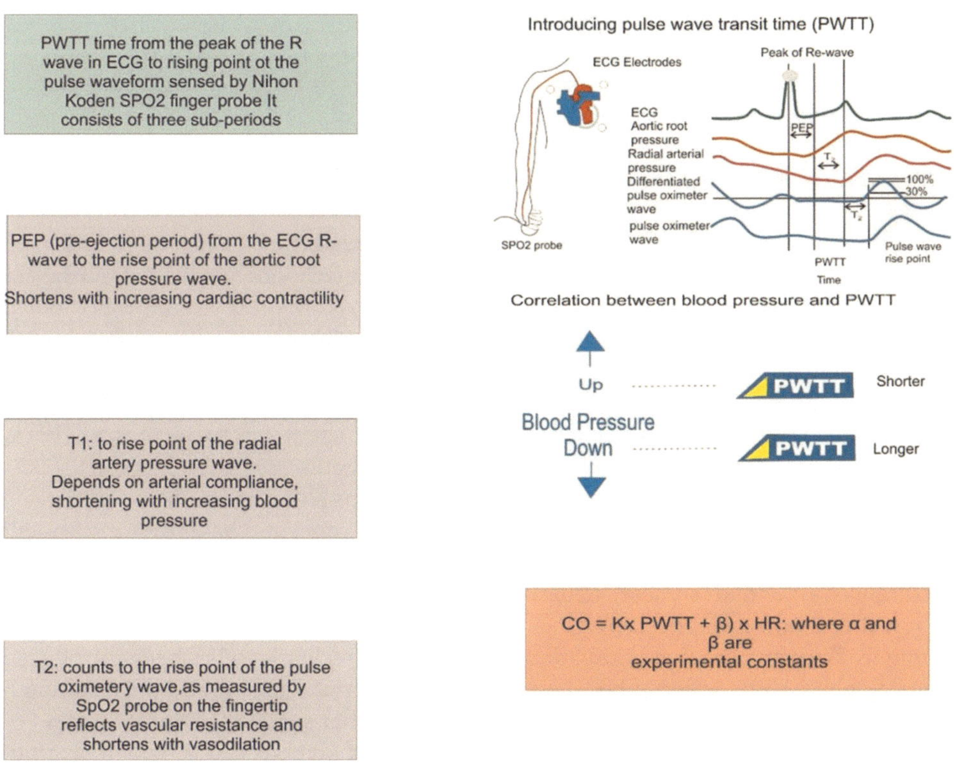

Figure 7.
The concept of pulse wave transit time, the time delay between the ECG, R wave and the pulse wave rise point, and the equation demonstrating how it is used to calculate the cardiac output.

5.10 Clinical validation and limitations of arterial waveform devices

Numerous studies have validated the precise and accurate nature of these systems in various clinical settings. The FloTrac/Vigileo system provides accurate and reliable cardiac output measurements in diverse clinical contexts. Giomarelli et al. found that the pressure recording analytical method (PRAM) is accurate for real-time cardiac output monitoring during coronary artery bypass graft (CABG) surgery and the post-operative period, when compared to pulmonary artery catheter (PAC) thermodilution [12]. Donati et al. compared PRAM, pulse contour cardiac output (PiCCO), and continuous PAC thermodilution in a mixed medical-surgical intensive care unit, showing good concordance between PRAM, PAC, and PiCCO in hemodynamically stabilized patients [38]. Romagnoli et al. investigated PRAM, FloTrac/Vigileo, and transthoracic echocardiography in vascular surgery patients, demonstrating good concordance between PRAM and echocardiographic measurements [39].

The Nexfin monitor has also been validated with positive results, while the PiCCOplus monitor has been shown to be reliable in pediatric patients, during one-lung ventilation, and in the setting of renal replacement therapy. Additionally, the EV1000/Volume View monitor has demonstrated superior calculation of global end-diastolic volume (GEDV) compared to the PiCCOplus monitor.

However, despite these advances, some studies have reported limitations and potential sources of error for these technologies. These include under- or over-damped arterial waveforms, various conditions that can distort the arterial pressure waveform, and reduced measurement accuracy in patients who are receiving significant inotropic or vasopressor support.

By understanding both the strengths and limitations of the arterial waveform method, clinicians can make informed decisions about its use in cardiac output monitoring and thereby optimize patient care.

5.11 Transthoracic impedance and bioreactance analysis

The realm of cardiac output monitoring has witnessed the emergence of innovative techniques, including impedance cardiography. This methodology, first described by Nyboer in 1950, involves the extrapolation of stroke volume (SV) using variations in transthoracic electrical impedance. The technique was later refined by Kubicek et al. [40] in 1966, paving the way for its clinical application.

Impedance cardiography operates on the principle of detecting changes in transthoracic voltage in response to an applied high-frequency current across the thorax. This is achieved through skin electrodes or electrodes mounted on a tracheal tube. The SV is calculated using a formula that takes into account various parameters, including the resistivity of blood, thoracic length, ventricular ejection time, and basal thoracic impedance. Despite its promise, it has limitations, including sources of error such as motion artifacts, electrical interferences, arrhythmias, and anatomical abnormalities, with a meta-analysis revealing a mean percentage error of 43% compared to the PAC thermodilution technique. To overcome these limitations, bioreactance technology has been introduced, analyzing phase shifts induced between an applied electrical current and the resulting voltage signal to calculate stroke volume, boasting a higher signal-to-noise ratio and reducing interference. Bioreactance provides a wealth of hemodynamic data, including cardiac output, heart rate, blood pressure, and thoracic fluid content, as well as clinical parameters like cardiac index and total peripheral resistance. While this technology holds promise, its accuracy during dynamic conditions remains debated. Further research is needed to validate the accuracy and reliability of impedance cardiography and bioreactance in various clinical settings, and as technology evolves, these methodologies are likely to play an increasingly important role in managing critically ill patients. A study published in the Journal of Clinical Monitoring and Computing found that bioreactance-based cardiac output monitoring was accurate and reliable in patients undergoing cardiac surgery. Another study published in Critical Care Medicine found that impedance cardiography was a useful tool for monitoring cardiac output in critically ill patients. However, other studies have raised concerns about the limitations and potential sources of error in these technologies. A meta-analysis published in the Journal of Critical Care found that impedance cardiography had a mean percentage error of 43% compared to the PAC thermodilution technique, highlighting the need for further validation. Another study published in the Journal of Cardiothoracic and Vascular Anesthesia found that bioreactance-based cardiac output monitoring was not accurate in patients undergoing cardiac surgery, particularly in the immediate postoperative period. Some studies have reported mixed results, suggesting that the accuracy of impedance cardiography and bioreactance may depend on specific patient populations or clinical contexts. For example, a study published in the Journal of Clinical Monitoring and Computing found that bioreactance-based cardiac output monitoring was accurate in patients with stable hemodynamics but not in those with dynamic changes in cardiac output. Overall, while some studies support the use of impedance cardiography and bioreactance in cardiac output monitoring, others highlight the need for further research to fully understand their limitations and potential applications (**Figure 8**).

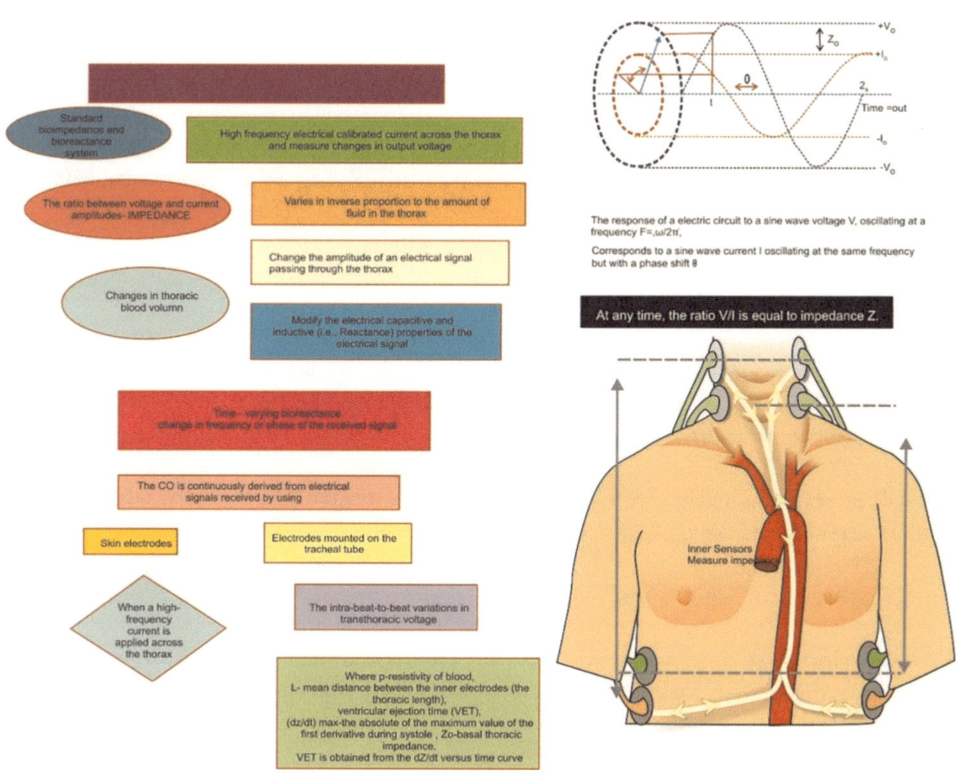

Figure 8.
A flowchart depicting the principle of bioreactance and impedance analysis, the mathematical equations involved and a picture depicting how the sensors are placed.

5.12 Transesophageal echocardiography and aortic Doppler

Transesophageal echocardiography (TEE) and *aortic Doppler* are advanced hemodynamic monitoring modalities that offer comprehensive insights into cardiac function and volume status, but their principles and clinical applications differ significantly [41].

5.12.1 Transesophageal echocardiography (TEE)

TEE is a sophisticated tool that provides detailed real-time information about cardiac structure, function, and hemodynamics. It utilizes an ultrasound probe placed in the esophagus, granting close proximity to the heart and excellent image quality, relatively uninhibited by chest wall, lung, or adipose tissue. TEE leverages Doppler technology to perform quantitative assessments of cardiac output and other hemodynamic parameters.

- Calculation of stroke volume (SV) and cardiac output (CO):
  - *Stroke volume (SV)* is determined using the Doppler velocity-time integral (VTI) and cross-sectional area (CSA) of the left ventricular outflow tract (LVOT):

$$\mathrm{SV} = \mathrm{VTI} \times \mathrm{CSA}$$

- VTI: Doppler velocity-time integral (cm)
- CSA: Cross-sectional area of LVOT (cm^2)
- *Cardiac output (CO)* is then calculated by multiplying SV by heart rate (HR):

$$\mathrm{CO} = \mathrm{SV} \times \mathrm{HR}$$

- Additional functional assessment:
  - TEE can evaluate ejection fraction (EF), estimate left ventricular end-diastolic area (LVEDA) as a surrogate for preload/volume status, and visualize wall motion or anatomical abnormalities.
  - It is highly sensitive for detecting right ventricular (RV) strain, which is valuable in cases of suspected pulmonary embolism.
- Validation and limitations:
  - Perrino et al. demonstrated that TEE yielded clinically acceptable agreement with thermodilution by pulmonary artery catheter during cardiac surgery [42].
  - However, Concha et al. noted significant discrepancies when comparing TEE to FloTrac/Vigileo in laparoscopic colon surgery, underscoring the need for context-specific interpretation and technique awareness [43].

- TEE is operator-dependent; high-quality images are essential for accuracy. Morbidity is rare but possible, as demonstrated by Kallmeyer et al., who reported a 0.2% complication rate (most commonly severe odynophagia) in over 7000 cardiac surgery patients [42].

5.12.2 Aortic Doppler

Aortic Doppler (also known as esophageal or transthoracic Doppler) provides a non-invasive or minimally invasive means of estimating cardiac output by measuring the velocity of red blood cells within the aorta—a surrogate for aortic blood flow.

- Doppler principle and calculation:
  - The Doppler equation for red cell velocity is: $Fd = 2Ft \cdot V \cdot \cos\theta / C$; $CFd = C2Ft \cdot V \cdot \cos\theta$

    - Fd: detected frequency shift

    - Ft: transmitted frequency

    - V: velocity of red blood cells

    - $\cos\theta$: correction factor for probe angle

    - C: Speed of sound in tissue

  - Conversion to flow (stroke volume):

    - The cross-sectional area (CSA) of the aorta is estimated via nomograms or M-mode ultrasound.

    - The integral of the velocity-time curve (stroke distance) is multiplied by CSA to yield stroke volume (SV).

  - Cardiac output calculation: $CO = SV \times HR$

- Clinical utility and limitations:

  - Aortic Doppler provides continuous beat-to-beat trend monitoring and is especially valuable in anesthetized or sedated patients where quick, minimally invasive assessment is needed.

  - Accuracy depends on appropriate probe positioning, correct angle of insonation, and appropriate patient selection for CSA estimation.

  - It does not provide detailed anatomical or structural information compared to TEE, but is less invasive and operator-dependent (**Figure 9**) [17].

The information gleaned from the cardiac output monitors can be analyzed in different ways. This can be better appreciated using a case scenario.

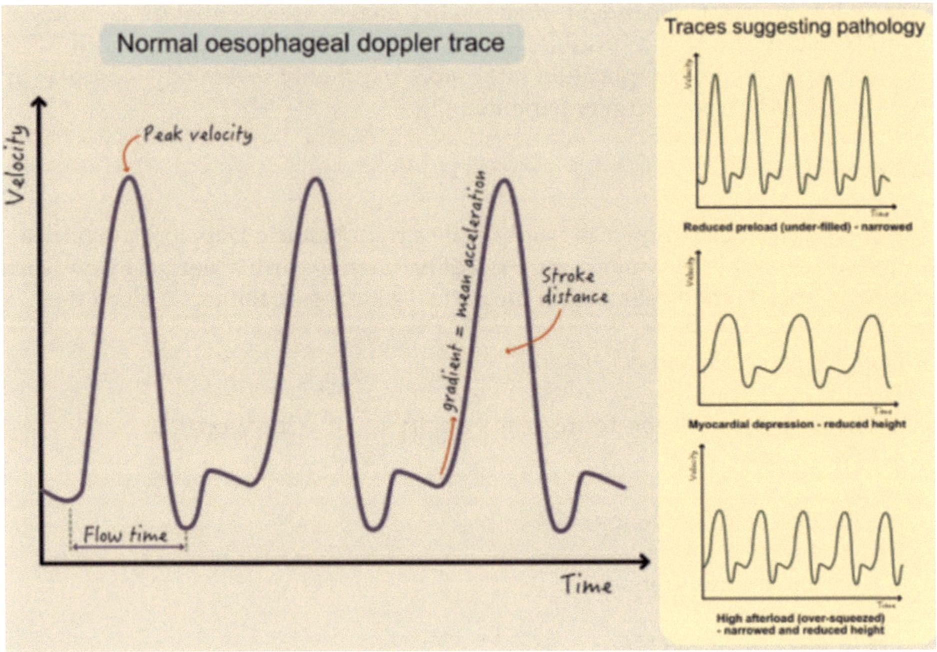

Figure 9.
Oesophagel Doppler monitoring of cardiac output devices. The diagram shows normal versus pathological traces.

5.13 Clinical application: Interpreting cardiac output monitor data: A case scenario

A 65-year-old male patient is admitted to the intensive care unit (ICU) with septic shock. He is mechanically ventilated and receiving vasopressor support. His hemodynamic parameters are as follows:

- Cardiac output (CO): 3.2 L/min
- Cardiac index (CI): 1.8 L/min/m^2
- Stroke volume (SV): 40 mL/beat
- Stroke volume index (SVI): 25 mL/m^2/beat
- Global end-diastolic volume index (GEDVI): 680 mL/m^2 (normal range: 600–800 mL/m^2)
- Extravascular lung water index (EVLWI): 12 mL/kg (normal range: 3–7 mL/kg)

5.13.1 Interpretation

- The patient's cardiac output and cardiac index are low, indicating decreased cardiac function.
- The stroke volume and stroke volume index are also low, suggesting decreased cardiac contractility.

- The GEDVI is within normal limits, suggesting adequate preload.
- The EVLWI is elevated, indicating pulmonary edema.

5.13.2 Management

- Administer fluids to optimize preload and cardiac output.
- Consider adding inotropes to support cardiac contractility.
- Titrate vasopressors to optimize blood pressure and perfusion.
- Implement strategies to reduce pulmonary edema, such as diuretics or ultrafiltration.

5.13.3 Goals

- Increase cardiac output and cardiac index to normal ranges.
- Improve stroke volume and stroke volume index.
- Reduce EVLWI to normal range.
- Optimize blood pressure and perfusion.

This case scenario illustrates the use of volumetric indices to guide hemodynamic management in a critically ill patient. By interpreting these indices, clinicians can make surmises about fluid therapy, vasopressor support, and other interventions to optimize cardiac function and patient outcomes. The pursuit of optimal cardiac output monitoring is a nuanced and multifaceted endeavor, with various devices and techniques vying for attention. Minimally invasive cardiac output monitoring (MICOM) devices aim to evaluate stroke volume (SV) and predict fluid responsiveness, but their utility is tempered by the complexity of individual patient needs and the limitations of each method.

6. Conclusion

In clinical practice, a goal-directed approach is essential, taking into account the unique characteristics and comorbidities of each patient. The Frank-Starling physiological model of the heart provides a framework for understanding the relationship between cardiac volume loading and stroke volume, but defining a "sustained response" and "an appropriate fluid challenge" can be challenging in real-world settings.

Derived indices, such as pulse pressure variation (PPV) and stroke volume variation (SVV), can offer valuable perspectives into fluid responsiveness, but their accuracy is influenced by factors like tidal volume and intrathoracic pressure. The clinician must therefore interpret these values in the context of the patient's overall clinical picture.

Despite these challenges, there is evidence to support the use of MICOM devices in improving patient outcomes, particularly in colorectal surgery and cardiac patients.

Goal-directed therapy protocols have been shown to reduce complications and length of stay in the ICU, but the exact mechanisms remain somewhat nebulous.

Ultimately, the effective use of MICOM devices requires a deep understanding of their limitations and the importance of individualized patient care. By acknowledging the complexities of cardiac output monitoring and embracing a nuanced approach, clinicians can harness the potential of these devices to improve patient outcomes and advance the field of critical care medicine.

Acknowledgements

The authors acknowledge the use of ChatGPT (OpenAI) for document template formatting, literature organization, and compilation of bibliographic references in Vancouver format. The authors assume full responsibility for all content presented.

Conflict of interest

The authors declare no conflict of interest.

Author details

Bhavya Naithani Dube[1*], Mallikarjun Dube[2] and Neeraj Kumar[3]

1 King George's Medical College, Lucknow, India

2 Command Hospital Eastern Command, Kolkata, India

3 All India Institute of Medical Sciences Patna, Bihar, India

*Address all correspondence to: doctorbhavyadube@gmail.com

References

[1] Rupérez M, López-Herce J, García C, Sánchez C, García E, Vigil D. Comparison between cardiac output measured by the pulmonary arterial thermodilution technique and that measured by the femoral arterial thermodilution technique in a pediatric animal model. Pediatric Cardiology. 2004;**25**(2):119-123. DOI: 10.1007/s00246-003-0450-2. Epub 2003 Dec 23

[2] Joosten A, Desebbe O, Suehiro K, Murphy LSL, Essiet M, Alexander B, et al. Accuracy and precision of non-invasive cardiac output monitoring devices in perioperative medicine: A systematic review and meta-analysis. British Journal of Anaesthesia. 2017;**118** (3):298-310. DOI: 10.1093/bja/aew461

[3] Pulmonary Artery Catheter: The Golden Way of Advanced Hemodynamic Monitoring. London, UK: IntechOpen. DOI: 10.1097/CCM.0b013e318298a41e. Available from: https://www.intechopen.com/online-first/1224367

[4] Sandham JD, Hull RD, Brant RF, Knox L, Pineo GF, Doig CJ, et al. A randomized, controlled trial of the use of pulmonary-artery catheters in high-risk surgical patients. The New England Journal of Medicine. 2003;**348**(1):5-14. DOI: 10.1056/NEJMoa021108

[5] Rajaram SS, Desai NK, Kalra A, Gajera M, Cavanaugh SK, Brampton W, et al. Pulmonary artery catheters for adult patients in intensive care. Cochrane Database of Systematic Reviews. 2013;**2013**(2):CD003408. DOI: 10.1002/14651858.CD003408.pub3

[6] De Backer D, Bakker J, Cecconi M, Hajjar L, Liu DW, Lobo S, et al. Alternatives to the Swan-Ganz catheter. Intensive Care Medicine. 2018;**44**(6): 730-741. DOI: 10.1007/s00134-018-5187-8. Epub 2018 May 3

[7] Delicce AV, Makaryus AN. Physiology, Frank Starling Law. In: StatPearls [Internet]. Treasure Island, FL: StatPearls Publishing; 2025. Available from: http://www.ncbi.nlm.nih.gov/books/NBK470295/

[8] Kumar A, Anel R, Bunnell E, Habet K, Zanotti S, Marshall S, et al. Pulmonary artery occlusion pressure and central venous pressure fail to predict ventricular filling volume, cardiac performance, or the response to volume infusion in normal subjects. Critical Care Medicine. 2004;**32**(3):691-699. DOI: 10.1097/01.ccm.0000114996.68110.c9

[9] Della Rocca G, Costa MG, Pietropaoli P. How to measure and interpret volumetric measures of preload. Current Opinion in Critical Care. 2007;**13**(3):297-302. DOI: 10.1097/MCC.0b013e32811d6ce3

[10] Demir ZA, Bingül ES, Dost B, Talih G, Aykut A, Aydın ME, et al. Foundations and advancements in hemodynamic monitoring: Part I-elements of hemodynamics. Turkish Journal of Anaesthesiology and Reanimation. 2025;**53**(3):87-97. DOI: 10.4274/TJAR.2025.251925. Epub 2025 Mar 27

[11] Kenaan M, Gajera M, Goonewardena SN. Hemodynamic assessment in the contemporary intensive care unit: A review of circulatory monitoring devices. Critical Care Clinics. 2014;**30** (3):413-445. DOI: 10.1016/j.ccc.2014.03.007

[12] Giomarelli P, Biagioli B, Scolletta S. Cardiac output monitoring by pressure recording analytical method in cardiac

surgery. European Journal of Cardio-Thoracic Surgery. 2004;**26**(3):515-520. DOI: 10.1016/j.ejcts.2004.05.025

[13] Jonas MM, Kelly FE, Linton RAF, Band DM, O'Brien TK, Linton NWF. A comparison of lithium dilution cardiac output measurements made using central and antecubital venous injection of lithium chloride. Journal of Clinical Monitoring and Computing. 1999;**15**(7): 525-528. DOI: 10.1023/a:1009914714769

[14] Saugel B, Kouz K, Scheeren TWL, Greiwe G, Hoppe P, Romagnoli S, et al. Cardiac output estimation using pulse wave analysis—physiology, algorithms, and technologies: A narrative review. British Journal of Anaesthesia. 2021;**126**(1):67-76. DOI: 10.1016/j.bja.2020.09.049

[15] Grensemann J. Cardiac output monitoring by pulse contour analysis, the technical basics of less-invasive techniques. Frontiers in Medicine (Lausanne). 2018;**5**:64. DOI: 10.3389/fmed.2018.00064

[16] Porter JM, Swain ID. Measurement of cardiac output by electrical impedance plethysmography. Journal of Biomedical Engineering. 1987;**9**(3):222-231. DOI: 10.1016/0141-5425(87)90006-9

[17] Ihlen H, Amlie JP, Dale J, Forfang K, Nitter-Hauge S, Otterstad JE, et al. Determination of cardiac output by Doppler echocardiography. British Heart Journal. 1984;**51**(1):54-60. DOI: 10.1136/hrt.51.1.54

[18] Li T, Cai H, Pan H, Pu Q. Cardiac output measurement using a modified carbon dioxide Fick method: Comparison analysis with pulmonary artery catheter method and pulse induced contour cardiac output method. International Journal of Clinical and Experimental Medicine. 2015;**8**(3):3530-3537. Available from: https://pubmed.ncbi.nlm.nih.gov/26064245/

[19] Blanch L, Fernández R, Benito S, Mancebo J, Calaf N, Net A. Accuracy of an indirect carbon dioxide Fick method in determination of the cardiac output in critically ill mechanically ventilated patients. Intensive Care Medicine. 1988;**14**(2):131-135. DOI: 10.1007/BF00257466

[20] Lai WW, Mertens LL, Cohen MS, Geva T, editors. Echocardiography in Pediatric and Congenital Heart Disease: From Fetus to Adult. Wiley-Blackwell; 2009. ISBN 978-1-444-30631-6

[21] Sánchez-Sánchez M, Herrero E, Cachafeiro L, Flores E, Agrifoglio A, Civantos B, et al. Main limitations of transpulmonary thermodilution: Set targets. Critical Care. 2017;**21**(1):242. DOI: 10.1186/s13054-017-1833-8

[22] Putko K, Erber J, Wagner F, Busch D, Schuster H, Schmid RM, et al. Accuracy of hemodynamic parameters derived by GE E-PiCCO in comparison with PiCCO® in patients admitted to the intensive care unit. Scientific Reports. 2023;**13**(1):6861. DOI: 10.1038/s41598-023-34141-8

[23] Monnet X, Teboul JL. Transpulmonary thermodilution: Advantages and limits. Critical Care. 2017;**21**(1):147. DOI: 10.1186/s13054-017-1739-5

[24] Sakka SG, Kozieras J, Thuemer O, van Hout N. Measurement of cardiac output: A comparison between transpulmonary thermodilution and uncalibrated pulse contour analysis. British Journal of Anaesthesia. 2007;**99**(3):337-342. DOI: 10.1093/bja/aem177

[25] Souto Moura T, Aguiar Rosa S, Germano N, Cavaco R, Sequeira T, Alves

M, et al. The accuracy of PiCCO® in measuring cardiac output in patients under therapeutic hypothermia: Comparison with transthoracic echocardiography. Medicina Intensiva (English Edition). 2018;**42**(2): 92-98. DOI: 10.1016/j.medin.2017.03.007. Epub 2017 May 25

[26] Iijima T, Aoyagi T, Iwao Y, Masuda J, Fuse M, Kobayashi N, et al. Cardiac output and circulating blood volume analysis by pulse dye-densitometry. Journal of Clinical Monitoring and Computing. 1997;**13**(2):81-89. DOI: 10.1023/a:1007339924083

[27] Imai T, Takahashi K, Goto F, Morishita Y. Measurement of blood concentration of indocyanine green by pulse dye densitometry–comparison with the conventional spectrophotometric method. Journal of Clinical Monitoring and Computing. 1998;**14**(7–8):477-484. DOI: 10.1023/a:1009948128543

[28] Costa MG, Della Rocca G, Chiarandini P, Mattelig S, Pomp L, Barriga MS, et al. Continuous and intermittent cardiac output measurement in hyperdynamic conditions: Pulmonary artery catheter vs. lithium dilution technique. Intensive Care Medicine. 2008;**34**(2):257-263. DOI: 10.1007/s00134-007-0878-6

[29] Jansen JR, Wesseling KH, Settels JJ, Schreuder JJ. Continuous cardiac output monitoring by pulse contour during cardiac surgery. European Heart Journal. 1990;**11**(Suppl I):26-32. DOI: 10.1093/eurheartj/11.suppl_i.26

[30] Pearse R, Dawson D, Fawcett J, Rhodes A, Grounds RM, Bennett ED. Early goal-directed therapy after major surgery reduces complications and duration of hospital stay. A randomised, controlled trial [ISRCTN38797445]. Critical Care. 2005;**9**(6):R687-R693. DOI: 10.1186/cc3887. Epub 2005 Nov 8

[31] Yamashita K, Nishiyama T, Yokoyama T, Abe H, Manabe M. Cardiac output by PulseCO is not interchangeable with thermodilution in patients undergoing OPCAB. Canadian Journal of Anaesthesia. 2005;**52**(5):530-534. DOI: 10.1007/BF03016534

[32] Belloni L, Pisano A, Natale A, Piccirillo MR, Piazza L, Ismeno G, et al. Assessment of fluid-responsiveness parameters for off-pump coronary artery bypass surgery: A comparison among LiDCO, transesophageal echochardiography, and pulmonary artery catheter. Journal of Cardiothoracic and Vascular Anesthesia. 2008;**22**(2):243-248. DOI: 10.1053/j.jvca.2007.07.007

[33] Hadian M, Kim HK, Severyn DA, Pinsky MR. Cross-comparison of cardiac output trending accuracy of LiDCO, PiCCO, FloTrac and pulmonary artery catheters. Critical Care. 2010;**14**(6): R212. DOI: 10.1186/cc9335. Epub 2010 Nov 23

[34] Schmidt AP, Bevilacqua Filho CT, Martinelli ES, de Moura VC. The pulmonary artery catheter in modern anesthesiology and intensive care: Indications, benefits, and limitations. Brazilian Journal of Anesthesiology. 2025;**75**(2):0-0. DOI: 10.1016/j.bjane.2025.844587

[35] Donati A, Loggi S, Preiser JC, Orsetti G, Münch C, Gabbanelli V, et al. Goal-directed intraoperative therapy reduces morbidity and length of hospital stay in high-risk surgical patients. Chest. 2007;**132**(6):1817-1824. DOI: 10.1378/chest.07-0621

[36] Wesseling KH, Jansen JR, Settels JJ, Schreuder JJ. Computation of aortic flow

from pressure in humans using a nonlinear, three-element model. Journal of Applied Physiology (1985). 1993;**74**(5):2566-2573. DOI: 10.1152/jappl.1993.74.5.2566

[37] Canty DJ, Kim M, Guha R, Pham T, Royse AG, Errey-Clarke S, et al. Comparison of cardiac output of both 2-dimensional and 3-dimensional transesophageal echocardiography with transpulmonary thermodilution during cardiac surgery. Journal of Cardiothoracic and Vascular Anesthesia. 2020;**34**(1):77-86. DOI: 10.1053/j.jvca.2019.06.007

[38] Donati A, Carsetti A, Tondi S, Scorcella C, Domizi R, Damiani E, et al. Thermodilution vs pressure recording analytical method in hemodynamic stabilized patients. Journal of Critical Care. 2014;**29**(2):260-264. DOI: 10.1016/j.jcrc.2013.11.003

[39] Romagnoli S, Ricci Z, Romano SM, Dimizio F, Bonicolini E, Quattrone D, et al. FloTrac/Vigileo(TM) (third generation) and MostCare(®)/PRAM versus echocardiography for cardiac output estimation in vascular surgery. Journal of Cardiothoracic and Vascular Anesthesia. 2013;**27**(6):1114-1121. DOI: 10.1053/j.jvca.2013.04.017. Epub 2013 Sep 19

[40] Kubicek WG, Karnegis JN, Patterson RP, Witsoe DA, Mattson RH. Development and evaluation of an impedance cardiac output system. Aerospace Medicine. 1966;**37**(12):1208-1212

[41] Torre DE, Pirri C. Point-of-care transesophageal echocardiography in emergency and intensive care: An evolving imaging modality. Biomedicine. 2025;**13**(11):2680. DOI: 10.3390/biomedicines13112680

[42] Perrino AC, Tuason D, O'Connor TZ. Transthoracic Doppler assessment of cardiac output during induction of anesthesia. Anesthesia & Analgesia. 1998;**86**(3):577-582. DOI: 10.1097/00000539-199803000-00025

[43] Concha MR, Mertz VF, Cortinez LI, Gonzalez KA, Butte JM. Pulse contour analysis and transesophageal echocardiography: A comparison of measurements of cardiac output during laparoscopic colon surgery. Anesthesia and Analgesia. 2009;**109**(1):114-118. DOI: 10.1213/ane.0b013e3181a491b8

Chapter 9

POCUS (Point of Care Ultrasound): Hemodynamic Monitoring of Future

Arshad H. Chanda, Shajahan Idayathulla, Hassam Zulfiqar, Mariyam Fatima, Abdelrahman Balal and Mojahid Mohammed Khaled Alhussein

Abstract

Hemodynamic monitoring is the cornerstone of modern critical care. It facilitates the early identification and management of hemodynamic instability, especially in complex conditions such as shock, heart failure, ARDS, and acute kidney injury. Monitoring techniques in ICU have evolved from basic bedside assessments to advanced invasive methods like PAC (PA catheter), minimally invasive methods like PiCCO (pulse contour analysis), and non-invasive modalities—especially point-of-care ultrasound (POCUS). This progress over the last five to six decades reflects the ongoing evolution of hemodynamic monitoring systems with a strong emphasis on patient safety and minimizing complications. POCUS is non-invasive, repeatable, and offers reliable sensitivity and specificity for organ-specific assessments (cardiac, respiratory, and renal) with the added advantage of no procedural risk. Dynamic and static physiological parameters derived from POCUS complement those obtained from conventional invasive devices such as PAC and PiCCO. Individualized management of fluid responsiveness and resuscitation endpoints can be achieved by integrating static and dynamic indices obtained from POCUS. The future of POCUS is promising as new modalities are emerging, such as VEXUS (Venous Excess Ultrasound) for detecting congestion, Doppler, and advanced cardiac ultrasound for detecting and quantifying both left and right ventricular function. Although there are technical challenges, especially steep learning curves associated with newer and more refined modalities, these can be overcome through training and regular incorporation of POCUS into advanced hemodynamic monitoring in the ICU setting.

Keywords: hemodynamic monitoring, critical care, point-of-care ultrasound (POCUS), pulmonary artery catheter (PAC), fluid responsiveness, cardiac output, preload and afterload, dynamic parameters

1. Introduction

1.1 Importance of hemodynamic monitoring in critical care

Hemodynamic monitoring is one of the most vital aspects of patient assessment and ongoing support in the ICU. It has been a cornerstone in the detection and management of shock, assisting in differentiating among various types of shock and guiding their specific treatments. Additionally, hemodynamic monitoring plays a crucial role in managing conditions such as heart failure, acute respiratory distress syndrome, and acute kidney injury. Focused hemodynamic evaluation enables clinicians to develop individualized management strategies, facilitating targeted interventions such as fluid administration, medication adjustment, and vasopressor titration. Traditionally, hemodynamic monitoring has been divided into basic and advanced methods. Although basic monitoring is important, it plays a limited role in the comprehensive care required in the ICU. Patients receiving organ support typically require advanced hemodynamic monitoring. Conventional advanced techniques include invasive methods such as arterial blood pressure monitoring, central venous pressure measurement, and the use of pulmonary artery catheters. These methods are either invasive or semi-invasive and have got both procedural and post-procedural complications, namely, the iatrogenic injuries and the postop procedural infection during the maintenance phase of the invasive lines [1].

With the advancement of research and critical care, there was always a surgery for non-invasive method of advanced hemodynamic monitoring in ICU. With the advances in ultrasound technology, portability of the ultrasound instruments and its advantages like safety, rapidity, reproducibility, and repeatability of point of care ultrasound was introduced into the ICU care. Studies have also demonstrated that POCUS has relative good sensitivity and specificity in detecting the cause of hemodynamic instability that his diagnostic accuracy and ultimately improving the outcome of the critically ill patients. In the last two decades, it has been seen that there are missed publications of literature on the use of point of care ultrasound and ICUs. Though there are some hurdles in focus like one time investment on quality ultrasound instrument, a steep learning curve, user dependent result with variability, maintenance of the instrument [2].

1.2 Evolution of monitoring techniques in the ICU

Hemodynamic monitoring in general, and particularly in the ICU, has witnessed remarkable evolution over the past five to six decades. It began with basic bedside, intermittent clinical assessments such as heart rate measurement, non-invasive blood pressure monitoring, and evaluation of perfusion signs like capillary refill, skin temperature, and urine output. During the 1953 polio epidemic, the first concept of the ICU was introduced, leading to the need for advanced monitoring techniques. Although invasive blood pressure monitoring was developed earlier in the 1900s, a landmark event came in the 1970s with the invention of the pulmonary artery catheter (PAC), which allowed direct and continuous monitoring of cardiac function and hemodynamics. However, the PA catheter was highly invasive; it was intermittent to begin with, later adding a few continuous, real-time features. The PA catheter was associated with significant procedural risks and complications without clear evidence of mortality benefit. This led to a search for less-invasive monitoring systems, such as arterial pressure waveform analysis. Around 2000, technologies using pulse contour and indicator dilution techniques were developed.

Over the last 15 years, the focus has shifted further toward minimally invasive and non-invasive modalities, including ultrasound-based methods like transthoracic and transoesophageal echocardiography and pulse contour analysis, as well as novel techniques like bio-impedance and bio-reactance [3].

The development of dynamic indices to predict fluid responsiveness, such as pulse pressure variation and stroke volume variation, has also improved the precision and clinical utility of monitoring. Today, point-of-care ultrasound (POCUS) allows for immediate bedside assessment of hemodynamics and organ function, establishing itself as an indispensable tool in the care of critically ill patients due to its acceptable accuracy in trained hands, safety, and repeatability. This continuous evolution reflects an ongoing effort to balance the need for accurate, clinically actionable information with the imperative to minimize risk and enhance patient comfort in the intensive care setting [1].

In this chapter, we will focus on the role of POCUS in hemodynamic monitoring in the ICU. We will compare the parameters used by POCUS with those of conventional invasive monitoring, highlighting the beneficial effects of POCUS while also acknowledging its disadvantages.

2. Physiological perspective of hemodynamic monitoring

2.1 Static and dynamic parameters

The term hemodynamics refers to the pumping of blood by the heart to the organs and the return of blood back to the heart. While assessing hemodynamics, there are methods that measure single time-point measurements referred to as static parameters. These can be pressures or volumes, for example, central venous pressure (CVP), pulmonary artery occlusion pressure (PAOP), and global end-diastolic volume, etc.

Parameters that are measured based on changes during the heart-lung interactions are called dynamic parameters. These changes normally occur during respiratory phases or volume challenges. These parameters are usually useful in guiding fluid management. Examples include pulse pressure variation (PPV) and changes in inferior vena cava (IVC) diameter during respiration [4].

2.2 Heart-lung interaction

This concept is very important to understand to derive dynamic parameters in hemodynamic monitoring. Heart-lung interaction refers to the physiological changes in heart function caused by phasic variations in intrathoracic pressure during inspiratory and expiratory cycles of respiration especially during the positive pressure ventilation. This is reflected both on the pressure and volumes of the circulatory system. Positive pressure inspiration increases intrathoracic pressure, leading to a decrease in venous return and subsequently reducing cardiac output. Inspiration will increase the lung volume and elevates the pulmonary vascular resistance, which impacts the right ventricular afterload and decreases the RV output which later (usually after three heart beats) will decrease the LV output. The increase in right atrial pressure causes distension of the vena cava. These interactions influence both the preload and afterload of the heart and play a crucial role in interpreting hemodynamic monitoring data. Many modern hemodynamic parameters, such as pulse pressure variation and stroke volume variation, rely on analyzing these heart-lung interactions to predict fluid responsiveness. Understanding this principle helps guide fluid management and optimizes cardiovascular support in critically ill patients.

This concept will also be briefly discussed when comparing parameters derived from different hemodynamic monitoring tools [5].

2.3 Classical hemodynamic parameters for assessment and management

Heart rate by continuous ECG monitoring, which has added advantage of rhythm and ST segment change monitoring. MAP can be assessed either by the NIBP or invasive arterial BP monitoring (**Table 1**).

2.4 Hemodynamic parameters monitored during management of a critically ill patient

The following classical parameters/indices are usually measured during the diagnosis and management of critically ill patients [6].

Cardiac output/index: Thermodilution via PAC, transpulmonary thermodilution by PiCCO, and estimated by Doppler or 2D ECHO in POCUS.

Preload and filling pressures: CVP (central venous pressure) and PCWP (pulmonary capillary wedge pressure) by PAC; GEDV (global end-diastolic volume) by PiCCO; and IVC diameter (inferior vena cava) and collapsibility in POCUS.

Contractility: Pressure waveform analysis in PAC, SVV (stroke volume variation) trends in PiCCO, and visual evaluation (eye balling) of ventricular function by POCUS.

Afterload: SVRI (systemic vascular resistance index) is calculated in PA Catheter and PiCCO data; POCUS estimates vascular resistance indirectly through ventricular function and Doppler assessments.

Volume responsiveness: Dynamic indices like PPV (pulse pressure variation) and SVV (stroke volume variation) from PiCCO and PAC; respiratory variation in IVC diameter – collapsibility and distensibility index by POCUS.

POCUS (point-of-care ultrasound) is a non-invasive tool for hemodynamic assessment in ICUs. It is used to identify shock and to classify shock. POCUS may help differentiate shock. It is also useful for assessing fluid responsiveness and for weaning from mechanical circulatory support like ECMO. Serial assessments are needed to guide fluid management.

Table 2 compares the parameters from standard monitoring by the PA catheter and PiCCO with those from POCUS [7, 8].

2.5 Preload

Preload is defined as the myocardial wall stress at the end of diastole, determined largely by ventricular filling volume and myocardial compliance. According to the

Parameter	Normal range/value	Data acquisition methods
Heart rate (HR)	60–100 beats/min	Measured directly (ECG, pulse)
Systolic blood pressure (SBP)	90–140 mmHg	Measured directly (arterial line, cuff)
Diastolic blood pressure (DBP)	60–90 mmHg	Measured directly (arterial line, cuff)
Mean arterial pressure (MAP)	70–105 mmHg	Measured directly (arterial line, cuff)

Table 1.
Basic hemodynamic parameters.

Parameter	PA catheter (PAC)	PiCCO	POCUS (Critical Care Echo)
Pressures – direct measurements			
Central venous pressure (CVP)	Yes	Optional (requires CVC)	Yes (estimate via IVC or SVC US)
Pulmonary artery pressure (PAP)	Yes	No	No (can suggest RVSP via Doppler)
Pulmonary capillary wedge pressure (PCWP)	Yes	No	No (estimate LA pressure via Doppler)
Volumes			
Preload (e.g., GEDV, ITBV, SVV)	No (uses CVP/PCWP)	Yes (GEDV, ITBV, SVV, PPV)	Yes (IVC, LV size, other indices)
Stroke volume/stroke volume index	Yes	Yes	Yes
Cardiac output/cardiac index	Yes (CO, CI, thermodilution)	Yes (TTP)	Yes (LVOT diameter × VTI)
Continuous cardiac output monitoring	Yes	Yes (pulse contour)	No (serial exams only)
Derived parameters			
Systemic vascular resistance (SVR/SVRI)	Yes (calculated)	Yes	No (calculated, less direct)
Contractility (e.g., dP/dt, CFI)	Limited (indirect)	Yes (dPmx, CFI, GEF)	Yes (visual/E-point septal separation)
Extravascular lung water (EVLW/ELWI)	No	Yes	No (can assess edema but not quantify)
Other functions			
Dynamic fluid responsiveness	No (static)	Yes (SVV, PPV)	Yes (IVC variation, LVOT VTI)
Oxygen saturation (SvO_2/$ScvO_2$)	Mixed venous O_2, yes	Central venous O_2, yes	No
Lung and other organ Assessment	No	No (parameters only)	Yes (lung, abdomen, pericardium, etc.)

Transpulmonary thermodilution.

Table 2.
Comparison of advanced hemodynamic parameters: PA catheter, PiCCO, and POCUS.

Frank–Starling principle, more preload usually increases stroke volume—up to a point. Beyond that point, extra filling does not improve output and may cause congestion. In the critically ill patients, the focus is not on the absolute value of preload but on fluid responsiveness, the capacity of the heart to increase stroke volume—typically by ≥10–15%—following a preload challenge [9].

Assessing preload is central to hemodynamic management, yet no single parameter perfectly reflects a patient's volume status. POCUS provides a powerful multimodal approach by integrating information from venous, cardiac, and pulmonary windows. The following sections outline the main POCUS-based parameters for preload assessment and fluid responsiveness.

2.6 Inferior vena cava (IVC) and internal jugular vein (IJV)

The most widely used approach is evaluation of the inferior vena cava (IVC). By measuring the IVC diameter and its variation with respiration, clinicians can estimate right atrial pressure and venous return. In spontaneously breathing patients, a marked inspiratory collapse of the IVC suggests low right atrial pressure and possible preload responsiveness, whereas a plethoric, non-collapsible IVC often indicates high filling pressures. In mechanically ventilated patients, the degree of cyclic distension of the IVC during positive-pressure breaths can reflect preload reserve. As an alternative when the IVC is technically difficult to visualize, ultrasound evaluation of the internal jugular vein (IJV) diameter and collapsibility has been explored, though it is less widely validated than IVC assessment [10].

The IVC is best visualized in the subcostal (subxiphoid) long-axis view using a low-frequency phased array or curvilinear probe (2–5 MHz). The probe is placed just below the xiphoid with the marker directed toward the patient's head. The IVC can be seen coursing into the right atrium. Measurements should be taken approximately 2 cm caudal to the junction of the IVC with the right atrium, avoiding the hepatic vein confluence. M-mode is often used for dynamic assessment of collapsibility or distensibility.

Parameters Measured [11]:

- IVC diameter (IVCd): The maximum and minimum diameters of the IVC are measured during the respiratory cycle.

- Collapsibility index (CI): For spontaneously breathing patients, CI = (IVCmax – IVCmin)/IVCmax × 100.

- Distensibility index (DI): For mechanically ventilated patients, DI = (IVCmax – IVCmin)/IVCmin × 100.12

- In spontaneously breathing patients:

    o IVCd <2.1 cm with >50% collapse → RAP ~0–5 mmHg (suggests low preload).

    o IVCd >2.1 cm with <50% collapse → RAP ~10–20 mmHg (suggests higher preload, possibly congestion).

- In mechanically ventilated patients [12]

    o A distensibility index >18% suggests fluid responsiveness.

1. *Left ventricular end-diastolic area (LVEDA)* [13].

2. The LVEDA, measured in the parasternal short-axis view, reflects left ventricular preload. An LVEDA <10 cm^2 is often taken as a marker of underfilling. A small LVEDA, particularly when associated with "kissing" of the ventricular walls during systole, is consistent with hypovolemia. Conversely, a dilated LV with poor contractile excursion suggests that the ventricle is operating on the flat portion of the Frank–Starling curve, where further fluid loading is unlikely to improve stroke volume.

3. *Right ventricular (RV) size and function* [14].

RV dimensions provide indirect clues to preload status and volume tolerance. A small, underfilled RV may indicate volume depletion, whereas a dilated RV (especially with septal shift) signals pressure overload or venous congestion. RV function should be considered in conjunction with IVC findings, since RV dysfunction may cause a distended IVC without true intravascular overload. Evaluating RV function at the bedside involves three primary parameters: tricuspid annular plane systolic excursion (TAPSE), RV outflow tract velocity-time integral (RVOT-VTI), and peak systolic tissue doppler velocity (S′). These measurements help determine how well the RV is contracting and pumping blood forward. TAPSE assesses the longitudinal movement of the tricuspid annulus, providing a simple measure of RV systolic function—values below 17 mm suggest dysfunction. RVOT-VTI reflects stroke volume across the RV outflow tract, with values <12 cm indicating reduced forward flow, particularly useful in shock states. S′, measured by tissue Doppler, detects subtle RV impairment when velocities fall below 10 cm/s, correlating well with mild RV dysfunction. While each parameter has strengths, they should be interpreted together—TAPSE and S′ are angle-dependent and load-sensitive, whereas RVOT-VTI better reflects hemodynamic impact. Integrating these with RV size and IVC dynamics helps distinguish between volume depletion, pressure overload, and intrinsic RV failure, guiding targeted clinical decisions.

4. *Lung ultrasound: B-lines*

Lung ultrasound complements cardiac assessment by revealing the downstream consequences of elevated filling pressures. Multiple bilateral B lines indicate extravascular lung water. When three or more B lines are visualized in a single intercostal space and this pattern is observed across multiple lung regions, it strongly suggests the presence of pulmonary edema, most commonly of cardiogenic origin. However, clinicians should maintain a broad differential diagnosis as similar findings may occur in ARDS, pulmonary fibrosis, or other diffuse parenchymal lung diseases. Moreover, in asymptomatic individuals, occasional B lines (1–2 per field) may be normal, particularly in dependent lung zones. It is pertinent to emphasize that lung ultrasound helps distinguish between a patient who is fluid responsive and one who may not be fluid tolerant. For example, a patient with a collapsible IVC but extensive B lines may improve cardiac output with fluids but at the cost of worsening pulmonary edema. Thus, integrating cardiac and lung ultrasound ensures safer hemodynamic management [14].

5. *Venous excess ultrasound (VEXUS)*

Traditional measures of fluid responsiveness, while useful for determining whether a patient will benefit from additional volume, fail to address the potential consequences of fluid administration on venous pressure and end-organ perfusion. This is where the venous excess ultrasound (VEXUS) protocol provides critical insight by interrogating organ-level venous flow disruptions, providing a direct window into congestion. The core principle of VEXUS rests on recognizing that elevated central venous pressure creates downstream pressure waves that propagate through the venous system, progressively altering normal blood flow patterns.

As right heart pressures increase, these abnormal hemodynamic forces transmit backward through the inferior vena cava to the hepatic, portal, and renal veins, transforming their characteristic Doppler waveforms from continuous forward flow to pulsatile or even reversed flow patterns. These sequential changes in venous Doppler signatures serve as a sensitive barometer of worsening congestion, where more distal venous abnormalities (like portal pulsatility or renal vein flow reversal) indicate increasingly severe venous hypertension and higher risk of end-organ damage. The protocol essentially maps this pressure cascade through standardized Doppler evaluation, converting abstract hemodynamic concepts into visible, gradable ultrasound findings that correlate with clinical outcomes. By shifting the clinical question from simple fluid responsiveness to a more sophisticated evaluation of fluid tolerance, VEXUS helps clinicians avoid the pitfalls of inappropriate fluid administration while optimizing organ perfusion in critical illness [15].

3. Left ventricular parameters

Dynamic parameters are particularly useful for predicting fluid responsiveness. POCUS can estimate stroke volume by measuring velocity-time integral (VTI) at the left ventricular outflow tract (LVOT). By repeating the VTI before and after a passive leg raise or a small fluid challenge, one can determine whether cardiac output increases meaningfully in response to increased venous return. An increase in VTI of more than 10–15% is usually considered a marker of preload responsiveness. Similarly, respirophasic changes in VTI or stroke volume in mechanically ventilated patients provide another dynamic window into preload dependence.

Trans-mitral Doppler and tissue Doppler imaging provide insights into left ventricular filling pressures. The ratio of early mitral inflow velocity (E) to early diastolic mitral annular velocity (e′) correlates with left atrial pressure. An elevated E/e′ ratio suggests impaired diastolic compliance and higher filling pressures, indicating that the patient is unlikely to tolerate further fluid loading. Although more complex to perform, this method adds valuable information, especially in patients with preserved or borderline LV systolic function.

No single parameter should be used in isolation. Instead, combining IVC or IJV assessment with LVEDA, RV assessment, lung POCUS, VEXUS, LVOT VTI, and E/e′ ratio provides a comprehensive view of preload and fluid responsiveness. POCUS thereby bridges the gap between static estimates of cardiac filling and dynamic evaluation of cardiac performance, allowing fluid administration to be tailored more safely and effectively at the bedside [16].

4. Measures of LV contractility

4.1 Ejection fraction

Ejection fraction is often employed as a surrogate measure to qualitatively or quantitatively estimate left ventricular performance or more commonly systolic function. At the bedside, there are various methods to estimate ejection fraction, namely, visual estimation of LV systolic function, E-point septal separation (EPSS), mitral annular plane systolic excursion (MAPSE), fractional shortening (FS), fractional area of change (FAC) or the Simpson's biplane method.

A rapid and accessible technique for estimating left ventricular ejection fraction (LVEF) is visual assessment, often called the "eyeball method." This approach is typically performed using the parasternal long-axis (PSLA), parasternal short-axis (PSSA), and apical 4-chamber (A4C) views. The clinician evaluates the motion of the mitral valve during diastole and assesses the movement of the left ventricular walls throughout the cardiac cycle. This competency can be acquired with minimal training, such as a one-day program and about 50 supervised POCUS examinations [17]. However, because this method is subjective, lacking quantitative analysis, it is not the most accurate in estimating ejection fraction.

The mitral E-point septal separation (EPSS) technique offers a rapid, quantitative method for assessing LV function and has been validated against cardiac MRI; while mitral annular plane systolic excursion (MAPSE) measures the longitudinal contraction of the left ventricle, a component responsible for approximately 60% of stroke volume. While MAPSE is specific for identifying a reduced LVEF, it lacks sensitivity. Therefore, combining MAPSE with both visual estimation and EPSS creates a more robust and accurate composite assessment than any single method used alone [18].

Fractional shortening (FS) is a measurement derived from the parasternal long-axis (PLAX) view, calculated by assessing the left ventricular end-diastolic diameter (LVEDD) and end-systolic diameter (LVESD). The formula FS (%) = [(LVEDD − LVESD)/LVEDD] × 100 quantifies the percentage change in the LV diameter between diastole and systole, serving as an estimate of the ventricle's contractile efficiency. However, this metric is a surrogate for ejection fraction (LVEF) and has significant limitations: it is highly dependent on preload and afterload, can appear artificially low in the presence of regional wall motion abnormalities, and has been demonstrated to underestimate LVEF in cases of concentric left ventricular hypertrophy [19].

Of all these methods, the Simpson's biplane method is recommended by the American Society of Echocardiography as a gold standard measure of LVEF by 2D echo. Owing to its operator-dependent nature and the practical difficulty of tracing endocardial borders in multiple views, this quantitative method is often bypassed in fast-paced clinical environments like the ICU. Consequently, many clinicians advocate for a more efficient approach that combines qualitative LVEF estimation with direct measurements of flow, such as the left ventricular outflow tract velocity time integral (LVOT VTI) [20].

4.2 Left ventricular velocity: Time integral (LVOT-VTI)

Left ventricular EF (LVEF) may not reliably reflect stroke volume (SV) or cardiac output (CO), and paradoxically a high LVEF can be associated with reduced SV, while a severely reduced LVEF can be associated with normal SV. A comprehensive hemodynamic assessment should include evaluating LVOT VTI variation in mechanically ventilated patients or performing a passive leg raise (PLR) test in spontaneously breathing patients to determine fluid responsiveness [20]. Measurement of SV and CO using LVOT diameter and LVOT-VTI provides real-time insight into the effectiveness of preload changes, such as those following a fluid bolus or passive leg raise test, as well as after interventions like inotropes. Cardiac Index obtained by indexing body surface area to cardiac output, provides a more refined assessment of hemodynamic status [14]. The LVOT diameter is measured in the PLAX view during mid-systole, when the aortic valve is fully open and the measurement is taken at the base of the aortic valve, and the LVOT area is then calculated using the formula:

$$\text{LVOT area} = 3.14 \times (\text{LVOT radius})^2 \quad (1)$$

The VTI represents the distance blood travels from the LVOT to the aorta, measured in centimeters and averaged over several cardiac cycles to account for beat-to-beat variability. It is obtained by placing the sample volume at the center of the LVOT and tracing the velocity curve in the apical five-chamber view using pulse-wave Doppler [14]. LV stroke volume can be calculated with the formula,

$$\text{LV stroke volume} = \text{LVOT area cm}^2 \times \text{LVOT VTI (cm)} \quad (2)$$

When combined with lactate measurements and blood pressure, the LVOT-VTI can also aid in determining the etiology of shock. A low VTI in the presence of hypotension and elevated lactate indicates a low-output shock (cardiogenic shock), whereas a high VTI with similar findings may point toward distributive shock (early sepsis). The normal LVOT-VTI range is 17–23 cm, and it serves as a surrogate marker for stroke volume. When interpreted alongside the overall clinical picture, VTI can be a valuable tool for longitudinal monitoring and has been associated with reduced duration of vasoactive agent use. The limitations of LVOT VTI should be recognized as conditions such as subaortic stenosis, dynamic LVOT obstruction from systolic anterior motion (SAM) of the mitral valve, significant aortic regurgitation, or the presence of a prosthetic aortic valve can lead to overestimation of stroke volume [20].

4.3 Left ventricular afterload

Echocardiography is a critical tool for assessing left ventricular afterload, particularly by identifying dynamic obstructions like left ventricular outflow tract obstruction (LVOTO). A peak gradient exceeding 30 mmHg indicates hemodynamically significant LVOTO, which has major implications for hemodynamic management. This condition often arises from systolic anterior motion (SAM) of the mitral valve or underlying pathologies such as hypertrophic or infiltrative cardiomyopathies. Importantly, critical illness states like hypovolemia, dehydration, and shock can precipitate or exacerbate LVOTO by reducing preload, even in structurally normal hearts. This load-sensitive nature means the condition often resolves with volume resuscitation and the cessation of inotropic support. The characteristic echocardiographic finding is a late-peaking, "dagger-shaped" continuous wave Doppler waveform across the LVOT, which is distinct from the symmetrical profile of fixed aortic stenosis. A key limitation of this bedside tool, however, is its inadequacy for ruling out acute aortic pathology due to difficulty in obtaining adequate views of the thoracic aorta [20].

5. Right ventricular function and contractility

5.1 RV to LV ratio

The RV-to-LV ratio is a simple qualitative indicator of RV dysfunction, as the RV which is normally smaller than the LV and shows an increased ratio when it becomes enlarged. In the Apical 4-Chamber View, freeze the image in end-diastole and divide the measurement of the RV diameter by the measurement of the LV diameter at the base of the heart [21].

- RV/LV Ratio of 0.67:1 to 1:1 is considered mildly dilated
- RV/LV Ratio of 1:1 to 1.5:1 is considered moderately dilated
- RV/LV Ratio of >1.5:1 is considered severely dilated

5.2 Tricuspid annular plane systolic excursion (TAPSE)

TAPSE, which correlates with RV ejection fraction, provides a regional assessment of RV systolic performance by evaluating longitudinal function. It measures the peak systolic excursion (in millimeters) of the tricuspid annulus from its end-diastolic position to its maximal systolic displacement toward the apex. This measurement is typically obtained using M-mode in the apical four-chamber view. A greater longitudinal displacement reflects better RV contractility, whereas a TAPSE value below 17 mm indicates RV systolic dysfunction, showing high specificity but low sensitivity [22].

5.3 Peak lateral tricuspid annular systolic velocity (S′ or systolic wave prime)

S′ is measured in the apical four-chamber view using tissue Doppler imaging (TDI) at the lateral tricuspid annulus. An S′ velocity below 10 cm/s is strongly associated with RV systolic dysfunction and may correlate more closely than TAPSE in cases ranging from normal RVEF to mild RVEF reduction. Specifically, an S′ of less than 11.5 cm/s corresponds to an RVEF below 45%, with 90% sensitivity and 85% specificity [11]. While simple and easy to perform, it shares the same limitations as TAPSE, being one-dimensional and dependent on load and angle.

- $S' \geq 10$ cm/s → normal RV systolic function
- $S' < 10$ cm/s → suggests RV systolic dysfunction
- Severely reduced S′ (< 7 cm/s) → may indicate significant RV failure

5.4 Right ventricular outflow tract velocity: Time integral (RVOT-VTI)

Like LVOT-VTI, RVOT-VTI reflects the distance blood travels through the RVOT during systole. Stroke volume is determined by multiplying the RVOT cross-sectional area by the RVOT-VTI. This parameter offers valuable information on both RV function and pulmonary vascular resistance, with values ≥12 cm generally considered normal [11].

6. Right ventricular afterload

6.1 Tricuspid regurgitation (TR) jet velocity

Tricuspid regurgitation (TR) jet velocity is a critical echocardiographic parameter used to estimate pulmonary artery systolic pressure (PASP), particularly in the screening and assessment of pulmonary hypertension (PH). A tricuspid regurgitation (TR) jet velocity exceeding 2.8 m/s serves as an independent predictor of pulmonary hypertension, whereas a velocity greater than 3.4 m/s is highly suggestive of it [23].

Pulmonary artery systolic pressure can be estimated using the modified Bernoulli equation:

$$\text{PASP} = 4\ (\text{TR velocity})^2 + \text{estimated right atrial pressure}\ (\text{RAP}) \qquad (3)$$

TR velocity is measured using continuous wave Doppler in the apical four-chamber or parasternal RV inflow view. RAP is estimated based on inferior vena cava (IVC) diameter and collapsibility.

- Normal RAP (0–5 mm Hg) – IVC diameter < 2.1 cm with >50% collapsibility
- High RAP (10–20 mmHg) – IVC diameter > 2.1 cm with <50% collapsibility

In combination with RVOT VTI, pulmonary vascular resistance (PVR) can be estimated with the formula:

$$\text{PVR} = (\text{TR velocity}) / \text{RVOT VTI} \times 10 + 0.16 \qquad (4)$$

PVR values >3 Wood units suggest elevated PVR and afterload.

6.2 Pulmonary artery acceleration time (PAAT)

PAAT is another measure to assess pulmonary hypertension. It is the time from the start of RV ejection to the peak of the RVOT VTI waveform. PAAT shortens as pulmonary hypertension worsens:

- Normal: >130 ms
- Borderline: ~100–130 ms
- Mild pulmonary hypertension: ~ 60–100 ms
- Severe pulmonary hypertension: < 60 ms

6.3 McConnell's sign

Hypokinesis or akinesis of the mid-right ventricular free wall with preserved apical contraction where the RV apex is hyperdynamic on POCUS is a well-established indicator of right heart strain, especially in the context of acute pulmonary embolism. This regional dysfunction is a marker of acute RV overload and has strong specificity for PE when present. While the pooled sensitivity is 22%, a specificity of 97% was noted in the setting of acute PE in a meta-analysis [24].

6.4 The 60/60 sign

A pulmonary acceleration time under 60 ms, when accompanied by a tricuspid regurgitant pressure gradient less than 60 mmHg, strongly suggests an acute rise in right ventricular afterload, often from pulmonary embolism. Though this finding is highly specific, it is not sensitive, and when combined with McConnell's sign, it has a sensitivity of 36% and a specificity of 94% [25].

6.5 The "D-sign"

D-sign is an indirect sign of elevated right ventricular afterload. In the parasternal short-axis view, the left ventricle may appear D-shaped as elevated right-sided pressure displaces the interventricular septum toward the left. This septal flattening is observed during both systole and diastole in the setting of pressure overload, indicating acute right ventricular strain. The eccentricity index (EI) is determined by comparing the left ventricular diameters measured parallel and perpendicular to the interventricular septum. In a normal heart, this ratio is approximately 1 while in the presence of pulmonary hypertension, elevated right ventricular pressure flattens the septum, resulting in an increased EI and a more D-shaped left ventricle that is associated with pulmonary hypertension, acute PE, and RV failure [22].

7. Conclusion

Advanced hemodynamic monitoring is an essential intervention for assessment and management in critical care. It helps guide the diagnosis and management of cardiovascular instability and other organ dysfunction, such as ARDS and AKI. The ongoing evolution of technology has led to the development of invasive, minimally invasive modalities, and non-invasive techniques like POCUS (point-of-care ultrasound), making cardiovascular monitoring safer and more cost-effective. POCUS is less time-consuming, easily available at the bedside, and offers the advantage of repeatability. It not only helps in assessing the cardiovascular system but also provides access to other organs such as the lungs, abdomen (FAST), and renal system (VEXUS). POCUS is a promising tool that has gained greater acceptance in the modern ICU, and new modalities are continually being discovered within this non-invasive platform.

Author details

Arshad H. Chanda[1*], Shajahan Idayathulla[1], Hassam Zulfiqar[2], Mariyam Fatima[3], Abdelrahman Balal[1] and Mojahid Mohammed Khaled Alhussein[1]

1 Surgical Intensive Care Unit, Hamad General Hospital, Doha, Qatar

2 Department of Anesthesiology, Hamad General Hospital, Doha, Qatar

3 Deccan College of Medical Sciences, Hyderabad, India

*Address all correspondence to: achanda@hamad.qa

References

[1] Rali AS, Butcher A, Tedford RJ, Sinha SS, Mekki P, Van Spall HG, et al. Contemporary review of hemodynamic monitoring in the critical care setting. US Cardiology Review. 28 Apr 2022;**16**:e12

[2] Huygh J, Peeters Y, Bernards J, Malbrain ML. Hemodynamic monitoring in the critically ill: An overview of current cardiac output monitoring methods. F1000Research. 16 Dec 2016:5-9

[3] Ramsingh D et al. Clinical review: Does it matter which hemodynamic monitoring technique is used? Critical Care. 2013;**17**:221

[4] Kan CFK, Skaggs JD. Current commonly used dynamic parameters and monitoring systems for perioperative goal-directed fluid therapy: A review. The Yale Journal of Biology and Medicine. 2023;**96**(1):107-123. DOI: 10.59249/JOAP6662

[5] Karamolegkos N, Albanese A, Chbat NW. Heart-lung interactions during mechanical ventilation: Analysis via a cardiopulmonary simulation model. IEEE Open Journal of Engineering in Medicine and Biology. 2021;**2**:324-341. DOI: 10.1109/OJEMB.2021.3128629

[6] Sakka SG. Hemodynamic monitoring in the critically ill patient - Current status and perspective. Frontiers in Medicine (Lausanne). 2015;**2**:44. DOI: 10.3389/fmed.2015.00044

[7] Uchino S, Bellomo R, Morimatsu H, Sugihara M, French C, Stephens D, et al. Pulmonary artery catheter versus pulse contour analysis: A prospective epidemiological study. Critical Care. 2006;**10**(6):R174. DOI: 10.1186/cc5126

[8] Andrei M, Dragoescu NA, Stanculescu A, Chiutu L, Dragoescu O, Istratoaie O. PiCCO or cardiac ultrasound? Which is better for hemodynamic monitoring in ICU? Medicina (Kaunas, Lithuania). 2024;**60**(11):1884. DOI: 10.3390/medicina60111884

[9] O'Keefe E, Singh P. Physiology, Cardiac Preload. In: StatPearls. Treasure Island (FL): StatPearls Publishing; 2025. Available from: https://www.ncbi.nlm.nih.gov/books/NBK541109/

[10] Berikashvili LB, Kuznetsov IV, Yadgarov MY, Ryzhkov PV, Polyakov PA, Yavorovskiy AG, et al. Assessment of fluid responsiveness via central venous ultrasound measurement: A network meta-analysis. Journal of Clinical Medicine. 2025;**14**(2):492. DOI: 10.3390/jcm14020492

[11] Rudski LG, Lai WW, Afilalo J, Hua L, Handschumacher MD, Chandrasekaran K, et al. Guidelines for the echocardiographic assessment of the right heart in adults: A report from the American Society of Echocardiography endorsed by the European Association of Echocardiography, a registered branch of the European Society of Cardiology, and the Canadian Society of Echocardiography. Journal of the American Society of Echocardiography. Jul 2010;**23**(7):685-713, quiz 786-788

[12] Sarıtaş A, Zincircioğlu Ç, Uzun Sarıtaş P, Uzun U, Köse I, Şenoğlu N. Comparison of inferior vena cava collapsibility, distensibility, and delta indices at different positive pressure supports and prediction values of indices for intravascular volume status. Turkish Journal of Medical Sciences.

2019;**49**(4):1170-1178. DOI: 10.3906/sag-1810-52

[13] Van der Mullen J, Wise R, Vermeulen G, Moonen PJ, Malbrain M. Assessment of hypovolaemia in the critically ill. Anestezjologia i Intensywna Terapia. 2018;**50**(2):152-161

[14] Noor A, Liu M, Jarman A, Yamanaka T, Kaul M. Point-of-care ultrasound use in hemodynamic assessment. Biomedicine. 2025;**13**(6):1426. DOI: 10.3390/biomedicines13061426

[15] Kattan E, Castro R, Miralles-Aguiar F, Hernández G, Rola P. The emerging concept of fluid tolerance: A position paper. Journal of Critical Care. 2022;**71**:154070

[16] La Via L et al. Prediction of fluid responsiveness in critical care: State of the art. Annals of Intensive Care. 2024;**14**(1):78

[17] Frederiksen CA, Juhl-Olsen P, Andersen NH, Sloth E. Assessment of cardiac pathology by point-of-care ultrasonography performed by a novice examiner is comparable to the gold standard. Scandinavian Journal of Trauma, Resuscitation and Emergency Medicine. 2013;**21**:87. DOI: 10.1186/1757-7241-21-87

[18] Schick AL, Kaine JC, Al-Sadhan NA, et al. Focused cardiac ultrasound with mitral annular plane systolic excursion (MAPSE) detection of left ventricular dysfunction. The American Journal of Emergency Medicine. 2023;**68**:52-58. DOI: 10.1016/j.ajem.2023.03.018

[19] Lang RM, Badano LP, Mor-Avi V, Afilalo J, Armstrong A, Ernande L, et al. Recommendations for cardiac chamber quantification by echocardiography in adults: An update from the American Society of Echocardiography and the European Association of Cardiovascular Imaging. Journal of the American Society of Echocardiography. 2015;**28**:1-39.e14

[20] Salinas P, Dieiev V. Critical care echocardiography: Assessing left and right ventricular function in the intensive care unit. Seminars in Ultrasound, CT, and MR. 2024;**45**(1):58-73. DOI: 10.1053/j.sult.2023.12.007. Epub 2023 Dec 12

[21] Slama M, Tribouilloy C, Maizel J. Left ventricular outflow tract obstruction in ICU patients. Current Opinion in Critical Care. 2016;**22**:260-266

[22] Nguyen C, Parfianowicz D, Bennett C. Point of care ultrasound and shock: The value in bedside diagnosis and hemodynamic assessment in undifferentiated shock patients. Journal of Translational Critical Care Medicine. 2024;**6**:e24-e00010

[23] Parasuraman S, Walker S, Loudon BL, Gollop ND, Wilson AM, Lowery C, et al. Assessment of pulmonary artery pressure by echocardiography-a comprehensive review. IJC Heart and Vasculature. 2016;**12**:45-51

[24] Fields JM, Davis J, Girson L, Au A, Potts J, Morgan CJ, et al. Transthoracic echocardiography for diagnosing pulmonary embolism: A systematic review and meta-analysis. Journal of the American Society of Echocardiography. 2017;**30**:714-723.e4

[25] Nasser MF, Jabri A, Limaye S, Sharma S, Hamade H, Mhanna M, et al. Echocardiographic evaluation of pulmonary embolism: A review. Journal of the American Society of Echocardiography. 2023;**36**:906-912

Chapter 10

Perioperative Hemodynamic Monitoring: Ensuring Stability and Improving Outcomes

Sana Saleem, Asreena Arayilakath Pattuvathil, Hamza Bin Saleem, Usama Bin Saleem, Roaa Naser Suleiman and Manal Faisal Alsharafi

Abstract

Perioperative hemodynamic monitoring plays a crucial role in guiding anesthetic management, maintaining cardiovascular stability, and improving surgical outcomes. This chapter provides a clinical overview of current monitoring methods, ranging from simple noninvasive tools to advanced technologies such as pulse contour analysis and transesophageal echocardiography (TEE). The objectives of monitoring throughout the perioperative phases are emphasized. Particular attention is paid to high-risk groups, such as the elderly and individuals suffering from cardiovascular disease. Smarter monitoring can have a quantifiable impact in a field where every second matters.

Keywords: perioperative, hemodynamic, intra-operative, invasive, noninvasive, anesthesia, monitoring, goal-directed therapy, stability, outcome

1. Introduction

Hemodynamic monitoring is central to anesthetic practice, particularly in the perioperative period, where patient physiology is challenged by significant stress—from anesthetic agents, surgical manipulation, fluid shifts, and underlying comorbidities. Major adverse consequences, such as myocardial damage, acute kidney injury, stroke, and delayed recovery, can result from even brief episodes of hypotension or impaired perfusion [1, 2]. As a result, meticulous hemodynamic parameter monitoring is an essential clinical duty rather than merely a technical one.

Technological developments in monitoring have broadened the anesthesiologist's toolkit beyond conventional measurements such as noninvasive blood pressure and central venous pressure. Real-time knowledge of cardiac output, volume responsiveness, and tissue perfusion can be obtained using devices such as bioimpedance systems, transesophageal echocardiography, and pulse contour analysis [3, 4].

As surgical populations age and case complexity rises, the function of hemodynamic monitoring has expanded beyond conventional parameters to include dynamic, goal-directed strategies that advise personalized patient management [4]. With an emphasis on when and how to employ different modalities during the preoperative, intraoperative, and postoperative phases, this chapter provides a clinical overview of perioperative hemodynamic monitoring. We go over the advantages and disadvantages of various devices, explore specialized strategies for high-risk groups, and take a look at how careful analysis of hemodynamic data can lessen complications and aid in the recovery process.

2. Goals of hemodynamic monitoring

The primary goal of perioperative hemodynamic monitoring is to maintain appropriate tissue perfusion and oxygen delivery during the surgical procedure. In order to direct prompt interventions, this entails not only monitoring cardiovascular parameters but also analyzing trends and changes in real time. Effective monitoring informs intraoperative decision-making regarding fluid administration, vasopressor support, and cardiac function optimization.

2.1 Detecting hemodynamic instability early

Hemodynamic instability is recognized as a complex syndrome involving many physiological parameters resulting in impaired circulation and oxygen delivery to vital organs. Blood pressure is the most widely used indicator of hemodynamic instability during the perioperative period. Clinically, hemodynamic instability is typically defined by abnormalities of blood pressure, heart rate/rhythm, cardiac output, stroke volume, and central venous pressure [5, 6].

According to the available data, even brief periods of hypotension and patient harm are strongly correlated [2, 5–7]. Additionally, there is proof that myocardial damage following noncardiac surgery is linked to variations in heart rate intraoperatively [1, 8]. Lastly, we know that hours of increasing hemodynamic instability precede the majority of in-hospital cardiac arrest events [9, 10].

2.2 Guiding fluid and vasoactive therapy

A major challenge in anesthesia is finding a balance between fluid resuscitation and avoiding fluid overload, which can lead to tissue edema, delayed wound healing, and pulmonary complications. It has been established that static measures such as central venous pressure (CVP) do not serve as very good indicators of fluid responsiveness. A systematic review showed that CVP and blood volume had a very poor relationship and that CVP/DeltaCVP could not predict the hemodynamic response to a fluid challenge [11].

Rather, goal-directed strategies use cardiac output monitoring and dynamic indices to optimize fluid and vasopressor use to the patient's needs, in particular, improving hemodynamic efficiency and outcomes [12].

2.3 Optimizing tissue perfusion and oxygen delivery

Enough oxygen, glucose, and other metabolites must be delivered to each cell, and the waste products of cell metabolism must be removed, in order for tissue perfusion

Goal	Monitoring focus	Intended clinical outcome
Early detection of instability	Continuous blood pressure, SVV, PPV, HR, and MAP	Prevention of myocardial injury, AKI, and stroke through prompt intervention
Tailored fluid and vasopressor therapy		
Optimizing perfusion and oxygen delivery	MAP ≥65 mmHg, $ScvO_2$, lactate, and urine output	Improved tissue oxygenation; reduced risk of ischemic complications
Intraoperative risk stratification	Trends in BP, CO, HR, lactate, and responsiveness to therapy	Early identification of deterioration; improved triage, and postoperative planning

SVV: Stroke volume variation, PPV: Pulse pressure variation, HR: Heart rate, MAP: Mean Arterial Pressure, ScvO2: Central Venous oxygen saturation, BP: Blood pressure, CO: Cardiac output.

Table 1.
Goals of hemodynamic monitoring and associated clinical outcomes [2, 5, 6, 8–11].

to occur. This is accomplished when each organ's flow at the microcirculation level is "adequate," a state that is impossible to evaluate with the monitoring tools we currently have. Thus, we focus on the primary factors that are most likely to produce sufficient microcirculatory blood flow: mean arterial pressure (MAP), central venous oxygen saturation ($ScvO_2$), and lactate levels. Thus, ideally, both instantaneous arterial pressure and beat-by-beat systemic blood flow should be monitored in addition to heart rate to "optimize" tissue perfusion [4].

2.4 Supporting risk stratification and prognostication

Monitoring data can inform intraoperative and postoperative risk assessment. Early warning systems are designed to provide a system for escalating care [10]. Communication, triage, and recovery planning are all enhanced when hemodynamic monitoring is incorporated into broader perioperative management strategies (**Table 1**) [3].

3. Monitoring modalities

Perioperative hemodynamic monitoring covers a wide range from simple, noninvasive methods to advanced technologies that can perform a thorough cardiovascular assessment. The patient's risk profile, the complexity of the surgery, and the requirement for real-time intervention all influence the modality selection. Three levels of monitoring strategies are distinguished in this section: basic, invasive, and advanced modalities.

3.1 Basic monitoring

Regardless of the length of time or location of anesthesia, the Association of Anaesthetists believes that it is imperative that minimum standards of monitoring be followed whenever a patient is put under anesthesia. The following, in our opinion, qualifies as minimal anesthesia monitoring [13]:

1. *Plethysmograph and pulse oximeter*: Arterial oxygen saturation can be continuously measured with this noninvasive device. By using the pleth variability index and waveform quality, it also offers indirect information about perfusion [13, 14].

2. *Noninvasive blood pressure*: NIBP, which is obtained sporadically using oscillometric cuffs, is crucial for monitoring trends but may overlook brief hypotension. When there are arrhythmias or inadequate perfusion, its accuracy decreases [13].

3. *ECG*: Arrhythmias, ischemia, and abnormal heart rates must all be identified with continuous ECG monitoring. For effective ischemic detection, Lead II and V5 are frequently utilized [14].

4. *Temperature*: Before anesthesia and every 30 min until the end of surgery.

5. *Capnography*: While primarily a respiratory monitor, it becomes a mandatory monitor during general anesthesia. EtCO2 levels reflect cardiac output, especially during low-flow states such as cardiac arrest or shock.

3.2 Invasive monitoring

The use of additional cardiovascular monitoring during anesthesia should be considered, for instance, due to cardiovascular comorbidity, frailty, the emergency or specific nature of the surgery; several methods exist. Invasive monitoring provides real-time, high-fidelity data critical for managing high-risk cases.

1. *Arterial catheterization*: Provides continuous beat-to-beat blood pressure measurements. Allows arterial blood gas sampling and advanced waveform analysis (e.g., dicrotic notch and PPV). Indicated in patients with anticipated hemodynamic fluctuations or major blood loss.

2. *Central venous pressure (CVP)*: Central venous pressure (CVP) is used almost universally to guide fluid therapy in hospitalized patients. Although recent studies have proven CVP to be an unreliable indicator [11], it is still useful for trend monitoring and for administering vasoactive drugs or total parenteral nutrition.

3. *Pulmonary artery catheter (PAC)*: Initially introduced in 1970, popularly known as the "Swan-Ganz" catheter, is used for measuring cardiac output (by the thermodilution technique), for right atrial and right ventricular pacing, and for measuring right-sided pressures, including pulmonary capillary wedge pressure [15]. While its use has declined over time due to invasiveness and associated complications, it remains valuable in select population (e.g., severe chronic heart failure and transplant cases) [12, 15].

3.3 Advanced monitoring technologies

Overall, the combination of technology development, expanding awareness of the goal-directed therapy (GDT) concept, and commercial interest in noninvasive monitoring has led to advanced monitoring modalities.

1. *Transesophageal echocardiography (TEE)*: The proximity of the esophagus to much of the heart and great vessels makes it an excellent ultrasonic window, so that TEE provides additional and more accurate information for several specific diagnoses and for many catheter-based cardiac interventions. Offers real-time

imaging of cardiac function, chamber size, volume status, and valve integrity. Requires interpretation and skill, but it is crucial for rapid identification of hemodynamic compromise [16].

2. *Pulse contour analysis (e.g., FloTrac/Vigileo, PiCCO, and LiDCO)*: Uses arterial waveform data to calculate stroke volume variation (SVV), cardiac output, and systemic vascular resistance. Uncalibrated PCS is a less invasive method to estimate CO. Effectiveness varies with patient condition and ventilation parameters [17].

3. *Esophageal Doppler*: Although the use of transthoracic echocardiography has become common for estimation of Stroke volume (SV), a small and simple-to-use handheld ultrasonic device is now available. Positioned in the sternal notch, a Doppler measure of ascending aortic blood flow velocity is obtained and referenced to a nomogram for aortic diameter, and these data are used for calculation of volume flow [12].

4. *Bioimpedance and bioreactance (e.g., NICOM):* When a high frequency/low voltage current is applied to the chest *via* surface electrodes, impedance to this current oscillates with cardiac filling and ejection. The amplitude of this oscillation is proportional to SV, and devices are available to estimate the proportionality constant and provide clinically useful information. As with bioimpedance, a current of constant frequency is applied. Unlike bioimpedance, bioreactance analyzes the phase difference between the applied current and the resultant voltage: oscillation of this phase difference is proportional to SV (**Table 2**) [12].

Modality	Category	Primary outputs	Typical usage indication
Noninvasive blood pressure	Basic	BP trends	All surgical patients
Echocardiography	Basic	HR, arrhythmia	All surgical patients
Pulse oximetry	Basic	SpO2, perfusion	All surgical patients
Capnography	Basic	ETCO2, perfusion	All under GA
Arterial line	Invasive	Continuos BP, ABG	Major surgery, unstable BP
Central venous pressure	Invasive	Preload estimate	Vasoactive therapy, volume status
Pulmonary artery catheter	Invasive	CO, PAP, ScvO2	Cardiac and transplant cases
Transesophageal Echocardiography	Advanced	Cardiac function and volume	Cardiac or complex noncardiac surgery
Pulse contour	Advanced	CO, SVV, and SVR	High-risk surgery and GDT protocol
Esophageal Doppler	Advanced	Aortic flow, SV	Fluid optimization
Bioimpedance	Advanced	CO (noninvasive)	Noninvasive CO trending

BP: Blood pressure, HR: Heart rate, SpO2: Oxygen saturation, ETCO2: End tidal CO_2, SV: Stroke Volume, SVV: Stroke volume variation, SVR: Systemic Vascular Resistance, ScvO2: Central venous oxygen saturation, CO: Cardiac output, PAP: Pulmonary artery pressure, GDT: Goal-Directed therapy, ABG: Arterial Blood Gas.

Table 2.
Monitoring modalities.

4. Perioperative phases and monitoring needs

Hemodynamic monitoring is a dynamic process that changes throughout the perioperative period in response to the patient's physiological needs. Every stage offers different obstacles and chances for action, and the type and level of monitoring should be in line with the changing risk profile.

4.1 Preoperative phase: Baseline risk and readiness

The goal of preoperative monitoring is not active management, but *risk stratification* and preparation. A thorough preoperative anesthesia assessment helps identify patients with cardiovascular vulnerabilities who may benefit from invasive or advanced monitoring intraoperatively. Consider preoperative echocardiography or stress testing in high-risk patients. Discussion with surgical and critical care teams regarding planned monitoring and resuscitation thresholds.

4.2 Intraoperative phase: Dynamic assessment and intervention

This is the most active phase for hemodynamic monitoring.

Focus areas:

Blood pressure stability and cardiac output.

Fluid responsiveness and ongoing losses.

Effects of anesthetic agents, positioning, and pneumoperitoneum.

Response to vasoactive medications.

The monitoring strategy includes basic monitoring for all patients (NIBP, ECG, SpO_2, and $EtCO_2$). An arterial line is used for high-risk cases or those with anticipated blood loss. CVP or cardiac output monitoring for fluid management in major procedures and use of dynamic indices (SVV and PPV) and/or TEE or pulse contour systems for real-time decision-making [14].

4.3 Postoperative phase: Surveillance and stabilization

Continuous monitoring during the first few hours after surgery enables the early identification of delayed decompensation, especially in high-risk patients or those who have persistent bleeding, residual vasodilation, or lingering anesthetic effects.

Phase	Primary goals	Monitoring needs
Preoperative	Risk stratification and optimization	NIBP, ECG, focused echo, discuss plan for invasive monitoring if needed
Intraoperative	Maintain stability, guide fluids/vasopressors	Full ASA monitors; ± A-line, CVP, SVV/PPV, TEE, CO monitor, and depending on complexity
Postoperative	Early detection of deterioration	Continuous ECG and BP; ± A-line, telemetry, output tracking, and ICU-level support

NIBP: noninvasive blood pressure, ECG: echocardiography, SpO_2: oxygen saturation, CVP: central venous pressure, SVV: stroke volume variation, PPV: pulse pressure variation, CO: cardiac output, TEE: transesophageal echocardiography.

Table 3.
Monitoring focus by perioperative phase [14].

DOI: http://dx.doi.org/10.5772/intechopen.1012309

Focus areas:
Rebound hypertension or hypotension.
Pain, agitation, or hypoxia-induced cardiovascular strain.
Persistent bleeding or third spacing.
Myocardial ischemia or arrhythmias.

The monitoring strategy includes continued ECG and BP monitoring in the PACU or ICU. The arterial line may be continued if still in place and the patient is unstable. Monitor urine output, lactate, and $ScvO_2$ if available.

Consider telemetry or step-down ICU monitoring for patients with intermediate risk (**Table 3**).

5. Guided hemodynamic strategies

The evolution of hemodynamic monitoring has shifted clinical practice from static assessment toward *goal-directed therapy (GDT), an individualized, responsive approach to fluid and cardiovascular management*. Rather than applying uniform protocols, guided strategies aim to match cardiovascular support with a patient's current physiological needs.

GDT extrapolates a patient's fluid responsiveness from measurable hemodynamic changes according to the Frank–Starling curve. It involves setting specific hemodynamic goals and using continuous monitoring to guide treatment decisions, most often in high-risk surgical patients. Core principles include:

1. Preload optimization: Guided by dynamic indices or response to fluid bolus.
2. Afterload management: Use of vasopressors or vasodilators to maintain target mean arterial pressure (MAP).
3. Contractility support: Use of inotropes when stroke volume or cardiac output remains low despite preload optimization.

Common targets include (summarized from literature) [18].

1. CVP 8–12 cm H_2O
2. MAP >65 mmHg
3. SvO_2 > 70%
4. $ScvO_2$ > 65%
5. Urine output >0.5 ml/kg/h
6. Hematocrit >30%

Guided strategies are only as effective as the data that inform them. GDT is best implemented using advanced monitoring modalities. Numerous studies have shown that intraoperative GDT reduces complications and shortens hospital stays, especially in high-risk surgeries.

6. Impact on outcomes

Effective hemodynamic monitoring contributes directly to improved perioperative outcomes by:

6.1 Enhancing surgical recovery

Meta-analysis concludes that the use of a preemptive strategy of hemodynamic monitoring and coupled GDT can reduce surgical mortality and morbidity [19].

6.2 Optimizing fluid management

Avoids both hypoperfusion and fluid overload, reducing risks of pulmonary edema and abdominal compartment syndrome.

Although the evidence base continues to evolve, trends support the integration of dynamic, individualized monitoring into routine anesthetic practice for high-risk patients (**Table 4**) [3, 4, 19].

The following outcome measures can be used to evaluate the effectiveness of hemodynamic monitoring.

7. Future of hemodynamic monitoring

As surgical care becomes more complex and personalized, the field of hemodynamic monitoring is evolving to meet new demands. Hemodynamic monitoring's future depends on more intelligent integration and decision support in addition to more advanced tools.

7.1 Artificial intelligence and predictive analytics

With appropriate algorithms, computers can learn to detect patterns and associations in large data sets. Preliminary studies show that AI-guided platforms can improve intraoperative blood pressure stability and reduce clinician workload [20].

7.2 Wearable and minimally invasive devices

The use of noninvasive cardiac output sensors, wireless patch monitors, and photoplethysmography (PPG) is enabling hemodynamic surveillance outside of the intensive care unit and operating room.

Outcome metric	Clinical relevance
Intraoperative hypotension episodes	Predictor of MI, AKI, stroke
Postoperative complication rate	Infection, ileus, pulmonary issues
Length of ICU and hospital stay	Resource use, recovery quality
30-day morbidity and mortality	Standard benchmark in surgical outcomes
Readmission and reoperation rates	Indicator of unresolved hemodynamic instability

MI: myocardial infarction, AKI: acute kidney injury.

Table 4.
Outcome measures to evaluate the effectiveness of hemodynamic monitoring.

7.3 Integration with electronic health records (EHR) and closed-loop systems

Health care organizations should organize care into a well-integrated and synergistic mesosystem that contains all of the microsystems throughout the patient's episode of care (preadmission, preoperative, intraoperative, postoperative, and recovery periods).

Centralized data platforms can enable accurate and efficient data collection, which can provide quality feedback to hospitals and individual clinicians.

8. Conclusion

Perioperative hemodynamic monitoring is a dynamic, decision-making process that has a direct impact on recovery paths, surgical outcomes, and patient safety. It is much more than a standard checklist. Anesthesiologists now have strong tools to evaluate and support cardiovascular function in real time, ranging from fundamental metrics like blood pressure and heart rate to sophisticated cardiac output monitoring and goal-directed therapy.

Individualized monitoring techniques are becoming more and more necessary as surgical care becomes more complex. Research keeps showing that careful, directed hemodynamic care improves outcomes, lowers morbidity, and shortens hospital stays, especially for high-risk patients. However, clinical judgment cannot be replaced by even the most sophisticated technology.

In the end, hemodynamic monitoring becomes more than just a tool when it is applied purposefully and intelligently; it becomes the foundation of safer, more intelligent anesthesia.

Acknowledgements

The author acknowledges the use of Grammarly AI for language polishing of the manuscript.

Author details

Sana Saleem[1*], Asreena Arayilakath Pattuvathil[1], Hamza Bin Saleem[1], Usama Bin Saleem[1], Roaa Naser Suleiman[1] and Manal Faisal Alsharafi[2]

1 Hamad Medical Corporation, Doha, Qatar

2 College of Medicine, Qatar University, Doha, Qatar

*Address all correspondence to: ssaleem4@hamad.qa

References

[1] Sessler DI, Meyhoff CS, Zimmerman NM, Mao G, Leslie K, Vásquez SM, et al. Period-dependent associations between hypotension during and for four days after noncardiac surgery and a composite of myocardial infarction and death: A substudy of the POISE-2 trial. Anesthesiology. 2018;**128**(2):317-327. DOI: 10.1097/ALN.0000000000001985

[2] Walsh M, Devereaux PJ, Garg AX, Kurz A, Turan A, Rodseth R, et al. Relationship between intraoperative mean arterial pressure and clinical outcomes after noncardiac surgery: Toward an empirical definition of hypotension. Anesthesiology. 2013;**119**(3):507-515. DOI: 10.1097/ALN.0b013e3182a10e26

[3] Saugel B, Vincent JL, Wagner JY. Personalized hemodynamic management. Current Opinion in Critical Care. 2017;**23**(4):334-341. DOI: 10.1097/MCC.0000000000000422

[4] Fellahi JL, Futier E, Vaisse C, et al. Perioperative hemodynamic optimization: From guidelines to implementation—An experts' opinion paper. Annals of Intensive Care. 2021;**11**:58. DOI: 10.1186/s13613-021-00845-1

[5] Scott MJ, the APSF Hemodynamic Instability Writing Group. Perioperative patients with hemodynamic instability: Consensus recommendations of the Anesthesia Patient Safety Foundation. Anesthesia & Analgesia. 2024;**138**(4):713-724. DOI: 10.1213/ANE.0000000000006789

[6] Abebe MM, Arefayne NR, Temesgen MM, Admass BA. Incidence and predictive factors associated with hemodynamic instability among adult surgical patients in the post-anesthesia care unit, 2021: A prospective follow up study. Annals of Medicine and Surgery (Lond). 2022;**74**:103321. DOI: 10.1016/j.amsu.2022.103321

[7] Bijker JB, van Klei WA, Kappen TH, van Wolfswinkel L, Moons KG, Kalkman CJ. Incidence of intraoperative hypotension as a function of the chosen definition: Literature definitions applied to a retrospective cohort using automated data collection. Anesthesiology. 2007;**107**(2):213-220. DOI: 10.1097/01.anes.0000270724.40897.8e

[8] Ruetzler K, Smilowitz NR, Berger JS, Devereaux PJ, Maron BA, Newby LK, et al. Diagnosis and management of patients with myocardial injury after noncardiac surgery: A scientific statement from the American Heart Association. Circulation. 2021;**144**(19):e287-e305

[9] Smith MEB, Chiovaro JC, O'Neil M, Kansagara D, Quiñones AR, Freeman M, et al. Early warning system scores for clinical deterioration in hospitalized patients: A systematic review. Annals of the American Thoracic Society. 2014;**11, no. 9**:1454-1465. DOI: 10.1513/AnnalsATS.201403-102OC. PubMed: 25296111

[10] Alam N, Hobbelink EL, van Tienhoven AJ, van de Ven PM, Jansma EP, Nanayakkara PWB. The impact of the use of the early warning score (EWS) on patient outcomes: A systematic review. Resuscitation. 2014;**85**(5):587-594. DOI: 10.1016/j.resuscitation.2014.01.013, ISSN 0300-9572

[11] Marik PE, Baram M, Vahid B. Does central venous pressure predict fluid

responsiveness? A systematic review of the literature and the tale of seven mares. Chest. 2008;**134**(1):172-178. DOI: 10.1378/chest.07-2331

[12] Meng L, Heerdt P. Perioperative goal-directed haemodynamic therapy based on flow parameters: A concept in evolution. BJA British Journal of Anaesthesia. 2016;**117**:3-17. DOI: 10.1093/bja/aew363

[13] Meidert AS, Saugel B. Techniques for non-invasive monitoring of arterial blood pressure. Frontiers in Medicine (Lausanne). 2018;**4**:231. DOI: 10.3389/fmed.2017.00231

[14] Klein AA, Meek T, Allcock E, Cook TM, Mincher N, Morris C, et al. Recommendations for standards of monitoring during anaesthesia and recovery 2021. Anaesthesia. 2021;**76**:1212-1223. DOI: 10.1111/anae.15501

[15] Chatterjee K. The swan-Ganz catheters: Past, present, and future: A viewpoint. Circulation. 2009;**119**(1):147-152

[16] Hahn RT, Abraham T, Adams MS, Bruce CJ, Glas KE, Lang RM, et al. Guidelines for performing a comprehensive transesophageal echocardiographic examination. Journal of the American Society of Echocardiography. 2013;**26**(9):921-964. DOI: 10.1016/j.echo.2013.07.009

[17] Grensemann J. Cardiac output monitoring by pulse contour analysis, the technical basics of less-invasive techniques. Frontiers in Medicine (Lausanne). 2018;**5**:64. DOI: 10.3389/fmed.2018.00064

[18] Rivers E, Nguyen B, Havstad S, Ressler J, Muzzin A, Knoblich B, et al. Early goal-directed therapy in the treatment of severe sepsis and septic shock. New England Journal of Medicine. 2001;**345**(19):1368-1377

[19] Hamilton MA, Cecconi M, Rhodes A. A systematic review and meta-analysis on the use of preemptive hemodynamic intervention to improve postoperative outcomes in moderate and high-risk surgical patients. Anesthesia & Analgesia. 2011;**112**(6):1392-1402. DOI: 10.1213/ANE.0b013e3181eeaae5

[20] Hatib F, Jian Z, Buddi S, Lee C, Settels J, Sibert K, et al. Machine-learning algorithm to predict hypotension based on high-fidelity arterial pressure waveform analysis. Anesthesiology. 2018;**129**(4):663-674. DOI: 10.1097/ALN.0000000000002300

Chapter 11

Pulmonary Artery Catheter: The Golden Way of Advanced Hemodynamic Monitoring

Jawdat Alali, Mahmoud Tabouni, Abdulmalik Jaber and Mohammad Hemadneh

Abstract

The pulmonary artery catheter (PAC), used first in the 1970s, remains an essential tool in advanced hemodynamic monitoring despite the presence of less invasive alternatives. This chapter provides an extensive review of the PAC's principles, clinical applications, and its role in critical care. It includes detailed anatomy and insertion technique of the PAC, focusing on its capability to provide real-time measurements of key parameters such as pulmonary artery pressure, pulmonary capillary wedge pressure, cardiac output, and mixed venous oxygen saturation. These measurements enable the accurate evaluation of volume status, cardiac function, and oxygen delivery, particularly in managing complex conditions such as shock, heart failure, and perioperative instability. The clinical utility of PAC in intensive care units and major surgeries is reinforced, along with its superiority in situations requiring detailed hemodynamic assessment. Despite risks associated with its use, including insertion-related complications and data misinterpretation, technological advancements and integration with personalized medicine continue to support its relevance. The PAC remains a gold standard for managing critically ill patients where high-precision, real-time cardiovascular parameters are essential for optimizing outcomes.

Keywords: pulmonary artery catheter (PAC), hemodynamic monitoring, cardiac output, pulmonary capillary wedge pressure (PCWP), critical care, heart failure, advanced monitoring, thermodilution

1. Introduction

1.1 Historical background

The pulmonary artery catheter (PAC) was first introduced by Dr. Swan and Dr. Ganz in the early 1970s, marking a significant milestone in the management of critically ill patients. Before this breakthrough, physicians had only a limited number of reliable tools to accurately assess hemodynamic status in patients with complex shock or heart failure. The PAC (**Figure 1**) allowed clinicians to measure intracardiac pressures, including pulmonary artery pressures (PAP) and pulmonary capillary

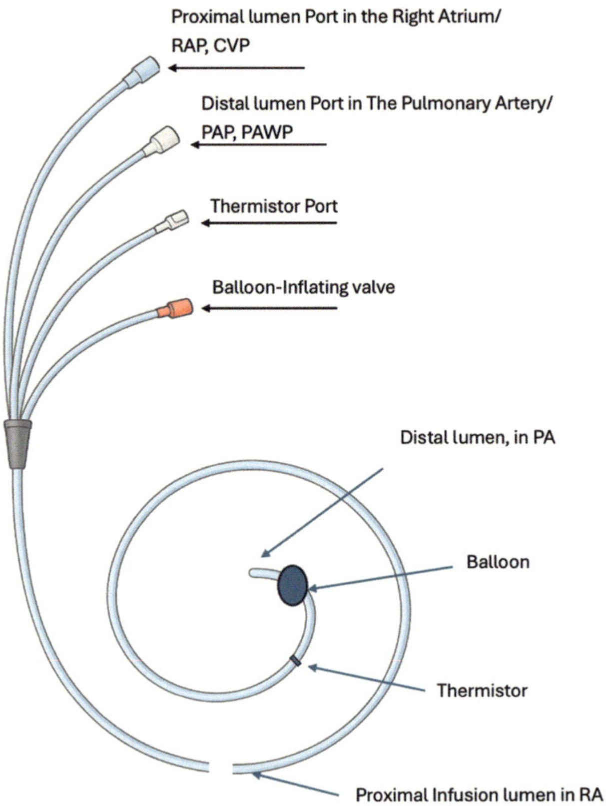

Figure 1.
Standard four-lumen pulmonary artery catheter.

wedge pressure (PCWP), as well as cardiac output (CO), in real time. This technology quickly gained widespread use in anesthesia and intensive care settings, enabling the precise monitoring of circulatory status [1]. The ability to assess both volume status and cardiac function facilitated decision-making, particularly for patients undergoing major surgeries or those in severe shock.

Though the start sparked excitement, the use of PAC has declined over the years, particularly due to the emergence of less invasive monitoring techniques and growing concerns about its potential complications. Nonetheless, research has repeatedly shown PACs' unparalleled capacity to deliver extensive hemodynamic data, especially for critically ill patients with multiple comorbidities or intricate hemodynamic profiles [2]. The historical background of PAC usage, along with its sustained clinical significance, validates its role as a core tool of advanced hemodynamic monitoring.

1.2 Overview of hemodynamic monitoring

Hemodynamic monitoring includes a range of techniques used to assess the cardiovascular system's function, focusing on parameters such as blood pressure, heart rate, cardiac output, systemic vascular resistance, and pulmonary pressures. It is of extreme importance in managing patients with acute cardiovascular compromise, especially in settings such as intensive care units (ICUs), postoperative care units, and emergency departments [3]. The primary purpose of hemodynamic monitoring is to assess perfusion, direct treatment strategies (fluid resuscitation, vasopressor use, etc.), and optimize organ function.

The PAC remains one of the most reliable techniques for hemodynamic monitoring. It provides continuous real-time data on parameters like cardiac output, pulmonary artery pressure, and mixed venous oxygen saturation (SvO_2), allowing clinicians to make evidence-based decisions depending on dynamic changes in physiology. Though newer technologies, such as noninvasive cardiac output monitoring or ultrasound-based assessments, have become popular, PAC continues to play a crucial role in complex cases, where these alternatives may not provide the level of detail required for appropriate intervention [4]. In this context, PAC is considered a 'gold standard' in advanced monitoring and is pivotal to the management of critically ill patients.

2. Principles of pulmonary artery catheterization

2.1 Anatomy and insertion technique

Insertion of the PAC is typically performed via the internal jugular vein, subclavian vein, or femoral vein, though the internal jugular central venous approach remains the most common. The catheter is advanced into the right atrium, then the right ventricle, and finally, the pulmonary artery. The catheter must be positioned properly within the pulmonary artery for accurate measurements. The process of catheter insertion is guided by either anatomical landmarks or ultrasound, which significantly reduces complications related to improper placement, such as arterial puncture, pneumothorax, and cardiac arrhythmias [5, 6].

The insertion of a PAC is generally performed under sterile conditions in an intensive care or operating room setting. Ultrasound guidance is used for the insertion of central venous access, providing real-time visualization of the vessels and improving the safety of catheter placement. After insertion, the catheter is connected to a pressure transducer, and the necessary hemodynamic parameters can be measured [7]. Additionally, the PAC can have various types of sensors and ports, including those that measure pressures (right atrial, right ventricular, pulmonary artery pressures) and those that allow for the blood sample extraction for analysis of mixed venous oxygen saturation (SvO_2). Correct positioning and regular monitoring of the catheter are essential to obtaining accurate and reliable readings.

2.2 Anatomy of the pulmonary artery catheter

The pulmonary artery catheter (PAC) is a 7-French catheter that typically is 110 cm in length, although shorter versions of approximately 90 cm are also available.

At its distal tip, the catheter features a single open lumen. This distal lumen has two functions: it allows for the measurement of pulmonary artery (PA) pressures and enables the sampling of venous blood for mixed venous oxygen saturation (SvO_2) analysis. Furthermore, an optical sensor is incorporated near the tip to enable continuous monitoring of mixed venous oxygen saturation (SvO_2).

The balloon is located at the very tip of the catheter and is designed to hold up to 1.5 ml of volume, which inflates it to a diameter of approximately 13 mm.

Approximately 4 cm proximal to the catheter tip, a thermistor is integrated into the catheter. This thermistor is responsible for sensing temperature changes in the pulmonary arterial blood as it flows past the catheter.

The thermistor is a small resistor that changes its resistance based on temperature, meaning that electrical resistance differs in response to changes in temperature. This feature allows for accurate thermal detection, which is essential for measuring cardiac output (**Table 1**).

2.3 Hemodynamic parameters measured

The primary hemodynamic variables assessed using the PAC include pulmonary artery pressure (PAP), pulmonary capillary wedge pressure (PCWP), cardiac output (CO), and mixed venous oxygen saturation (SvO_2). These measurements generate a valuable understanding of both the heart's ability to pump blood and the lungs' ability to oxygenate blood.

- *Pulmonary artery pressure (PAP)*: PAP is an important parameter for assessing pulmonary hypertension and diagnosing left-sided heart failure. It is measured directly through the catheter's distal lumen and can be used to determine whether elevated pressures in the pulmonary arteries are due to intrinsic lung pathology or left-sided heart dysfunction [3].

- *Pulmonary capillary wedge pressure (PCWP)*: PCWP is a surrogate for left atrial pressure and is essential in evaluating fluid status and distinguishing between cardiogenic and non-cardiogenic pulmonary edema (**Figure 2**) [8]. An elevated PCWP suggests left-sided heart failure, whereas a normal PCWP in the presence of pulmonary edema suggests other causes, such as acute respiratory distress syndrome (ARDS) (**Figure 3**) [9].

- *Cardiac output (CO)*: Using the thermodilution method, the PAC provides accurate real-time data on cardiac output (**Figure 4**). This measurement is critical for assessing the heart's pumping efficiency and is used to guide therapy in

Port/Lumen	Location	Function
Proximal port/Blue	RA	Measures *central venous pressure (CVP)* and allows for injection of fluid or cold saline for thermodilution cardiac output measurement.
Distal port/Yellow	PA	Measures *PAP* and samples mixed venous blood.
Balloon inflation port/Red	Connects to the balloon near the catheter tip	Inflates a small balloon to help float the catheter into place and to measure *PAWP*.
Thermistor port/ White	Near the distal tip	Measures blood temperature for *cardiac output* determination via thermodilution.
Proximal infusion port	RA	Used for fluid or medication infusion.

Table 1.
Standard pulmonary artery catheter ports/lumens.

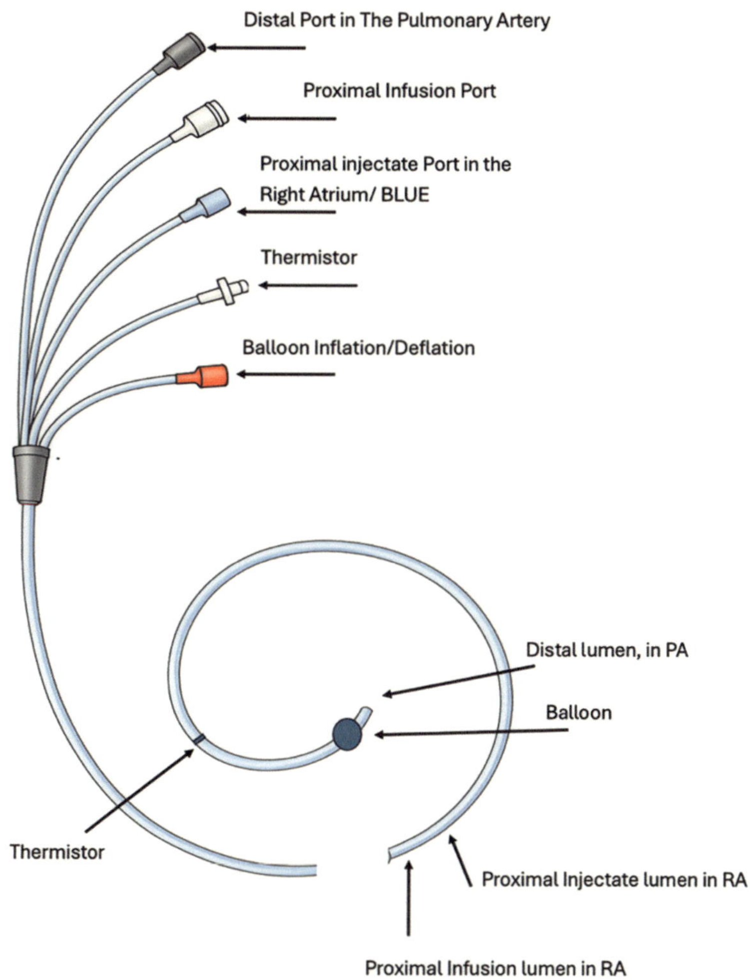

Figure 2.
Standard pulmonary artery catheter ports/lumens.

patients with shock [7]. The most recent version of pulmonary artery catheters (PACs) implements a pulsed heated thermodilution method to measure cardiac output in a continuous fashion, known as Thermodilution Continuous Cardiac Output (TDCCO). In this technique, a small amount of heat is released from a thermal filament located in the right ventricular segment of the catheter. The resulting temperature change is detected by a thermistor at the catheter tip and processed through a modified Stewart-Hamilton equation to calculate TDCCO in real time [10].

- *Mixed venous oxygen saturation (SvO_2)*: SvO_2 reflects the balance between oxygen delivery and consumption. It is measured through the catheter and provides critical information in managing patients with systemic shock, sepsis, or multi-organ failure [11].

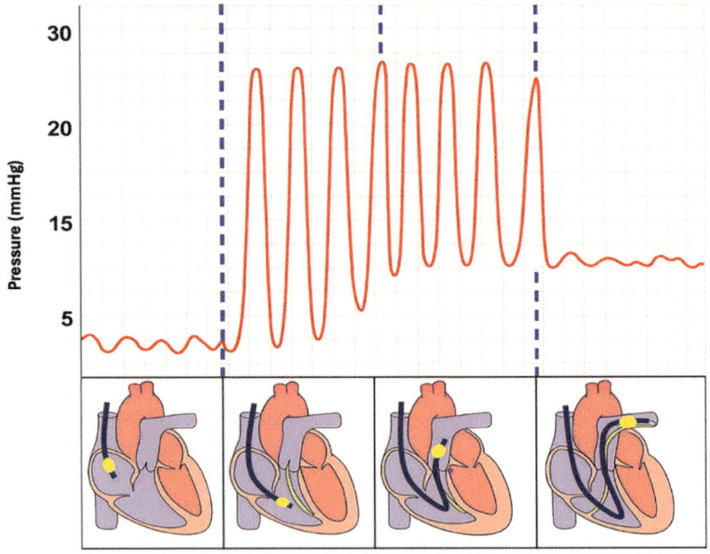

Right Atrium	Right Ventricle	Pulmonary Artery	Pulmonary Artery Wedge
0–6 mmHg	25/0 mmHg	15–30 / 5–15 mmHg	2–10 mmHg

Figure 3.
The PAC displayed pressure waveforms/values from the right atrium, right ventricle, pulmonary artery, and wedge (PCWP) positions.

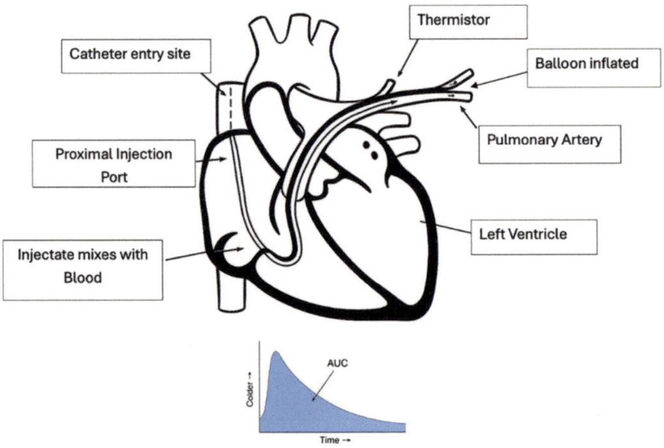

The equation is:

$$\text{Cardiac Output (CO)} = \frac{V \cdot (T_b - T_i) \cdot K}{\int \Delta T(t)dt}$$

Where:

- V = Volume of injectate (mL)
- T_b = Blood temperature
- T_i = Injectate temperature
- $\Delta T(t)$ = Change in blood temperature over time
- K = Constant that incorporates the specific heat and density of blood and injectate

Figure 4.
The temperature change versus time graph applied to the Stewart-Hamilton equation.

3. Clinical applications

3.1 Use in critical care

The use of the PAC in critical care settings has become standard practice for managing patients with severe cardiovascular or respiratory compromise. Its ability to provide continuous real-time data makes it invaluable for managing critically ill patients, particularly those with shock, severe heart failure, and multi-organ dysfunction [11, 12]. PAC monitoring is beneficial in situations where clinical examination by itself is inadequate for making decisions, such as in cases of acute decompensated heart failure, sepsis, and postoperative management following major surgery. For example, in shock states such as cardiogenic, septic, and hypovolemic shock, the PAC supplies vital data to differentiate between causes of hypotension and guide interventions. In these settings, monitoring both cardiac output and right atrial pressure can help clinicians adjust fluid therapy, vasopressors, and inotropes, ultimately optimizing the patient's hemodynamics and maximizing treatment effectiveness [13].

3.2 Role in cardiogenic shock and heart failure

PAC has been particularly valuable in the management of cardiogenic shock and heart failure, where the understanding of preload, afterload, and contractility is important for determining the optimal treatment approach. In cardiogenic shock, the PAC provides real-time data on right and left heart function, helping distinguish between fluid overload and low cardiac output states. It has been shown to guide the use of inotropes, diuretics, and vasopressors to optimize hemodynamics in patients with severe heart failure [14, 15].

In patients with decompensated heart failure, especially those in need of advanced therapies like mechanical circulatory support or heart transplantation, PAC data have been indispensable in guiding management strategies [16, 17]. The ability to monitor pulmonary pressures, CO, and SvO_2 in these complex cases has led to improved decision-making and outcomes in this critically ill patient population [11, 18].

3.3 Application in major surgeries

PAC is commonly employed in major surgeries, particularly cardiac surgery, where managing fluid balance, cardiac output, and pulmonary pressures is necessary. It is also used in high-risk noncardiac surgeries where the patient's hemodynamic status is subject to acute changes and instability. For example, in cardiac surgery, PAC monitoring is essential to ensure adequate perfusion pressures and to prevent ischemia during periods of impaired cardiac function or perfusion [19, 20].

During major surgeries, continuous monitoring of the right ventricle (RV) and left ventricle (LV) performance, along with PAP and CO, helps ensure the heart can cope with the hemodynamic demands of the surgery. This monitoring enables the anesthesia and surgical teams to take immediate action to any changes in the patient's condition and to adjust interventions promptly [3]. Additionally, PAC data aids in postoperative recovery, ensuring that the patient is stabilized and lowering the incidence of complications.

4. Interpretation of hemodynamic data

4.1 Pulmonary artery pressure

Pulmonary artery pressure is an important indicator of the pressure load in the right side of the heart and the pulmonary circulation. Elevated PAP can be a sign of pulmonary hypertension, which may be secondary to left-sided heart failure, pulmonary embolism, or intrinsic lung disease. Accurate interpretation of PAP in conjunction with PCWP and CO is essential to identify the underlying cause of pulmonary hypertension [21, 22]. For instance, high PAP in the presence of elevated PCWP suggests cardiogenic causes, while normal or low PCWP with elevated PAP indicates primary pulmonary disease [14].

In patients with complex shock or right ventricular failure, continuous PAP monitoring is invaluable for adjusting fluid management and vasoactive therapies [19, 23].

4.2 Cardiac output and mixed venous oxygen saturation

Cardiac output measurement using the PAC is crucial for assessing the heart's ability to pump oxygenated blood into vital organs. Decreased CO can indicate heart failure, sepsis, or other shock states, and appropriate interventions (e.g., fluid resuscitation, inotropes) are often guided by CO measurements [7]. Additionally, monitoring mixed venous oxygen saturation (SvO_2) provides information about the balance between oxygen delivery and consumption. A low SvO_2 can signal inadequate perfusion or an increase in metabolic demand, both of which may require interventions like increasing cardiac output or correcting oxygenation deficits [11].

4.3 Pulmonary capillary wedge pressure

PCWP is considered one of the most accurate indirect measures of left atrial pressure and is a vital diagnostic aid in differentiating between cardiogenic and non-cardiogenic pulmonary edema. High PCWP in the context of pulmonary edema often implies left-sided heart failure, whereas normal PCWP with pulmonary edema is suggestive of ARDS or other non-cardiogenic causes [9]. The continuous monitoring of PCWP helps guide fluid management and diuretic therapy in patients with heart failure, improving clinical outcomes and avoiding volume overload.

5. Benefits of pulmonary artery catheter use

5.1 Precision in volume status assessment

PAC facilitates precise measurement of right atrial pressure (RAP), pulmonary artery pressures, and cardiac output, which together provide a thorough assessment of a patient's volume status. These measurements are far more accurate than depending exclusively on clinical examination or more basic hemodynamic parameters like central venous pressure (CVP) [24]. The ability to assess preload, afterload, and cardiac contractility in real-time ensures that fluid therapy and vasopressor use are optimized, minimizing the risk of under-resuscitation or fluid overload [13]. This is particularly critical in patients with complex shock or heart failure, where traditional markers often fail to provide adequate guidance.

5.2 Guiding vasopressor and fluid therapy

In critically ill patients, titration of vasopressors, inotropes, and fluids plays a central role in enhancing hemodynamic status and preventing multi-organ failure. PAC's ability to measure cardiac output, pulmonary pressures, and SvO_2 allows clinicians to dynamically adjust therapy in response to changes in the patient's condition. For example, a drop in SvO_2 could prompt the use of inotropes or increased fluid resuscitation, while elevated pulmonary pressures may suggest the need for diuretics or adjustments in afterload reduction [8, 25].

6. Risks and complications

6.1 Insertion-related risks

Although the pulmonary artery catheter is a high-impact modality for hemodynamic monitoring, its insertion carries intrinsic hazards. The most common complications include vascular injury, arrhythmias, pneumothorax, and catheter-related infections. Vascular injury can occur during central venous catheterization, particularly if the procedure is performed in an emergency or with inadequate training or supervision [26]. Arterial puncture, hematoma formation, or even inadvertent arterial cannulation can lead to bleeding or vessel injury, especially if proper technique is not employed. Furthermore, the placement of the catheter may lead to arrhythmias, particularly during catheter passage through the right atrium and ventricle [6].

The risk of pneumothorax is especially worrisome when the catheter is inserted via the subclavian vein or when the catheter is advanced too far, leading to perforation of the vessel and subsequent leakage of air into the pleural space. This can cause significant complications, requiring immediate management, including thoracostomy [5]. Other less common but life-threatening complications include catheter misplacement and damage to heart structures, leading to arrhythmias, tamponade, or perforation of the myocardium [7]. To minimize these risks, using ultrasound-guided catheter placement has become a widely adopted practice in many centers, improving safety and success rates [6].

6.2 Misinterpretation and over-reliance

A prevailing challenge associated with PAC use is the potential for misinterpretation of data, particularly if the measured values are not considered within the broader clinical context. For example, evaluating elevated pulmonary pressures without accounting for patient factors such as fluid status, lung compliance, or systemic vascular resistance can lead to suboptimal therapeutic decisions, such as unnecessary diuresis or overuse of inotropes. Similarly, PAC data should never be the sole determinant of therapeutic interventions; clinical judgment remains foundational in guiding patient management [5, 15].

Over-reliance on PAC can also be problematic. In recent years, there has been a growing recognition of the importance of integrating PAC data with other monitoring tools, such as echocardiography, pulse index continuous cardiac output (PiCCO), and clinical examination. Failure to incorporate other aspects of patient evaluation can lead to inadequate responses to changes in the patient's condition [8]. For example, a patient may exhibit a normal CO but still be clinically unstable due to other factors such as sepsis or arrhythmias, which require specific management beyond the scope of PAC measurements [5].

7. Alternatives and comparisons

7.1 Comparison with less invasive techniques

The advent of less invasive hemodynamic monitoring techniques, such as PiCCO (pulse index continuous cardiac output) and echocardiography, has prompted comparison with the PAC. PiCCO, which uses transpulmonary thermodilution, provides continuous cardiac output monitoring without the need for central venous catheter placement, making it a promising alternative for certain patients [27]. Similarly, echocardiography, both transthoracic and transesophageal, offers real-time visualization of cardiac anatomy and function and can be used to estimate cardiac output, assess ventricular function, and detect abnormalities such as valvular disease or intraventricular thrombus [6].

These less invasive alternatives have the advantages of avoiding the risks associated with PAC insertion, such as infection, pneumothorax, and arrhythmias. However, they also have limitations. PiCCO requires a catheter to be placed in a central vein, and while it does not need to enter the pulmonary circulation, it still requires invasive access. Furthermore, echocardiography, while providing dynamic and comprehensive data on cardiac function, is operator-dependent and may not always provide accurate measurements in critically ill patients, particularly those with poor echogenicity or challenging anatomy [27].

Despite these alternatives, the PAC remains the most comprehensive tool available for measuring pulmonary pressures, cardiac output, and mixed venous oxygen saturation, all critical parameters in the management of complex shock and heart failure [26]. The decision to use a PAC versus an alternative method depends on the clinical context, the patient's condition, and the available expertise.

7.2 When PAC is superior

While less invasive methods have their place in clinical practice, PAC remains superior in certain situations. In critically ill patients with severe right heart failure, pulmonary hypertension, or complex shock, the ability to measure direct pulmonary artery pressures and accurately assess cardiac output is essential for making rational therapeutic decisions [28]. Additionally, in patients undergoing major cardiac surgery, the PAC provides continuous real-time monitoring, which is vital for promoting ideal hemodynamic management and avoiding adverse outcomes [15].

Moreover, the PAC's ability to simultaneously evaluate multiple hemodynamic parameters—including right atrial pressure, pulmonary artery pressure, cardiac output, and mixed venous oxygen saturation—makes it an indispensable tool in cases where detailed, multifactorial hemodynamic assessment is needed [29]. For patients with severe multi-organ failure or who are undergoing complex surgical procedures, the comprehensive data provided by the PAC allows clinicians to manage these high-risk situations more effectively, minimizing the risk of adverse outcomes.

8. Recent advances and future perspectives

8.1 Technological improvements

The PAC has experienced substantial technological improvements over the past several decades. One remarkable advance is the incorporation of fiber-optic sensors, enabling more precise and continuous measurements of hemodynamic parameters, including cardiac output and pulmonary artery pressures. These sensors offer enhanced resistance to interference and provide real-time data with higher precision, which is essential for handling complex clinical situations [26].

Furthermore, newer PACs are equipped with integrated temperature sensors that improve the accuracy of thermodilution-based cardiac output measurements. These advances have improved the overall value of the PAC, particularly in high-risk patients, through enhanced data reliability and minimal calibration demands. Moreover, the improvement of more user-friendly PAC systems, with developed graphical interfaces and automated data processing, has simplified data interpretation for clinicians, even in busy ICU settings [29].

Wireless data transmission is an emerging advancement, allowing for remote monitoring of patients in critical care settings. This could transform the management of patients, particularly in telemedicine or in environments with high nurse-to-patient ratios. As a result of these technological advancements, the PAC may continue to serve a key function in advanced hemodynamic monitoring sustainably over time.

8.2 Evolving role in personalized medicine

As personalized medicine becomes more embedded within clinical practice, the role of the PAC is projected to develop further. Within the framework of precision medicine, where treatments are adapted based on an individual's genetic makeup, underlying diseases, and response to therapy, PAC monitoring will provide important data to guide patient-specific interventions. For example, in patients with heart failure or pulmonary hypertension, understanding their individual hemodynamic profile will enable more precise titration of medications such as inotropes, diuretics, and vasopressors, decreasing the risk of treatment failure or adverse reactions.

Moreover, in the context of organ transplantation (such as heart, lung, or kidney transplants), PAC monitoring may assist in directing early postoperative management, guaranteeing that perfusion pressures and cardiac output are optimized during the critical early days after surgery. Continuous assessment of the patient's hemodynamic status will enable clinicians to modify therapies as needed, enhancing long-term outcomes and reducing the risk of graft rejection or organ failure [27].

9. Conclusion

9.1 Summary of clinical value

The pulmonary artery catheter is still considered the gold standard for advanced hemodynamic monitoring, affording comprehensive, real-time data on critical parameters such as pulmonary artery pressure, cardiac output, and mixed venous oxygen saturation. Its role in assessing both the right and left sides of the heart, along with the pulmonary circulation, provides clinicians with an extensive understanding of a patient's hemodynamic status. Such detailed information is invaluable in managing complex, critically ill patients, most significantly those with severe shock, heart failure, or undergoing major surgeries [27]. The PAC plays a critical role in settings where other monitoring tools may be inadequate, such as in cases of severe right heart failure, pulmonary hypertension, or multi-organ dysfunction.

9.2 Recommendations for practice

While the use of the PAC is associated with some risks, such as insertion-related complications and the potential for misinterpretation of data, these can be mitigated with proper technique, intensive monitoring, and extensive insight into the clinical context. Clinicians need to incorporate PAC data with other diagnostic tools, such as echocardiography, laboratory results, and clinical examination, to ensure that management decisions are based on a holistic view of the patient's condition.

Given its precision and depth of information, PAC remains a cornerstone in the management of critically ill patients, despite the availability of less invasive alternatives. In settings where detailed hemodynamic monitoring is essential, the PAC offers unparalleled value and is likely to continue evolving with advancements in technology, enhancing its role in personalized and precision medicine.

Conflict of interest

The authors declare no conflict of interest.

Author details

Jawdat Alali[1*], Mahmoud Tabouni[2], Abdulmalik Jaber[3] and Mohammad Hemadneh[2]

1 Surgical Intensive Care Unit, Hamad Medical Corporation (HMC), Doha, Qatar

2 Internal Medicine Department, Hamad Medical Corporation (HMC), Doha, Qatar

3 Anesthesia and Intensive Care Department, Hamad Medical Corporation (HMC), Doha, Qatar

*Address all correspondence to: jalali1@hamad.qa

References

[1] Gnaegi A, Feihl F, Perret C. Intensive care physicians' insufficient knowledge of right-heart catheterization at the bedside: Time to act? Critical Care Medicine. 1997;**25**(2):213-220

[2] Iberti TJ, Fischer EP, Leibowitz AB, Panacek EA, Silverstein JH, Albertson TE. A multicenter study of physicians' knowledge of the pulmonary artery catheter. Pulmonary Artery Catheter Study Group. JAMA. 1990;**264**(22):2928-2932

[3] Bootsma IT, Boerma EC, de Lange F, Scheeren TWL. The contemporary pulmonary artery catheter. Part 1: Placement and waveform analysis. Journal of Clinical Monitoring and Computing. Feb 2022;**36**(1):5-15. DOI: 10.1007/s10877-021-00662-8. Epub 2021 Feb 10. PMID: 33564995; PMCID: PMC8894225

[4] McGee WT, Young C, Frazier JA, editors. Edwards Clinical Education Quick Guide to Cardiopulmonary Care. 4th ed. Edwards Critical Care Education: Irvine; 2018

[5] Sun Q, Rogiers P, Pauwels D, Vincent JL. Comparison of continuous thermodilution and bolus cardiac output measurements in septic shock. Intensive Care Medicine. 2002;**28**(9):1276-1280

[6] Saugel B, Scheeren TWL, Teboul JL. Ultrasound-guided central venous catheter placement: A structured review and recommendations for clinical practice. Critical Care. 2017;**21**(1):225

[7] Marino PL. Marino's the ICU Book. 4th ed. Philadelphia: Lippincott Williams and Wilkins; 2013

[8] Rajaram SS, Desai NK, Kalra A, Gajera M, Cavanaugh SK, Brampton W, et al. Pulmonary artery catheters for adult patients in intensive care. Cochrane Database of Systematic Reviews. 2013;**2013**(2):CD003408

[9] Lamia B, Maizel J, Ochagavia A, Chemla D, Osman D, Richard C, et al. Echocardiographic diagnosis of pulmonary artery occlusion pressure elevation during weaning from mechanical ventilation. Critical Care Medicine. 2009;**37**(5):1696-1701

[10] Ameloot K, Meex I, Genbrugge C, Jans F, Malbrain M, Mullens W, et al. Accuracy of continuous thermodilution cardiac output monitoring by pulmonary artery catheter during therapeutic hypothermia in post-cardiac arrest patients. Resuscitation. 2014;**85**(9):1263-1268

[11] Nishikawa T, Dohi S. Errors in the measurement of cardiac output by thermodilution. Canadian Journal of Anaesthesia. 1993;**40**(2):142-153

[12] Renner LE, Morton MJ, Sakuma GY. Indicator amount, temperature, and intrinsic cardiac output affect thermodilution cardiac output accuracy and reproducibility. Critical Care Medicine. 1993;**21**(4):586-597

[13] Stevenson LW, Perlof JK. The limited reliability of physical signs for estimating hemodynamics in chronic heart failure. JAMA. 1989;**261**(6):884-888

[14] Rossello X, Vila M, Rivas-Lasarte M, Ferrero-Gregori A, SansRoselló J, Duran-Cambra A, et al. Impact of pulmonary artery catheter use on short- and long-term mortality in patients with cardiogenic shock. Cardiology. 2017;**136**(1):61-69

[15] Lim HS. Cardiac power output revisited. Circulation. Heart Failure. 2020;**13**(10):e007393

[16] Naeije R, Badagliacca R. The overloaded right heart and ventricular interdependence. Cardiovascular Research. 2017;**113**(12):1474-1485

[17] Lim HS, Gustafsson F. Pulmonary artery pulsatility index: Physiological basis and clinical application. European Journal of Heart Failure. 2020;**22**(1):32-38

[18] Nadeau S, Noble WH. Limitations of cardiac output measurements by thermodilution. Canadian Anaesthetists' Society Journal. 1986;**33**(6):780-784

[19] Grønlykke L, Couture EJ, Haddad F, Amsallem M, Ravn HB, Raymond M, et al. Preliminary experience using diastolic right ventricular pressure gradient monitoring in cardiac surgery. Journal of Cardiothoracic and Vascular Anesthesia. 2020;**34**(8):2116-2125

[20] Raymond M, Grønlykke L, Couture EJ, Desjardins G, Cogan J, Cloutier J, et al. Perioperative right ventricular pressure monitoring in cardiac surgery. Journal of Cardiothoracic and Vascular Anesthesia. 2019;**33**(4):1090-1104

[21] Simonneau G, Montani D, Celermajer DS, Denton CP, Gatzoulis MA, KrowkaM,et al.Haemodynamicdefinitions and updated clinical classification of pulmonary hypertension. European Respiratory Journal. 2019;**53**(1):1801913

[22] Deaño RC, Glassner-Kolmin C, Rubenfre M, Frost A, Visovatti S, McLaughlin VV, et al. Referral of patients with pulmonary hypertension diagnoses to tertiary pulmonary hypertension centers: The multicenter RePHerral study. JAMA Internal Medicine. 2013;**173**(10):887-893

[23] Mehmood M, Biederman RWW, Markert RJ, McCarthy MC, Tchorz KM. Right heart function in critically ill patients at risk for acute right heart failure: A description of right ventricular-pulmonary arterial coupling, ejection fraction and pulmonary artery pulsatility index. Heart, Lung & Circulation. 2020;**29**(6):867-873

[24] Teboul JL, Saugel B, Cecconi M, De Backer D, Hofer CK, Monnet X, et al. Less invasive hemodynamic monitoring in critically ill patients. Intensive Care Medicine. 2016;**42**(9):1350-1359

[25] Gayat E, Mebazaa A. Pulmonary hypertension in critical care. Current Opinion in Critical Care. 2011;**17**(5):439-448

[26] American Society of Anesthesiologists Task Force on Pulmonary Artery Catheterization. Practice guidelines for pulmonary artery catheterization: An updated report by the American Society of Anesthesiologists Task Force on pulmonary artery catheterization. Anesthesiology. 2003;**99**(4):988-1014

[27] Mermel LA, McCormick RD, Springman SR, Maki DG. The pathogenesis and epidemiology of catheter-related infection with pulmonary artery swan-Ganz catheters: A prospective study utilizing molecular subtyping. The American Journal of Medicine. 1991;**91**(3B):197S-205S

[28] Robitaille A, Denault AY, Couture P, Bélisle S, Fortier A, Guertin MC, et al. Importance of relative pulmonary hypertension in cardiac surgery: The mean systemic-to-pulmonary artery pressure ratio. Journal of Cardiothoracic and Vascular Anesthesia. 2006;**20**(3):331-339

[29] Cohen Y, Fosse JP, Karoubi P, Reboul-Marty J, Dreyfuss D, Hoang P, et al. The "hands-of" catheter and the prevention of systemic infections associated with pulmonary artery catheter: A prospective study. American Journal of Respiratory and Critical Care Medicine. 1998;**157**(1):284-287

Chapter 12

Non-Invasive Cardiac Output Monitoring in Perioperative Medicine

Ashok Kandasamy

Abstract

Hemodynamic monitoring is a key aspect in intensive care, which enables the tailoring of fluid and vasoactive drug therapy. Non-invasive monitoring has the advantage of low invasiveness and fewer complications, when compared to invasive methods. This chapter will offer a short overview of the various techniques of non-invasive CO monitoring, associated principles, validation data and limitations. Methods reviewed are electrical bioimpedance and bioreactance, respiratory-based CO monitoring, pulse wave transit time, radial artery applanation tonometry and ultrasound CO monitoring. Although numerous techniques are already in use, additional work is required to develop devices that are sufficiently accurate for routine, non-invasive measurements.

Keywords: non-invasive cardiac output monitoring, hemodynamic, bioimpedance, bioreactance, pulse wave transit time, radial artery applanation tonometry, ultrasound

1. Introduction

Cardiac output measurement is an integral part of hemodynamic monitoring in perioperative care. In addition to the Swan-Ganz pulmonary artery catheter (PAC) and transpulmonary thermodilution, less invasive methods for CO determination like pulse contour analysis and esophageal Doppler are already in widespread use. Completely non-invasive methods like electrical bioimpedance, bioreactance, pulse wave transit time, radial artery applanation tonometry and ultrasound are now available for CO monitoring.

In this review, we will discuss these non-invasive methods for CO estimation.

1.1 Use of non-invasive cardiac output monitoring in perioperative medicine

For patients undergoing surgery, goal-directed optimization of hemodynamic variables reduces both postoperative morbidity and improves patient outcomes [1–3]. There is evidence from Cochrane Systematic Review including more than 5000 patients from 31 studies, that goal-directed measures to augment global blood flow result in an overall reduction in postoperative complications and hospital stay [4]. Moreover, a recent meta-analysis of cardiac surgical patients revealed improved outcomes in terms of postoperative complications and length of hospital stay in cardiac

IntechOpen

surgery patients using goal-directed hemodynamic therapy [5]. There is a lot of data to show that goal-directed optimization of oxygen delivery and cardiac index can reduce postoperative complications and mortality in selected high-risk surgical patients [6].

1.2 Critical illness

In critically ill patients, monitoring of cardiac output, oxygen delivery and tissue oxygenation plays a decisive role in differentiating shock states [7, 8]. Monitoring of cardiac output is also vital in identifying which patients may benefit from volume expansion (fluid responders—patients who can increase their stroke volume after administration of a fluid challenge) [9, 10]. Close monitoring of the patient's volume status (preload) and cardiac function (cardiac output) is of utmost importance in patients with severe sepsis, distributive shock and septic cardiomyopathy [11].

2. Methods of non-invasive cardiac output measurement

2.1 Electrical bioimpedance

2.1.1 Technical details

Electrical bioimpedance is based on the assumption that impedance of thorax varies with thoracic fluid content. Based on a circulatory system model, variation in aortic blood volume during cardiac cycle (Qi) results in changes in aortic impedance (Za). This can be assessed by application of a high-frequency current to thorax and estimating the difference between applied and detected voltage. Transthoracic impedance (Z_o) can be obtained from the applied voltage and amplitude. Stroke volume is the product of peak flow and ventricular ejection time (VET). Stroke volume (SV) can also be determined by the multiplying maximal rate of change of Z_o (dZ_o/dt_{max}) with ventricular ejection time (**Figure 1**) (VET)—Eq. (1).

$$[SV = dZ_o/dt_{max} X\, VET] \tag{1}$$

Electrical bioimpedance principles have been described by Kubicek and colleagues for clinical application in 1966 and by Bernstein et al. in 1986 [12, 13]. In the

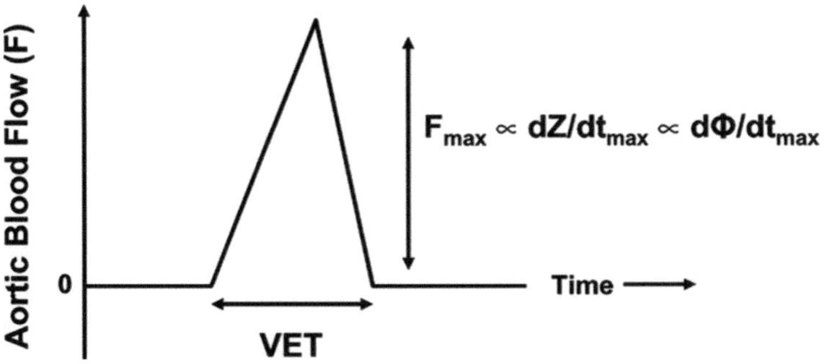

Figure 1.
Diagram depicting aortic flow as a function of time to estimate SV from bioimpedance (dZ_{max}/dt) or phase shifts ($d\Phi/dt_{max}$, bioreactance). Stroke volume is proportional to the product of peak flow (F_{max}) and ventricular ejection time (VET)—Reprinted with permission—Copyright © 2007 by the American Physiological Society.

meantime, many devices have emerged that employ electrodes that are placed on patients' skin for quantifying thoracic electrical bioimpedance [14]. Several systems utilizing these principles have been commercialized or are under development, including 'electrical velocimetry', which uses a modified equation based on the maximum rate of change of impedance to assess aortic flow and stroke volume [15].

A modification of the thoracic bioimpedance method by placing electrodes on the endotracheal tube, close to the aorta (ECOM; ConMed Corp), is available. This method of signal recording first appeared in experiments on animal models (swine) in 2000 [16].

2.1.2 Review of literature

Many studies have been carried out across different patient populations to study the performance of thoracic bioimpedance in a variety of patient and clinical settings [17]. Thoracic bioimpedance has undergone further testing using upgraded software for measurement of CO. On the one hand, in cardiac surgical patients, studies showed encouraging results when comparing thoracic bioimpedance with Swan Ganz thermodilution catheter (TDC) measurement [18–21]. On the other hand, studies revealed high bias and wide limits of agreement when comparing thoracic bioimpedance with Swan Ganz thermodilution catheter (TDC) measurement in cardiac surgical and mixed ICU patients [22, 23].

Electrical velocimetry (which utilizes bioimpedance technology) showed low accuracy and precision when compared with pulmonary artery thermodilution in cardiac surgery patients [24]. Clinical studies on electrical bioimpedance with electrodes attached to an endotracheal tube demonstrated low precision and high percentage error in cardiac surgical patients when compared with Swan-Ganz thermodilution [25–28].

2.1.3 Limitations

Measurement of thoracic bioimpedance is highly dependent on the position of electrodes and is limited by electrocauterization, pleural effusion, pulmonary congestion, changes in vascular resistance and cardiac Arrhythmias [29–32].

3. Thoracic bioreactance

3.1 Technical details

Bioreactance represents the phase shift in voltage across the thorax (**Figure 2**). It is assumed that the phase shift depends on pulsatile flow and that the bioreactance signal is more closely related to aortic blood flow and less dependent on intra and extravascular lung water [33]. Non-invasive CO monitoring, Cheetah Medical (NICOM) (Portland, OR, USA) utilizes four electrodes and calculates CO for the right and left side of the body (independently) with the final CO being the average of these two values [33].

The pulsatile changes in frequency (due to flow) combined with the changes in voltage across the thorax are determined by the bioreactance principle. Of note, the bioreactance eliminates the impact of extraneous artifacts on CO measurement. Non-invasive CO monitoring, Cheetah Medical (NICOM) has shown good agreement with other CO monitoring systems using arterial waveform analysis, as well as Swan Ganz thermodilution in multidisciplinary ICU and cardiac surgical patients.

3.2 Review of literature

The NICOM bioreactance system for measuring cardiac output was first described in 2007, and later evaluated in 110 ICU patients after cardiac surgery, with average bias (standard deviation) +0.06 liter min^{-1} (0.71 liter min^{-1}) [34, 35]. In a multicentre analysis comparing the NICOM bioreactance method in 111 patients (mixed ICUs and cardiac catheterization laboratories) with PA catheter-derived cardiac output, the authors observed a low bias of −0.09 liter min^{-1} and wide 95% limits of agreement of −2.5 liter min^{-1} to +2.3 liter min^{-1} for ICU patients [36]. Consistent results were obtained in studies performed in post-cardiac surgical patients when using CO

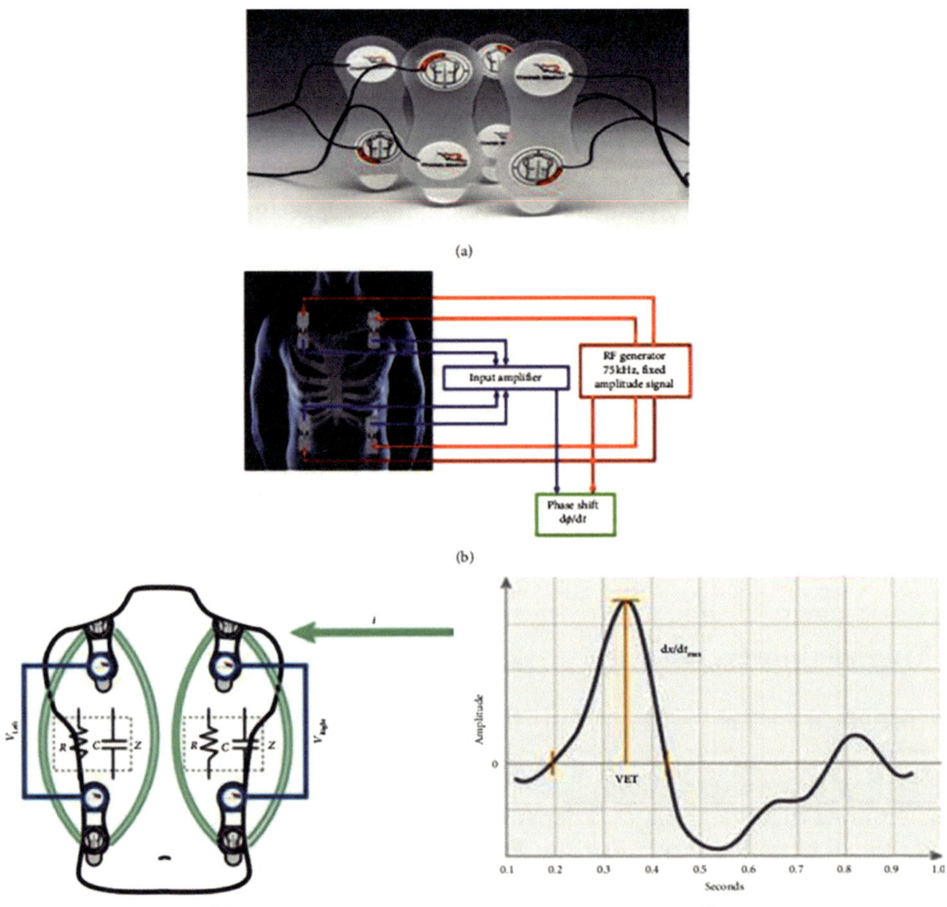

Figure 2.
NICOM principle (a) Electrodes are placed on the thorax. (b and c) Voltages are recorded between two inner electrodes after passing a high-frequency current between two outer electrodes. The phase shift (ϕ) and rate of change of phase (dϕ/dt) between these signals are used to estimate stroke volume (SV). RF radio frequency (d) representations of flow in the aorta as a function of time underlying the basic principle for estimation of stroke volume from changes in phase shifts (dx/dt_{max}) and ventricular ejection time (VET). (Crit Care Res Pract. 2020 *Sep 15;2020: 748181. Reprinted with permission—Copyright © 2020 Sanjeev Sivakumar and Christos Lazaridis).*

measurements from transpulmonary thermodilution and calibrated pulse contour analysis [37] or with PA thermodilution as the criterion standard [38]. A study in surgical patients treated for ovarian cancer revealed that thoracic bioreactance does not provide an acceptable cardiac index when compared with transpulmonary thermodilution [39].

3.3 Limitations

The present bioreactance technology is not free of weaknesses. Like bioimpedance, bioreactance recordings can be influenced by electrical interference. Bioreactance does not indicate rapid variations in cardiac output, as it provides measurements that are averaged over a minute. This approach can be particularly useful in the presence of mild arrhythmias (as it is an averaged value).

4. Respiratory-derived cardiac output (CO) monitoring

Fick principle is used to calculate cardiac output from oxygen consumption (VO_2) and the difference between arterial and venous blood oxygen content (CaO_2 - CvO_2). This technique was originally described in intubated, sedated and ventilated patients (without severe gas-exchange abnormality), using exhaled oxygen (O_2) or carbon dioxide (CO_2) exhaled gas, and requires invasive arterial and mixed venous blood sampling, applying the following equations [40]:

$$\mathrm{CO} = \mathrm{VO_2} / \mathrm{CaO_2} - \mathrm{CvO_2}$$

$$\mathrm{CO} = \mathrm{VCO_2} / \mathrm{CaCO_2} - \mathrm{CvCO_2} \tag{2}$$

A non-invasive tool based on the slope of the CO_2 dissociation curve (S) and the end-tidal carbon dioxide (S. $etCO_2$) as a surrogate for $CaCO_2$ has been introduced. As $CvCO_2$ is cumbersome to measure, it is estimated based on separate time intervals: normal respiration (*n*) and a 30-second period of rebreathing (*r*). If CO and the $CvCO_2$ are unchanged during both time intervals, the equation can be extrapolated as:

$$\mathrm{CO} = \Delta\,\mathrm{VCO_2} / \Delta(\mathrm{S.etCO_2}) \tag{3}$$

It is feasible to measure $etCO_2$ in expired gas with a tight-fitting facemask. Rebreathing permits estimation of CO without the need for invasive vascular access. This necessitates an extra loop of the ventilatory circuit to create a temporary partial rebreathing system (**Figure 3**).

The NICO-sensor (Philips Respironics, Eindhoven, the Netherlands) and INNOCOR (Innovision ApS, Denmark) are designed based on the partial rebreathing principle [42, 43]. However, there are several limitations like (i) minimal changes in CO_2 can cause significant differences in CO measurements, that is, even minimal leaks in face mask can induce measurement bias, (ii) may not be applicable in ICU setting, as these devices require the patient to be in a steady respiratory state, (c) differences between VCO_2 and end-tidal CO_2 reflect only the fraction of the lung that is ventilated; therefore, contribution of atelectasis or intrapulmonary shunting

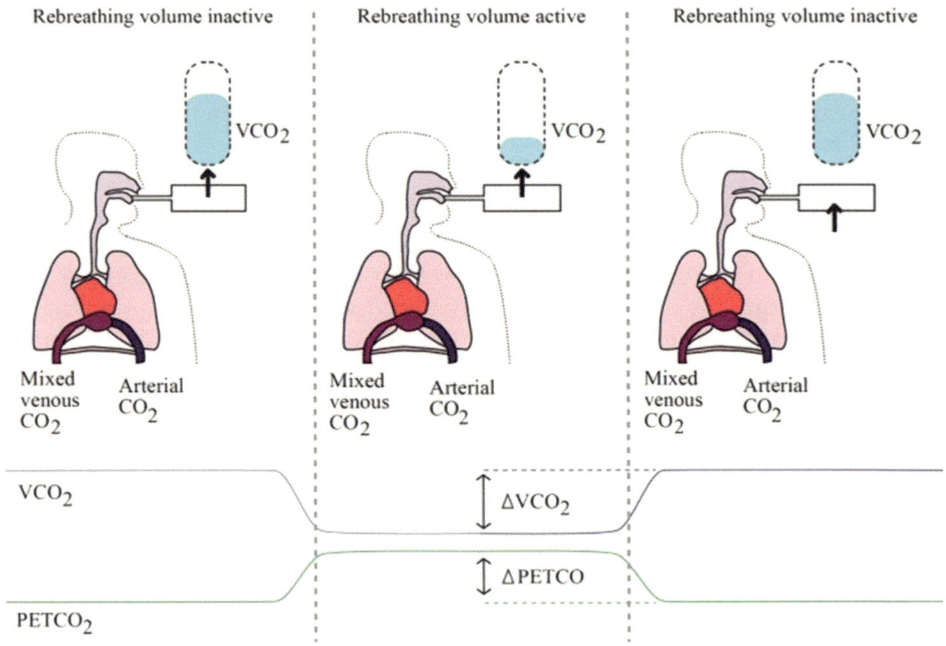

Figure 3.
Partial rebreathing principle. Left (baseline)—rebreathing valve is off—parameters at baseline. Middle (early rebreathing)—valve is on—decrease of VCO_2 with simultaneous rise in $PaCO_2$ and $PETCO_2$. Right panel (late rebreathing)—valve is off—parameters return to baseline levels, whereas mixed venous PCO_2 has varied. (Reprinted with permission: [41].)

has to be taken into account, which is difficult in the ICU where patients can present with more than one lung pathology [44–46]. Two recent articles studied the partial rebreathing principle with thermodilution. Neither of these could demonstrate equivalence between the two methods [47, 48].

A recent retrospective cohort study compared thermodilution and the Fick principle in over 12,000 patients who underwent right heart catheterization. This study revealed an acceptable systematic bias of 0.4% but poor limits of agreement from −1.31 to +1.27 l/min, and a measurement difference of more than 20% for CO in 40% of patients [49].

Thus, partial CO_2-rebreathing is not yet simple enough for routine use in critical care, but developments like improved rebreather-face interface to optimize mask seal and algorithms that can take into account the variations in end-tidal CO_2 are applicable in critical care. In fact, the latter issue appears intractable since respiratory disorders like pulmonary edema, pneumonia and acute exacerbations of COPD are the most frequent causes for ICU admission.

5. Pulse wave transit time

5.1 Technical details

When applied to non-invasive CO monitoring, pulse wave transit time (PWTT) is the time interval between the R-wave in the ECG and pulse wave rise-point measured by pulse oximetry. The esCCO method (Nihon Kohden, Japan) provides non-invasive

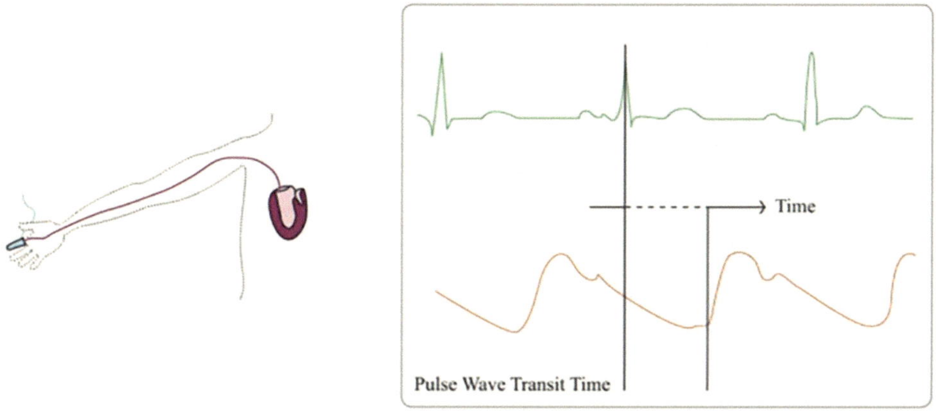

Figure 4.
PWTT is the delay between the generation of stroke volume (orange) and the generation of the R-wave of an ECG (green). Reprinted with permission—Copyright © 2017 Nguyen and Squara.

CO measurement by analysis of ECG, pulse oximeter waveform, and arterial pressure. Simplified methodology for monitoring of CO in this regard is based on the assumed negative relationship between the PWTT and stroke volume (**Figure 4**).

5.2 Review of literature

There is a paucity of literature on this innovative technology. Yamada and co-workers in 2004 evaluated the esCCO system in comparison with continuous PAC thermodilution (multicentre study, 213 surgical and ICU patients) and revealed a bias of 0.13 liter min^{-1} with 95% limits of agreement of –2.13 liter min^{-1} to +2.39 liter min^{-1} and a percentage error of 54% [50, 51]. In another study of 35 cardiac surgical patients, a bias of 0.80 liter min^{-1} (95% limits of agreement of –2.00 liter min^{-1} to +3.61 liter min^{-1}; percentage error 53%) was observed [52].

5.3 Limitations

One of the drawbacks to the esCCO system was the need for a reference cardiac output value at the time of the first measurement for adjustment [53]. Although a calibration model based on patient demographic features and cardiovascular variables including heart rate, pulse pressure, and pulse wave transit time was reported, it was not thoroughly tested and likely requires refinement [53, 54].

6. Radial artery applanation tonometry

6.1 Technical details

Radial artery applanation tonometry allows continuous non-invasive measurement of the arterial pressure waveform [55–61]. This concept was first reported in 1963 [62, 63]. Many of these devices required arterial pressure values obtained from cuff oscillometry for the purpose of calibration [64–68]. The T-Line (Tensys Medical Inc., USA) has developed its own algorithm for continuous arterial waveform analysis

[57]. After placing the sensor on the radial artery, its position is adjusted using an electromechanical system. From the arterial pressure signal measured in the optimal 'applanation' state (Transmural pressure of the artery equals zero), mean arterial pressure can be calculated. The arterial waveform is scaled using a proprietary algorithm based on biometrical data, from which systolic and diastolic blood pressure can be derived (**Figure 5**).

6.2 Review of literature

A recently developed auto-calibrating algorithm for non-invasive continuous CO monitoring using radial artery applanation tonometry was validated in a pilot study [69]. It is possible to measure CO by monitoring the arterial pressure waveform at the root of the radial artery with the use of applanation tonometry using this algorithm if the harmonic analysis of the arterial pressure waveform is accomplished with a non-linear mathematical model using physiological and biometrical input of the patient [69]. In this proof-of-concept study, cardiac output values recorded by means of radial artery applanation tonometry and pulse contour analysis in real-time, calibrated by transpulmonary thermodilution, were recorded simultaneously [69]. A CO bias of +0.1 L/min (0.8 L/min), 95% limits of agreement of −1.5 to +1.7 L/min, and percentage error of 23% indicated good accuracy and precision in this study.

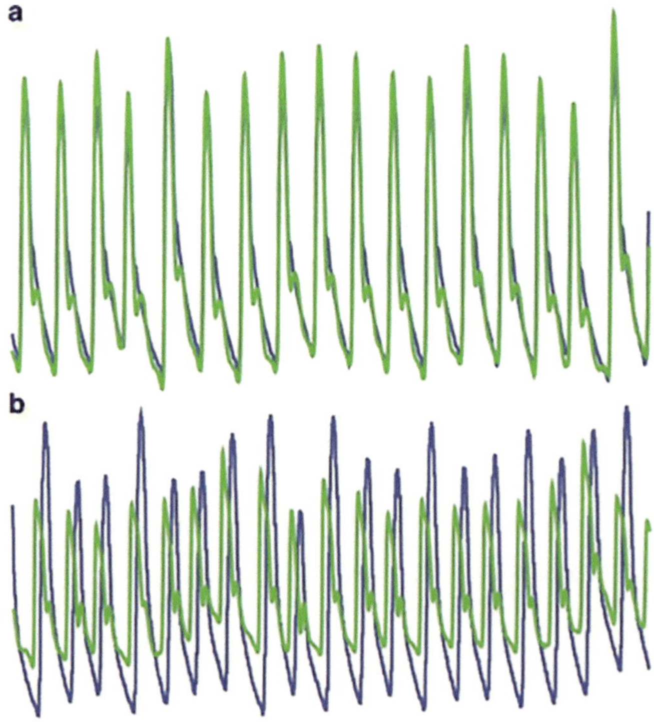

Figure 5.
Arterial pressure waveforms: Prior to incorporating the arterial waveform analysis, the pressure curve for each patient (green) was visually verified to overlay with the corresponding arterial catheter-based tracings (blue). An illustration for an impeccable (a) and not impeccable (b) waveform is provided above.

6.3 Limitations

Radial artery applanation tonometry is dependent on the quality of the arterial waveform. Under these circumstances, the most important prerequisite is the proper placement of the sensor over the radial artery. Rapid movement of the patient's arm can influence the accuracy of waveform analysis and thus CO determination.

7. Ultrasonic methods

7.1 Key concept

Cardiac output can be determined from aortic flow velocity and cross-sectional area of the aorta. Velocity of the flow of blood can be determined by the application of Doppler ultrasound:

$$SV = VTI \times CSA \tag{4}$$

VTI = aortic velocity time integral, CSA = cross-sectional area of aorta. Therefore, a non-invasive estimation of CO measurement requires a device continuously measuring aortic flow velocity, in a constant manner (**Figure 6**).

The ultrasonic cardiac output-monitoring (USCOM) device requires pre-calculation of the aortic valve area based on the patient's age and body weight. In addition, the ICU environment does not appear suitable for performing USCOM [70–72]. Limitations are (i) difficulty in maintaining a steady Doppler probe position in critically ill patients [73] (ii) poor echo window in post-cardiac surgical patients, and (iii) lack of accuracy of the valve area estimation with increasing age

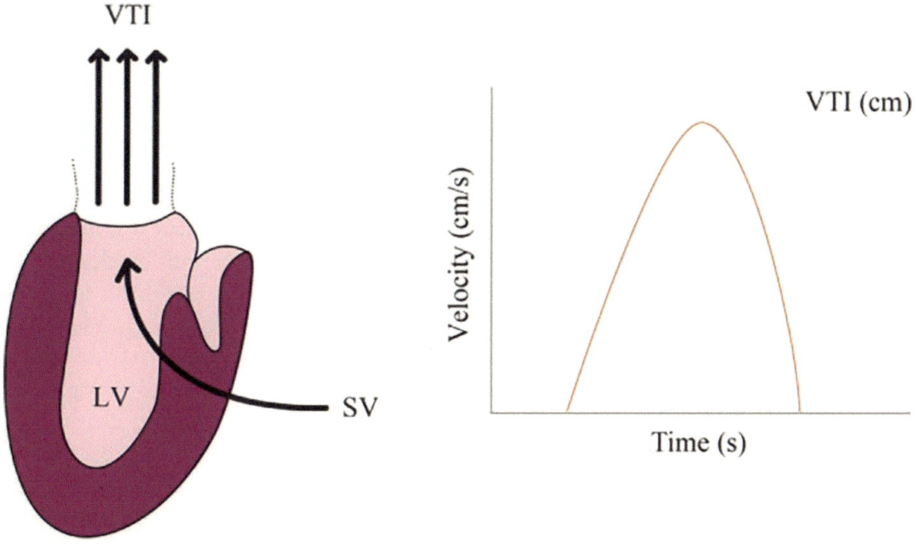

Figure 6.
Echocardiographic cardiac output measurement. Velocity time integral (VTI) multiplied by cross-sectional area (CSA) of the aorta allows estimation of stroke volume (SV). Reprinted with permission—Copyright © 2017 Nguyen and Squara.

group. Few studies highlight the utility of USCOM in critical care, with a systematic bias of −0.36 L/min. Nonetheless, the limits of agreement were not acceptable, ranging from −2.34 to 1.62 l/min, and the reported percentage error (29%) seemed too high for daily use [74].

POCUS for hemodynamic monitoring has become very popular in the ICU, but not so for continuous echocardiographic monitoring of CO by USCOM. In fact, a very high error, related to valve area estimate error and/or probe displacement, renders it difficult to use in a routine way. Nevertheless, the initial calibration from echocardiography-determined valve area and standard signal-quality controls might optimize this approach.

8. Non-invasive CO monitoring in critically ill patients

Assessment of CO is vital in the hemodynamic monitoring of critically ill patients. The 'clinical reference standard' for CO monitoring has been assessed by thermodilution with a pulmonary artery catheter (TDPAC). Due to the concerns regarding the safety of Pulmonary artery catheters, semi-invasive and non-invasive methods to estimate CO have been developed. In elective postoperative ICU patients, the non-invasive methods perform reasonably well and appear to be better as trend-monitoring devices (rather than for determination of the absolute CO) [75].

9. Conclusions

In summary, cardiac output measurement is of fundamental importance in perioperative medicine. Several totally non-invasive technologies are in use for haemodynamic optimization. They are easy to handle, operator-independent and have a better safety profile. These technologies constitute potentially valuable non-invasive tools to quantify the heart-lung interaction at the bedside and can be integrated for use at various stages in the perioperative care. They also enable goal-directed strategies in low or intermediate-risk surgical patients and those undergoing proecdures like endoscopy. Furthermore, these technologies might allow non-invasive real-time monitoring of therapeutic maneuvers like the fluid challenge or the passive leg raising test.

A note of caution: Cardiac output estimates are obtained with high accuracy and precision by several technologies under experimental conditions, but not necessarily so in the real world. However, for most devices, there is contradictory evidence about the measurement quality. Thus, it is important to investigate the potential improvement of various technologies in terms of signal recording and processing. Moreover, there are limitations to each technology for clinical application. Despite their apparent ease of application, however, for every available non-invasive CO monitoring device, there are clinical situations where CO measurement can be challenging, if not impossible. These settings must be established in detail for each application in research and in clinical practice. More research and development are required to enhance the practicability and clinical application of non-invasive CO monitoring techniques.

Author details

Ashok Kandasamy
Hamad Medical Corporation, Doha, Qatar

*Address all correspondence to: ashokkandasamy76@gmail.com

References

[1] Gurgel ST, do Nascimento P Jr. Maintaining tissue perfusion in high-risk surgical patients: A systematic review of randomized clinical trials. Anesthesia and Analgesia. 2011;**112**:1384-1391

[2] Hamilton MA, Cecconi M, Rhodes A. A systematic review and meta-analysis on the use of preemptive hemodynamic intervention to improve postoperative outcomes in moderate and high-risk surgical patients. Anesthesia and Analgesia. 2011;**112**:1392-1402

[3] Cecconi M, Corredor C, Arulkumaran N, et al. Clinical review: Goal-directed therapy-what is the evidence in surgical patients? The effect on different risk groups. Critical Care. 2013;**17**:209

[4] Grocott MP, Dushianthan A, Hamilton MA, et al. Perioperative increase in global blood flow to explicit defined goals and outcomes after surgery: A Cochrane systematic review. British Journal of Anaesthesia. 2013;**111**:535-548

[5] Aya HD, Cecconi M, Hamilton M, Rhodes A. Goal-directed therapy in cardiac surgery: A systematic review and meta-analysis. British Journal of Anaesthesia. 2013;**110**:510-517

[6] Lees N, Hamilton M, Rhodes A. Clinical review: Goal-directed therapy in high-risk surgical patients. Critical Care. 2009;**13**:231

[7] Pinsky MR. Hemodynamic evaluation and monitoring in the ICU. Chest. 2007;**132**:2020-2029

[8] Vincent JL, De Backer D. Circulatory shock. New England Journal of Medicine. 2014;**370**:583

[9] Cecconi M, Parsons AK, Rhodes A. What is a fluid challenge? Current Opinion in Critical Care. 2011;**17**:290-295

[10] Monnet X, Teboul JL. Passive leg raising. Intensive Care Medicine. 2008;**34**:659-663

[11] Vincent JL. Cardiovascular alterations in septic shock. The Journal of Antimicrobial Chemotherapy. 1998;**41**(Suppl A):9-15

[12] Kubicek WG, Karnegis JN, Patterson RP, Witsoe DA, Mattson RH. Development and evaluation of an impedance cardiac output system. Aerospace Medicine. 1966;**37**:1208-1212

[13] Bernstein DP. A new stroke volume equation for thoracic electrical bioimpedance: Theory and rationale. Critical Care Medicine. 1986;**14**:904-909

[14] Critchley LA, Lee A, Ho AM. A critical review of the ability of continuous cardiac output monitors to measure trends in cardiac output. Anesthesia and Analgesia. 2010;**111**:1180-1192

[15] Raue W, Swierzy M, Koplin G, Schwenk W. Comparison of electrical velocimetry and transthoracic thermodilution technique for cardiac output assessment in critically ill patients. European Journal of Anaesthesiology. 2009;**26**:1067-1071

[16] Wallace AW, Salahieh A, Lawrence A, Spector K, Owens C, Alonso D. Endotracheal cardiac output monitor. Anesthesiology. 2000;**92**:178-189

[17] Raaijmakers E, Faes TJ, Scholten RJ, Goovaerts HG, Heethaar RM. A

meta-analysis of three decades of validating thoracic impedance cardiography. Critical Care Medicine. 1999;**27**:1203-1213

[18] Spiess BD, Patel MA, Soltow LO, Wright IH. Comparison of bioimpedance versus thermodilution cardiac output during cardiac surgery: Evaluation of a second-generation bioimpedance device. Journal of Cardiothoracic and Vascular Anesthesia. 2001;**15**:567-573

[19] Sageman WS, Riffenburgh RH, Spiess BD. Equivalence of bioimpedance and thermodilution in measuring cardiac index after cardiac surgery. Journal of Cardiothoracic and Vascular Anesthesia. 2002;**16**:8-14

[20] Gujjar AR, Muralidhar K, Banakal S, Gupta R, Sathyaprabha TN, Jairaj PS. Non-invasive cardiac output by transthoracic electrical bioimpedance in post-cardiac surgery patients: Comparison with thermodilution method. Journal of Clinical Monitoring and Computing. 2008;**22**:175-180

[21] Chakravarthy M, Rajeev S, Jawali V. Cardiac index value measurement by invasive, semi-invasive and non-invasive techniques: A prospective study in postoperative off pump coronary artery bypass surgery patients. Journal of Clinical Monitoring and Computing. 2009;**23**:175-180

[22] Simon R, Desebbe O, Henaine R, Bastien O, Lehot JJ, Cannesson M. Comparison of ICG thoracic bioimpedance cardiac output monitoring system in patients undergoing cardiac surgery with pulmonary artery cardiac output measurements. Annales Françaises d'Anesthèsie et de Rèanimation. 2009;**28**:537-541

[23] Engoren M, Barbee D. Comparison of cardiac output determined by bioimpedance, thermodilution, and the Fick method. American Journal of Critical Care. 2005;**14**:40-45

[24] Heringlake M, Handke U, Hanke T, et al. Lack of agreement between thermodilution and electrical velocimetry cardiac output measurements. Intensive Care Medicine. 2007;**33**:2168-2172

[25] Ball TR, Culp BC, Patel V, Gloyna DF, Ciceri DP, Culp WC Jr. Comparison of the endotracheal cardiac output monitor to thermodilution in cardiac surgery patients. Journal of Cardiothoracic and Vascular Anesthesia. 2010;**24**:762-766

[26] Maus TM, Reber B, Banks DA, Berry A, Guerrero E, Manecke GR. Cardiac output determination from endotracheally measured impedance cardiography: Clinical evaluation of endotracheal cardiac output monitor. Journal of Cardiothoracic and Vascular Anesthesia. 2011;**25**:770-775

[27] Moller-Sorensen H, Hansen KL, Ostergaard M, Andersen LW, Moller K. Lack of agreement and trending ability of the endotracheal cardiac output monitor compared with thermodilution. Acta Anaesthesiologica Scandinavica. 2012;**56**:433-440

[28] van der Kleij SC, Koolen BB, Newhall DA, et al. Clinical evaluation of a new tracheal impedance cardiography method. Anaesthesia. 2012;**67**:729-733

[29] Critchley LA, Calcroft RM, Tan PY, Kew J, Critchley JA. The effect of lung injury and excessive lung fluid, on impedance cardiac output measurements, in the critically ill. Intensive Care Medicine. 2000;**26**:679-685

[30] Critchley LA, Peng ZY, Fok BS, James AE. The effect of peripheral

resistance on impedance cardiography measurements in the anesthetized dog. Anesthesia and Analgesia. 2005;**100**:1708-1712

[31] Sathyaprabha TN, Pradhan C, Rashmi G, Thennarasu K, Raju TR. Non-invasive cardiac output measurement by transthoracic electrical bioimpedance: Influence of age and gender. Journal of Clinical Monitoring and Computing. 2008;**22**:401-408

[32] Chamos C, Vele L, Hamilton M, Cecconi M. Less invasive methods of advanced hemodynamic monitoring: Principles, devices, and their role in the perioperative hemodynamic optimization. Perioperative Medicine. 2013;**2**:19

[33] Marik PE. Non-invasive cardiac output monitors: A state-of the-art review. Journal of Cardiothoracic and Vascular Anesthesia. 2013;**27**:121-134

[34] Keren H, Burkhoff D, Squara P. Evaluation of a non-invasive continuous cardiac output monitoring system based on thoracic bioreactance. American Journal of Physiology. Heart and Circulatory Physiology. 2007;**293**:H583-H589

[35] Squara P, Denjean D, Estagnasie P, Brusset A, Dib JC, Dubois C. Non-invasive cardiac output monitoring (NICOM): A clinical validation. Intensive Care Medicine. 2007;**33**:1191-1194

[36] Raval NY, Squara P, Cleman M, Yalamanchili K, Winklmaier M, Burkhoff D. Multicenter evaluation of noninvasive cardiac output measurement by bioreactance technique. Journal of Clinical Monitoring and Computing. 2008;**22**:113-119

[37] Squara P, Rotcajg D, Denjean D, Estagnasie P, Brusset A. Comparison of monitoring performance of bioreactance vs. pulse contour during lung recruitment maneuvers. Critical Care. 2009;**13**:R125

[38] Marque S, Cariou A, Chiche JD, Squara P. Comparison between flotrac-vigileo and bioreactance, a totally non-invasive method for cardiac output monitoring. Critical Care. 2009;**13**:R73

[39] Kober D, Trepte C, Petzoldt M, et al. Cardiac index assessment using bioreactance in patients undergoing cytoreductive surgery in ovarian carcinoma. Journal of Clinical Monitoring and Computing. 2013;**27**:621-627

[40] Lee AJ, Cohn JH, Ranasinghe JS. Cardiac output assessed by invasive and minimally invasive techniques. Anesthesiology Research and Practice. 2011;**2011**:1-17. DOI: 10.1155

[41] Nguyen LS, Squara P. Non-invasive monitoring of cardiac output in critical care medicine. Front Med (Lausanne). 2017;**4**:200

[42] Kotake Y, Yamada T, Nagata H, Suzuki T, Serita R, Katori N, et al. Improved accuracy of cardiac output estimation by the partial CO_2 rebreathing method. Journal of Clinical Monitoring and Computing. 2009;**23**:149-155

[43] Dong L, Wang JA, Jiang CY. Validation of the use of foreign gas rebreathing method for non-invasive determination of cardiac output in heart disease patients. Journal of Zhejiang University. Science. B. 2005;**6**:1157-1162

[44] Benatar SR, Hewlett AM, Nunn JF. The use of iso-shunt lines for control of oxygen therapy. British Journal of Anaesthesia. 1973;**45**:711-718

[45] de Abreu MG, Geiger S, Winkler T, Ragaller M, Pfeiffer T, Leutheuser D, et al. Evaluation of a new device for

noninvasive measurement of nonshunted pulmonary capillary blood flow in patients with acute lung injury. Intensive Care Medicine. 2002;**28**:318-323

[46] Rocco M, Spadetta G, Morelli A, Dell'Utri D, Porzi P, Conti G, et al. A comparative evaluation of thermodilution and partial CO_2 rebreathing techniques for cardiac output assessment in critically ill patients during assisted ventilation. Intensive Care Medicine. 2004;**30**:82-87

[47] Lang CC, Karlin P, Haythe J, Tsao L, Mancini DM. Ease of noninvasive measurement of cardiac output coupled with peak VO_2 determination at rest and during exercise in patients with heart failure. The American Journal of Cardiology. 2007;**99**:404-405

[48] Palmers PJ, Vidts W, Ameloot K, Cordemans C, Van Regenmortel N, De Laet I, et al. Assessment of three minimally invasive continuous cardiac output measurement methods in critically ill patients and a review of the literature. Anaesthesiology Intensive Therapy. 2012;**44**:188-199

[49] Opotowsky AR, Hess E, Maron BA, Brittain EL, Baron AE, Maddox TM, et al. Thermodilution vs estimated fick cardiac output measurement in clinical practice: An analysis of mortality from the veterans affairs clinical assessment, reporting, and tracking (VA CART) program and Vanderbilt University. JAMA Cardiology. 2017;**2**(10):1090-1099

[50] Ishihara H, Okawa H, Tanabe K, et al. A new non-invasive continuous cardiac output trend solely utilizing routine cardiovascular monitors. Journal of Clinical Monitoring and Computing. 2004;**18**:313-320

[51] Yamada T, Tsutsui M, Sugo Y, et al. Multicenter study verifying a method of non-invasive continuous cardiac output measurement using pulse wave transit time: A comparison with intermittent bolus thermodilution cardiac output. Anesthesia and Analgesia. 2012;**115**:82-87

[52] Ball TR, Tricinella AP, Kimbrough BA, et al. Accuracy of non-invasive estimated continuous cardiac output (esCCO) compared to thermodilution cardiac output: A pilot study in cardiac patients. Journal of Cardiothoracic and Vascular Anesthesia. 2013;**27**:1128-1132

[53] Ishihara H, Sugo Y, Tsutsui M, et al. The ability of a new continuous cardiac output monitor to measure trends in cardiac output following implementation of a patient information calibration and an automated exclusion algorithm. Journal of Clinical Monitoring and Computing. 2012;**26**:465-471

[54] Bataille B, Bertuit M, Mora M, et al. Comparison of esCCO and transthoracic echocardiography for non-invasive measurement of cardiac output intensive care. British Journal of Anaesthesia. 2012;**109**:879-886

[55] Janelle GM, Gravenstein N. An accuracy evaluation of the T-line tensymeter (continuous non-invasive blood pressure management device) versus conventional invasive radial artery monitoring in surgical patients. Anesthesia and Analgesia. 2006;**102**:484-490

[56] Szmuk P, Pivalizza E, Warters RD, Ezri T, Gebhard R. An evaluation of the T-line tensymeter continuous non-invasive blood pressure device during induced hypotension. Anaesthesia. 2008;**63**:307-312

[57] Dueck R, Goedje O, Clopton P. Non-invasive continuous beat-to-beat radial artery pressure via TL-200

applanation tonometry. Journal of Clinical Monitoring and Computing. 2012;**26**:75-83

[58] Saugel B, Fassio F, Hapfelmeier A, Meidert AS, Schmid RM, Huber W. The T-line TL-200 system for continuous non-invasive blood pressure measurement in medical intensive care unit patients. Intensive Care Medicine. 2012;**38**:1471-1477

[59] Meidert AS, Huber W, Hapfelmeier A, et al. Evaluation of the radial artery applanation tonometry technology for continuous non-invasive blood pressure monitoring compared with central aortic blood pressure measurements in patients with multiple organ dysfunction syndrome. Journal of Critical Care. 2013;**28**:908-912

[60] Saugel B, Meidert AS, Hapfelmeier A, Eyer F, Schmid RM, Huber W. Non-invasive continuous arterial pressure measurement based on radial artery tonometry in the intensive care unit: A method comparison study using the T-line TL-200 pro device. British Journal of Anaesthesia. 2013;**111**:185-190

[61] Meidert AS, Huber W, Muller JN, et al. Radial artery applanation tonometry for continuous non-invasive arterial pressure monitoring in intensive care unit patients: Comparison with invasively assessed radial arterial pressure. British Journal of Anaesthesia. 2014;**112**:521-528

[62] Pressman GL, Newgard PM. A transducer for the continuous external measurement of arterial blood pressure. IEEE Transactions on Biomedical Engineering. 1963;**10**:73-81

[63] Drzewiecki GM, Melbin J, Noordergraaf A. Arterial tonometry: Review and analysis. Journal of Biomechanics. 1983;**16**:141-152

[64] Kemmotsu O, Ueda M, Otsuka H, Yamamura T, Winter DC, Eckerle JS. Arterial tonometry for non-invasive, continuous blood pressure monitoring during anesthesia. Anesthesiology. 1991;**75**:333-340

[65] Kemmotsu O, Ueda M, Otsuka H, et al. Blood pressure measurement by arterial tonometry in controlled hypotension. Anesthesia and Analgesia. 1991;**73**:54-58

[66] Sato T, Nishinaga M, Kawamoto A, Ozawa T, Takatsuji H. Accuracy of a continuous blood pressure monitor based on arterial tonometry. Hypertension. 1993;**21**:866-874

[67] Siegel LC, Brock-Utne JG, Brodsky JB. Comparison of arterial tonometry with radial artery catheter measurements of blood pressure in anesthetized patients. Anesthesiology. 1994;**81**:578-584

[68] Searle NR, Gauthier J, Sahab P. An evaluation of the N-CAT, a new arterial tonometer. Canadian Journal of Anaesthesia. 1995;**42**:526-531

[69] Saugel B, Meidert AS, Langwieser N, et al. An auto-calibrating algorithm for non-invasive cardiac output determination based on the analysis of an arterial pressure waveform recorded with radial artery applanation tonometry: A proof-of-concept pilot analysis. Journal of Clinical Monitoring and Computing. 2014;**28**:357-362

[70] Thom O, Taylor DM, Wolfe RE, Cade J, Myles P, Krum H, et al. Comparison of a supra-sternal cardiac output monitor (USCOM) with the pulmonary artery catheter. British Journal of Anaesthesia. 2009;**103**:800-804

[71] Boyle M, Steel L, Flynn GM, Murgo M, Nicholson L, O'Brien M, et al. Assessment of the clinical utility of an ultrasonic monitor of cardiac output (the USCOM) and agreement with thermodilution measurement. Critical Care and Resuscitation. 2009;**11**:198-203

[72] Nguyen HB, Banta DP, Stewart G, Kim T, Bansal R, Anholm J, et al. Cardiac index measurements by transcutaneous Doppler ultrasound and transthoracic echocardiography in adult and pediatric emergency patients. Journal of Clinical Monitoring and Computing. 2010;**24**:237-247

[73] Via G, Hussain A, Wells M, Reardon R, ElBarbary M, Noble VE, et al. International evidence-based recommendations for focused cardiac ultrasound. Journal of the American Society of Echocardiography. 2014;**27**(683):e1-e33

[74] Horster S, Stemmler HJ, Strecker N, Brettner F, Hausmann A, Cnossen J, et al. Cardiac output measurements in septic patients: Comparing the accuracy of USCOM to PiCCO. Critical Care Research and Practice. 2012;**2012**:270631

[75] Kerstens MK, Wijnberge M, Geerts B, Vlaar A, Veelo D. Non-invasive cardiac output monitoring techniques in the ICU. Netherlands Journal of Critical Care. 2018;**26**:104-110

Chapter 13

Hemodynamic and Monitoring in Pregnancy

Seema Nahid, Fateen Shareef, Umm E. Amara, Salma Mehjabeen, Umme Nashrah, Roshan Afsha, M. Abdul Wasay and Azha Fatima

Abstract

This chapter reviews the physiological changes of pregnancy, their impact on maternal hemodynamics, and the role of invasive and non-invasive monitoring techniques. It integrates evidence-based recommendations from ASA, AHA, ESC, and WHO to connect physiological understanding with clinical monitoring strategies. Pregnancy produces major cardiovascular adaptations, including expanded plasma volume, increased cardiac output through enhanced stroke volume and heart rate, and reduced systemic vascular resistance. Aortocaval compression further modifies preload, afterload, and venous return, influencing overall perfusion. These adaptations may mimic or mask disease, complicating the interpretation of vital signs, laboratory findings, and imaging results. A structured, risk-based approach tailors monitoring intensity to maternal condition across antenatal, intrapartum, perioperative, and postpartum stages. Core noninvasive modalities—blood pressure, ECG, pulse oximetry, and capnography—form the foundation of safe obstetric anesthesia practice, while bedside echocardiography refines the evaluation of ventricular function, filling status, and pulmonary pressures without radiation exposure. When greater precision is required, invasive arterial lines enable beat-to-beat pressure measurement and arterial blood gas analysis. Central venous and pulmonary artery catheters are reserved for complex cardiopulmonary disease or refractory shock. Advanced hemodynamic systems, such as arterial waveform analysis and transpulmonary thermodilution, provide the continuous assessment of cardiac output, preload, and afterload, guiding individualized fluid and vasopressor therapy in severe preeclampsia, obstetric hemorrhage, or cardiomyopathy. Effective collaboration among anesthesiologists, obstetricians, and intensivists ensures accurate interpretation and timely response to evolving physiology. Integrating physiological insight with guideline-based monitoring enhances early recognition of deterioration and optimizes maternal and neonatal outcomes.

Keywords: pregnancy, hemodynamic monitoring, obstetric anesthesia, cardiovascular adaptations, maternal outcomes, fetal outcomes

1. Introduction

Pregnancy is associated with significant physiological changes in blood pressure, heart rate, and cardiac output, requiring tailored hemodynamic monitoring in pregnancy for the early detection and management of maternal cardiovascular compromise, as well as improved maternal and fetal outcomes. Some of the physiological adaptations of normal pregnancy can unmask or worsen preexisting disease, confounding the diagnosis of heart disease. Thus, an understanding of pregnancy adaptations is essential to avoid misinterpretation. Women with underlying cardiac disease may not always accommodate these changes, and ventricular dysfunction leads to cardiogenic heart failure [1].

Traditionally, anesthesia practice has been grounded in vigilance and continuous clinical assessment of the patient. The term "monitoring" itself comes from the Latin monere, meaning to warn, remind, or caution. Although there is limited high-grade evidence that electronic monitors alone reduce morbidity and mortality, modern monitoring devices do not replace the clinician's responsibility. Instead, they complement it by providing clinical information more rapidly, more frequently, and with greater quantitative precision than physical examination alone.

The purpose of monitoring is to enhance the anesthesiologist's situational awareness, enabling timely recognition and management of clinical problems while guiding therapy. The value of any monitoring method lies in its ability to help maintain the patient's physiology within safe limits. However, the benefits of each technique must be weighed against its costs and potential risks, as invasive monitoring may expose patients to iatrogenic complications if not appropriately justified.

Pregnancy-induced hypervolemia serves multiple purposes: it supports the metabolic demands of the enlarged uterus and its expanded vasculature, ensures adequate nutrients for the growing placenta and fetus, protects against reduced venous return in supine or upright positions, and provides a safety margin against blood loss during delivery.

Over a century ago, Williams noted that pregnancy in women with significant heart disease carries serious risks, including decompensation and death. Today, cardiovascular disease contributes to nearly 26% of pregnancy-related maternal deaths, highlighting the critical importance of careful hemodynamic monitoring. Some women with life-threatening cardiac abnormalities can undergo corrective surgery, after which pregnancy carries a significantly reduced risk. Heart disease in pregnancy remains the leading non-obstetric cause of maternal mortality.

Gestational changes begin soon after the cessation of the bleeding tear drop, when the ovum is fertilized, and pregnancy changes continue throughout, stimulated by the placenta and fetus, which modify every organ system to accommodate the growing fetus.

Physiological changes during gestation are adaptive and necessary to ensure the well-being of both the mother and fetus throughout pregnancy, as well as to prepare the mother to meet the increasing metabolic and circulatory demands. The journey of three trimesters involves every organ system undergoing alteration to facilitate fetal growth and prepare for the delivery and breastfeeding of the newborn beyond the amniotic sac.

2. Background

Pregnancy involves extensive physiological adaptations that affect multiple organ systems, where values considered abnormal outside of gestation may represent normal changes during pregnancy. These modifications can obscure the recognition of underlying medical disorders or intensify their clinical expression. Cardiovascular alterations, particularly changes in preload, afterload, and cardiac function, are central to these adaptations and may significantly influence the course of preexisting heart disease, thereby increasing maternal and fetal risk.

Heart failure symptoms may manifest in pregnant mothers with severe cardiac dysfunction when pregnancy-related increases in blood volume and cardiac output reach their maximum.

Most healthy women are able to adapt easily to these physiological changes, but women with significant heart disease may develop new symptoms or worsening of pre-existing symptoms as they struggle to adapt cardiovascularly. A healthy heart has sufficient reserve to manage the increased load, whereas a diseased heart may fail to compensate.

In women with severe cardiac dysfunction, heart failure may occur as pregnancy-induced hypervolemia and cardiac output peak, most often peripartum, when labor, delivery, or complications such as preeclampsia, hemorrhage, anemia, or sepsis impose additional strain.

The incidence of cardiovascular disease is increasing among women of childbearing age and during pregnancy, driven by factors such as corrected congenital heart disease in women reaching reproductive age and the more frequent diagnosis of new cardiac conditions with advancing medical care. In some cases, life-threatening cardiac abnormalities can be corrected surgically, making subsequent pregnancies considerably safer.

During labor, cardiac output (CO) increases by ~10% due to autotransfusion and pain-induced catecholamines and further rises in the second stage with maternal pushing. It peaks at up to 80% immediately after delivery, resulting from autotransfusion and the relief of aortocaval compression, and then returns to pre-labor levels within one hour.

3. Role of hemodynamic monitoring in pregnancy

Hemodynamic monitoring during pregnancy is crucial for distinguishing physiological changes from pathology, detecting complications early, guiding management in high-risk conditions, and ensuring both maternal stability and fetal well-being [2].

The pursuit of safer anesthetic techniques characterized the late nineteenth and early twentieth centuries. The introduction of electrocardiography, pulse oximetry, blood gas analysis, capnography, and neuromuscular monitoring transformed anesthesia practice, significantly reducing morbidity and mortality. These monitors provided early warning of acute physiological deterioration, allowing intervention before irreversible harm occurred.

The emergence of more advanced and sophisticated monitoring technologies does not diminish the anesthesiologist's responsibility to apply sound clinical judgment. On the contrary, it demands a thorough understanding of these devices to ensure they are utilized safely, accurately, and appropriately.

3.1 Physiological adaptation monitoring

Pregnancy induces significant cardiovascular adaptations, including increased blood volume, elevated cardiac output, reduced systemic vascular resistance,

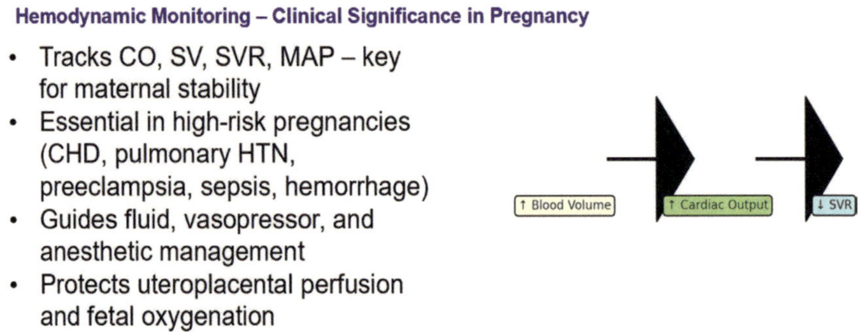

Figure 1.
Hemodynamic monitoring and clinical significance in pregnancy.

and positional hemodynamic effects (**Figure 1**). Careful monitoring is essential to differentiate these normal physiological changes from early manifestations of underlying pathology.

3.2 Early detection of complications

Hemodynamic monitoring in pregnancy plays a pivotal role in differentiating physiological adaptations from pathological changes. It enables the early detection of hypertensive disorders such as gestational hypertension, preeclampsia, and eclampsia, ensuring timely intervention to prevent maternal and fetal morbidity. Monitoring also helps in identifying hypotension, which may occur due to conditions like supine hypotension syndrome or as a complication of neuraxial anesthesia. Furthermore, it assists in recognizing early signs of heart failure, arrhythmias, or decompensation, particularly in women with preexisting structural or acquired heart disease, thereby safeguarding maternal cardiovascular stability and fetal well-being.

3.3 Guidance in high-risk pregnancies

Hemodynamic monitoring is crucial in high-risk pregnancies, particularly in women with congenital or acquired heart disease, pulmonary hypertension, severe preeclampsia, sepsis, or obstetric hemorrhage, where even minor circulatory imbalances can result in significant maternal or fetal compromise. In such cases, monitoring provides essential information to guide individualized fluid therapy, optimize vasopressor use, and titrate medications with precision. This targeted approach not only supports maternal hemodynamic stability but also preserves uteroplacental perfusion, thereby reducing the risk of adverse outcomes for both mother and fetus.

3.4 Intrapartum and perioperative safety

Continuous hemodynamic monitoring during labor, cesarean delivery, and critical care is essential to ensure maternal stability and maintain adequate fetal perfusion. Pregnancy and delivery are characterized by rapid and sometimes dramatic cardiovascular changes, particularly during uterine contractions, the stress of delivery, and the immediate postpartum period when autotransfusion from the contracted uterus significantly increases circulating blood volume. Early detection of these

Hemodynamic monitoring in pregnancy	
Indications	**Contraindications/limitations**
• Track physiological adaptations (↑CO, ↑volume, and ↓SVR) • Early detection of complications (HTN, preeclampsia, hypotension, heart failure, and arrhythmias) • High-risk pregnancies (CHD, pulmonary HTN, severe preeclampsia, sepsis, and hemorrhage) • Intrapartum and perioperative monitoring (labor, cesarean, and critical illness) • Guide fluids, vasopressors, and anesthetic drugs • Protect maternal stability and uteroplacental perfusion	• No absolute contraindications – type depends on modality (invasive vs. noninvasive) • Invasive monitoring limited by infection risk, coagulopathy, and vascular complications

Table 1.
Hemodynamic monitoring in pregnancy.

hemodynamic shifts allows timely interventions to prevent maternal decompensation, optimize fluid (**Table 1**) and drug therapy, and safeguard uteroplacental blood flow, thereby protecting both maternal and fetal outcomes.

3.5 Protecting maternal and fetal outcomes

It ensures optimal maternal circulation, which is vital for maintaining adequate uteroplacental blood flow and supporting fetal oxygenation, while also minimizing the risk of adverse events through early recognition and timely intervention [3].

4. Monitoring standards

ASA standards mandate continuous basic anesthetic monitoring by qualified personnel, with specific requirements for oxygenation, ventilation, circulation, and temperature to ensure patient safety. Specifically, arterial blood pressure and heart rate must be assessed at least every five minutes in all anesthetized patients.

Intermittent noninvasive blood pressure monitoring typically meets this standard, but continuous monitoring may be necessary in patients with significant comorbidities or during high-risk surgeries.

The American Society of Anesthesiologists (ASA) first issued monitoring standards in 1986, reflecting advances in technology and practice [4]. The current version (effective July 1, 2011) emphasizes regular and frequent monitoring [5], the integration of clinical judgment, and awareness of circumstances that may impact the accuracy or applicability of monitoring systems [6].

Standard I

Qualified anesthesia personnel must be present in the operating room during general anesthesia, regional anesthesia, or monitored anesthesia care. These providers are responsible for continuously monitoring the patient, adjusting anesthetic care, and responding to physiological changes resulting from surgery or drug therapy.

Standard II

Continuous evaluation of the patient's oxygenation, ventilation, circulation, and temperature is required. Key requirements include the following:

1. Oxygenation: During general anesthesia, inspired oxygen concentration should be continuously monitored with an analyzer equipped with a low-concentration alarm, while pulse oximetry provides a quantitative assessment of blood oxygenation, ensuring patient safety throughout anesthesia care.

2. Ventilation [7]: Ventilation must be continuously assessed in all anesthetics, using clinical signs and, whenever possible, capnography with tidal volume monitoring in general anesthesia. In regional or local anesthesia, clinical observation is sufficient, while moderate or deep sedation requires both clinical assessment and exhaled CO_2 monitoring, unless technically limited. Clinical signs and the detection of expired CO_2 should always confirm proper placement of the airway device. Mechanical ventilation must include a device to detect breathing system disconnections, ensuring patient safety.

3. *Circulation* [8]: Circulatory monitoring requires continuous ECG display with blood pressure and heart rate measured at least every five minutes, while overall circulatory function should be continually assessed using methods such as pulse palpation, heart sound auscultation, intra-arterial pressure tracing, peripheral pulse ultrasound, plethysmography, or oximetry.

4. Temperature: Continuous temperature monitoring must always be available during anesthesia and is mandatory in situations where significant temperature changes are intended, anticipated, or suspected, ensuring early detection and management of hypothermia, hyperthermia, or malignant hyperthermia to maintain patient safety.

4.1 Monitoring goals

- Early detection of hypotension, hypovolemia, or cardiac decompression [9]
- Fluid therapy
- Vasoactive drug administration
- Adequate maternal and fetal perfusion
- Minimize perioperative and peripartum complications

4.2 Monitoring parameters

- Heart rate, blood pressure, and oxygen saturation
- Cardiac output and stroke volume
- Central venous pressure with a central venous catheter [10]
- Pulmonary artery pressure (in selected cardiac cases)
- Indirect perfusion monitors (urine output and Lactate)

5. Hemodynamic changes in pregnancy and clinical significance

5.1 Cardiovascular system

Anatomical changes: The gravid uterus elevates the diaphragm, displacing the heart upward, outward, and slightly rotated on its long axis to the left. The apex beat shifts to the fourth intercostal space, ~2.5 cm lateral to the midclavicular line. Pregnancy utilizes a mixture of eccentric and concentric ventricular remodeling (**Figure 2**).

5.2 Physiological changes

Cardiac output – An increase in cardiac output from the fifth week of gestation until term is reflected as reduced systemic vascular resistance with increased stroke volume and heart rate, ensuring adequate perfusion of maternal organs and fetoplacental circulation. The rise in cardiac output during pregnancy results from expanded blood volume and the higher oxygen demand driven by increased metabolic activity. These adaptations may be profound in multiple gestations [12].

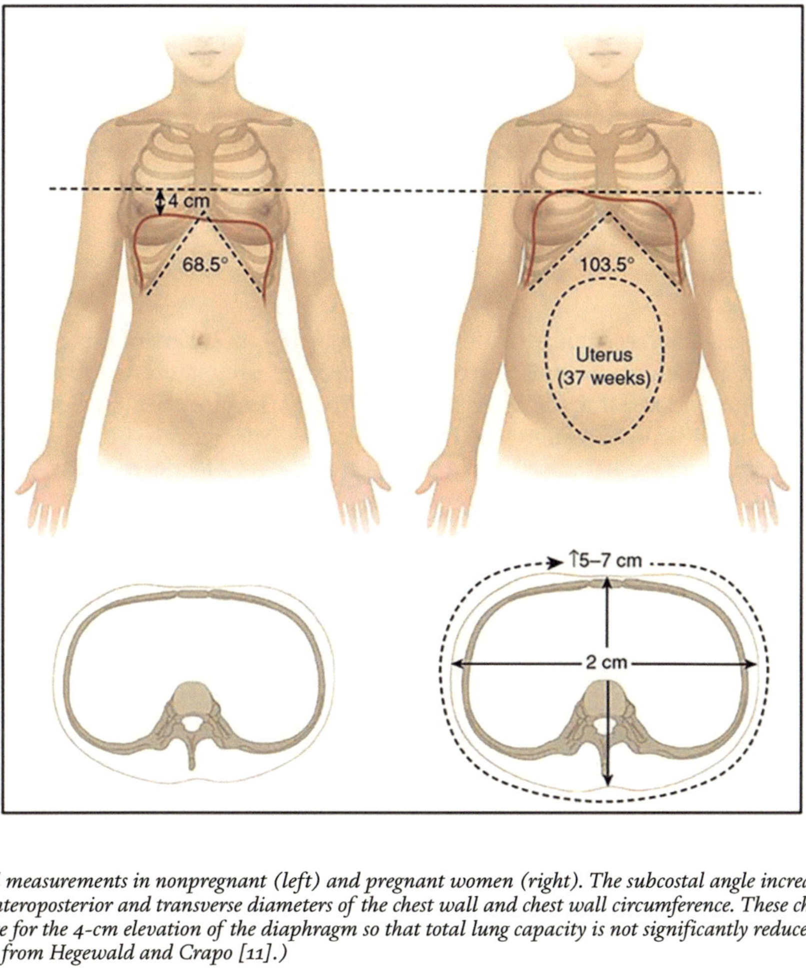

Figure 2.
Chest wall measurements in nonpregnant (left) and pregnant women (right). The subcostal angle increases, as does the anteroposterior and transverse diameters of the chest wall and chest wall circumference. These changes compensate for the 4-cm elevation of the diaphragm so that total lung capacity is not significantly reduced. (Redrawn from Hegewald and Crapo [11].)

Cardiac output	Gestational age
CO starts to increase	Fifth week of gestation
Peaks	30–34 weeks
Term gestation	Stable till delivery (lateral recumbent)
Labor	• 50% ↑ from baseline • With an additional increase of 15–30% during contractions • Autotransfusion of blood from the placenta occurs in the third stage of labor
Immediate postpartum	70% ↑ from baseline (autotransfusion +↑MAP)
Postpartum	• 1-hour postpartum returns to prelabor level • 4 weeks return to pre-pregnant level

Table 2.
Physiological adaptations in pregnancy.

Blood volume: increases throughout pregnancy by 45–50% greater than pre-pregnancy values at term. This represents an increase in both red cell volume and relatively greater plasma volume, resulting in physiological anemia.

Systemic vascular resistance is reduced due to peripheral vasodilatation mediated by progesterone, estrogen, and prostacyclin (**Table 2**).

Central venous and pulmonary artery pressures are unchanged during pregnancy, although central venous pressure is increased during labor and may remain elevated for a few hours postpartum.

5.3 Blood pressure

Systemic vascular resistance (SVR) decreases by about 21% in pregnancy, primarily due to the smooth muscle-relaxing effects of progesterone, nitric oxide, prostaglandins, and atrial natriuretic peptide (ANP). Despite the significant rise in cardiac output (**Table 3**), maternal blood pressure falls because BP = CO × SVR. Consequently, diastolic BP and mean arterial pressure (MAP) decrease by 5–10 mmHg, mirroring the reduction in SVR.

Hemodynamic changes in pregnancy		
Parameters	**Increased**	**Decreased**
Cardiac output	+40%	
Stroke volume	+27%	
Heart rate	+17%	
Venous pressure	+100%	
Systemic vascular resistance (SVR)		−21%
Pulmonary vascular resistance		−34%

Table 3.
Hemodynamic changes of pregnancy.

DOI: http://dx.doi.org/10.5772/intechopen.1013589

5.4 Venous pressure

Antecubital venous pressure remains unchanged during pregnancy, whereas femoral venous pressure rises significantly, particularly in the later months. This increase is caused by the compression of the common iliac veins by the gravid uterus, which is more pronounced on the right side due to uterine dextrorotation. Femoral venous pressure rises from 8 to 10 cm H_2O in the nonpregnant state to about 25 cm H_2O in the lying position and up to 80–100 cm H_2O when standing [13].

5.5 Central hemodynamics

Despite increases in blood volume, cardiac output, and heart rate during pregnancy, there is no significant change in CVP, MAP, or PCWP. This stability is due to a marked reduction in systemic vascular resistance (SVR), pulmonary vascular resistance (PVR), and colloid osmotic pressure.

6. Monitoring modalities

Non-invasive (**Table 4**)

- Blood pressure

Comparison of monitoring modalities in pregnancy	
ECG monitoring	*Pulse oximetry*
• Detects arrhythmias (SVT, AF, ectopics, and blocks) • Essential in high-risk women (CHD, cardiomyopathy, and valves) • Guides therapy (QT, ischemia, pacing, and cardioversion) • Evaluates palpitations, syncope, chest pain • Intrapartum/postpartum safety	• Monitors maternal oxygenation • Early hypoxemia detection (PE, asthma, pneumonia, and cardiac disease) • Intrapartum and perioperative monitoring • Critical care use (cardiac, pulmonary, and sepsis) • Supports fetal well-being via maternal oxygenation
NIBP monitoring	*Hemodynamic monitoring*
• Routine BP checks (antenatal, labor, and postpartum) • Detects hypertension, preeclampsia, and eclampsia • Essential in high-risk (chronic HTN, renal, diabetes, and cardiac) • Intrapartum safety (hypotension after neuraxial and surges) • Guides fluids, anti-hypertensives, and anesthetics • Protects maternal-fetal perfusion	• Tracks physiological adaptations (↑ CO, ↑ volume, and ↓ SVR) • Detects complications (HTN, preeclampsia, HF, and arrhythmias) • High-risk: CHD, pulmonary HTN, sepsis, and hemorrhage • Intrapartum/periop: guides fluids, drugs, and vasopressors • Ensures maternal stability and uteroplacental perfusion

Table 4.
Monitoring modalities in pregnancy.

- o Manual
- o Automated
- ECG (heart rate and rhythm) [14]
- Oxygen saturation (SpO2)
- Doppler (non-invasive cardiac output monitoring)
- Exercise testing
- Holter monitoring

Invasive monitoring

- Arterial line for continuous blood pressure monitoring and oxygen saturation
- Central venous pressure monitoring (CVP)
- Pulmonary artery catheter (in severe cardiac disease) [15]
- Right heart catheterization
- Advanced hemodynamic monitors (e.g., FloTrac, PiCCO)
- Edwards monitor
- Cardioversion
- Cardiopulmonary bypass

6.1 Non-invasive blood pressure monitoring in pregnancy (NIBP)

NIBP monitoring in pregnancy is a simple, safe, and an essential tool for early detection of hypertensive disorders, guiding therapy, and ensuring maternal and fetal well-being.

Noninvasive blood pressure monitoring is appropriate for patients with medical comorbidities who do not necessitate continuous blood pressure monitoring. The measurement interval should be tailored to the patient's clinical condition and the appropriate size cuff (**Figure 3**) [16].

Role of non-invasive blood pressure (NIBP) monitoring in pregnancy:

Noninvasive blood pressure monitoring is a safe, simple, and widely used tool for routine surveillance during antenatal care, labor, and the postpartum period. It allows early detection of hypertensive disorders such as gestational hypertension (**Table 5**), preeclampsia, and eclampsia and is essential in high-risk women with chronic hypertension, renal disease, diabetes, or cardiac conditions. During labor, it enhances safety by detecting hypotension after neuraxial block or hypertensive surges, while also guiding therapy through the titration of antihypertensives, fluids, and anesthetic drugs. Ultimately, it protects both mother and fetus by ensuring adequate uteroplacental perfusion and oxygenation [17].

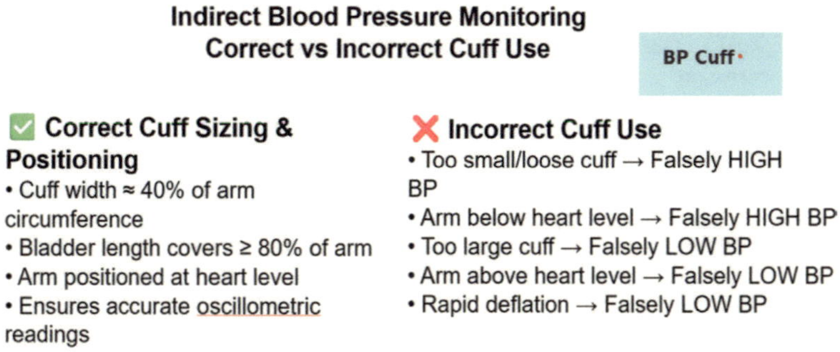

Figure 3.
Blood pressure cuff sizing.

Role of non-invasive blood pressure (NIBP) monitoring in pregnancy
Routine surveillance
Monitors BP during antenatal visits, labor, and postpartum
Early detection
Identifies gestational hypertension, preeclampsia, and eclampsia
High-risk monitoring
Essential for chronic HTN, renal disease, diabetes, and cardiac conditions
Intrapartum safety
Detects hypotension after neuraxial block or hypertensive surges
Guides therapy
Assists in titration of antihypertensives, fluids, and anesthetic agents
Maternal and fetal protection
Maintains uteroplacental perfusion and fetal oxygenation

Table 5.
Non-invasive blood pressure monitoring in pregnancy.

Non-invasive blood pressure (NIBP) monitoring can be performed using automated oscillometric devices for continuous, user-friendly measurements, or manual auscultatory methods for confirmation and accuracy in selected cases (**Table 6**).

6.1.1 Indications

Periods of marked hemodynamic variability may necessitate more frequent blood pressure measurements to ensure optimal management. In prolonged surgical cases, repositioning the blood pressure cuffs every few hours is advisable to minimize the risk of neuropraxia or skin injury.

6.1.2 Contraindications

Noninvasive blood pressure cuffs can cause iatrogenic injury even in healthy limbs. Repeated cycling during prolonged surgery may result in skin abrasions or contusions, which can be reduced by placing a light dressing under the cuff. The radial

Manual vs. automated NIBP monitoring	
Manual BP measurement	**Automated NIBP (oscillometric)**
Estimates systolic BP by palpating the return of an arterial pulse while cuff deflates.	Uses oscillometric method to detect arterial wall oscillations and estimate BP.
Relies on clinician skill, simple equipment, useful when oscillometry is not reliable.	Provides automated, repeatable readings, widely used in perioperative care.

Table 6.
NIBP monitoring manual vs. automated.

nerve, which spirals around the humerus, is also vulnerable to neuropraxia from prolonged (**Table 7**) mechanical compression. To minimize these risks, relocating the cuff every few hours during lengthy procedures is advisable [18].

6.1.3 Clinical significance of blood pressure monitoring

Mean arterial pressure in pregnancy (MAP)

- $MAP \approx DBP + 1/3\ (SBP - DBP)$
- Represents average arterial pressure during a single cardiac cycle
- Reflects tissue perfusion more accurately than SBP or DBP alone
- Normal in pregnancy: slightly reduced in mid-pregnancy due to ↓SVR
- Critical for maintaining uteroplacental perfusion

6.1.4 Physiological pulse pressure in pregnancy

Pregnancy is characterized by an increase in stroke volume and cardiac output, accompanied by a reduction in systemic vascular resistance (SVR) [19]. These hemodynamic adaptations result in a slight widening of pulse pressure compared to

Non-invasive blood pressure (NIBP) monitoring	
Indications	**Contraindications/limitations**
• Routine surveillance (antenatal visits, labor, and postpartum) • Early detection of gestational hypertension, preeclampsia, and eclampsia • High-risk women (chronic HTN, renal disease, diabetes, and cardiac disease) • Intrapartum safety (neuraxial-induced hypotension and hypertensive surges) • Guides fluid, antihypertensive, and anesthetic therapy • Maternal-fetal protection (maintains uteroplacental perfusion)	• Few limitations – safe and noninvasive • Inaccurate in arrhythmias (e.g., AF) • Frequent cycling may cause discomfort

Table 7.
Indications and contraindications of non-invasive blood pressure monitoring.

the non-pregnant state, reflecting the physiological adjustments required to support maternal and fetal circulation.

6.1.4.1 Widened pulse pressure (>60 mmHg)

A widened pulse pressure may indicate conditions such as aortic regurgitation, hyperthyroidism, anemia, or patent ductus arteriosus, as well as other high-output states, including normal physiological changes during pregnancy. While a modest increase in pulse pressure is expected during pregnancy (**Table 8**), an excessive widening beyond physiological limits should raise concern for underlying pathology and prompt further evaluation.

6.1.4.2 Narrow pulse pressure (<25 mmHg)

A narrowed pulse pressure may indicate serious conditions such as hypovolemia, hemorrhage, shock, cardiac tamponade, or severe heart failure. In obstetric practice, it is particularly significant as a narrowing pulse pressure can serve as an early marker of hypovolemia, most notably in cases of postpartum hemorrhage, allowing for prompt (**Table 8**) recognition and intervention [20].

6.1.5 Monitoring

Pulse pressure (PP) serves as a valuable parameter for assessing stroke volume and arterial compliance, providing insight into cardiovascular function. When interpreted in conjunction with mean arterial pressure (MAP), it helps determine the adequacy of tissue perfusion. In high-risk pregnancies, such as those complicated by preeclampsia or underlying cardiac disease, continuous arterial line monitoring enables real-time PP analysis, facilitating timely interventions to optimize maternal hemodynamics and safeguard fetal well-being (**Figure 4**).

6.2 ECG adaptations in pregnancy

ECG monitoring in pregnancy is vital for detecting arrhythmias, guiding treatment, ensuring perioperative and intrapartum safety, and protecting both mother and fetus in high-risk conditions [21].

Normal pregnancy causes an alteration in the electrocardiogram, with an average 15-degree left-axis deviation, as the diaphragm is elevated, which alters the

Significance in pregnancy
• SVR = (MAP - CVP) × 80/CO
• Reflects resistance offered by systemic circulation
• Pregnancy: ↓SVR due to progesterone, NO, and prostaglandins
• Helps explain ↓MAP despite ↑CO
• Low SVR is critical to accommodate ↑blood volume without hypertension
• Abnormal rise in SVR → preeclampsia and hypertension

Table 8.
Significance of pulse pressure in pregnancy.

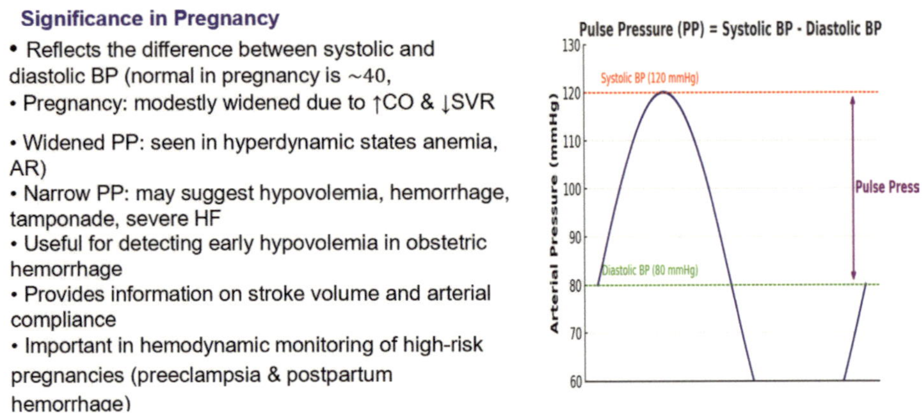

Figure 4.
Pulse pressure graph.

heart's position; however, it does not alter ECG voltage. These physiological changes (**Figure 5**) necessitate a cautious approach when diagnosing heart disease in pregnancy.

- Reduced mean PR interval
- Increased heart rate
- Left axis deviation

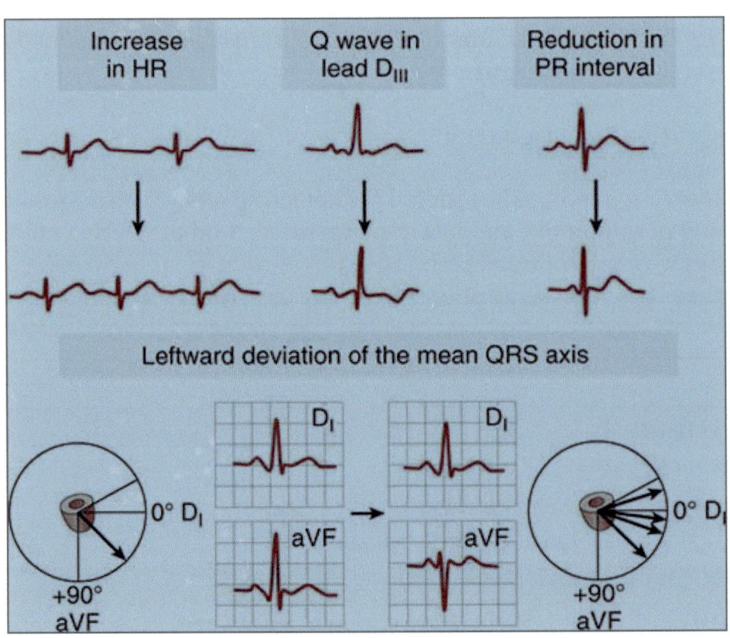

Figure 5.
Normal electrocardiograph (ECG) adaptations during pregnancy, including a reduced mean PR interval, increased heart rate, left axis deviation, inverted or flattened T waves, and a Q wave in lead DIII. (Reproduced with permission from [22, 23].)

- Inverted or flattened T waves in lead III and V1–V3
- Q wave in lead II and III and avF

The incidence of arrhythmias increases during pregnancy in women with or without structural heart disease. This is mainly attributed to atrial and ventricular stretch from increased intravascular volume and a higher resting heart rate. Autonomic and hormonal changes of pregnancy may also contribute. Holter monitoring frequently shows premature atrial and ventricular contractions (**Table 9**).

ECG monitoring facilitates early detection of atrial fibrillation in pregnant women with stenotic valvular lesions (such as aortic or mitral stenosis) or with hypertrophic cardiomyopathy and associated diastolic dysfunction leading to significant hemodynamic compromise, especially in pregnant women with stenotic valvular lesions (such as aortic or mitral stenosis) or with hypertrophic cardiomyopathy and associated diastolic dysfunction.

6.2.1 ECG monitoring – Clinical significance in pregnancy

6.2.1.1 Detection of arrhythmias

Pregnancy increases the risk of arrhythmias such as atrial and ventricular ectopics, supraventricular tachycardia, atrial fibrillation, and conduction abnormalities [24]. Continuous ECG monitoring is therefore essential, as it enables the early identification of rhythm disturbances and allows for timely intervention to protect maternal and fetal outcomes (**Table 10**).

6.2.1.2 Evaluation of high-risk patients

ECG monitoring is essential in women with congenital heart disease, cardiomyopathies, valvular disease, or pulmonary hypertension, as it facilitates the early detection of rhythm or conduction abnormalities and allows for the prompt recognition of cardiovascular decompensation.

Role of ECG monitoring in pregnancy
Detection
Identifies arrhythmias (SVT, AF, ventricular ectopics, and blocks)
High-risk use
Essential in congenital/structural heart disease, cardiomyopathy, and prosthetic valves
Guiding Management
Monitors QT, conduction, ischemia; guides drugs, pacing, and cardioversion
Symptom evaluation
Assesses palpitations, syncope, chest pain, and dyspnea
Labour and postpartum
Continuous ECG ensures early detection of decompensation or arrhythmias

Table 9.
Role of ECG monitoring in pregnancy.

ECG monitoring in pregnancy	
Indications	**Contraindications/limitations**
• Detection of arrhythmias (SVT, AF, ectopics, and blocks) • High-risk women (CHD, cardiomyopathy, and prosthetic valves) • Guides therapy (QT, ischemia, pacing, and cardioversion) • Evaluation of palpitations, syncope, chest pain, and dyspnea • Continuous monitoring during labour and postpartum in high-risk women	• No absolute contraindications (safe and noninvasive) • Artifacts due to motion, poor electrode contact • Misinterpretation due to normal pregnancy-related ECG changes

Table 10.
Indications and contraindications of ECG monitoring in pregnancy.

6.2.1.3 Guidance in therapy

Continuous ECG monitoring is invaluable for assessing the effects of antiarrhythmic medications, guiding electrolyte management, and evaluating the outcomes of interventions such as pacing or cardioversion. It also facilitates the early detection of QT prolongation, ischemia, or conduction delays, enabling clinicians to promptly adjust therapy and minimize the risk of complications in both mother and fetus (**Table 11**).

6.2.1.4 Perioperative and intrapartum monitoring

Continuous ECG monitoring during labor, cesarean section, or anesthesia in high-risk pregnancies is vital for enhancing maternal safety, as it enables the rapid detection of arrhythmia or ischemic changes and allows for immediate intervention [25].

6.2.1.5 Protects maternal-fetal outcomes

Early detection and prompt correction of maternal cardiac instability help maintain uteroplacental perfusion and minimize fetal risk.

6.3 Pulse oximeter monitoring in pregnancy hemodynamics

Pulse oximetry is indicated in almost all pregnant women requiring monitoring (**Table 12**), especially high-risk or critically ill patients. It has no absolute contraindications; however, certain technical and physiological factors may affect its reliability.

ECG Monitoring – clinical significance in pregnancy
• Detection of arrhythmias: ectopics, SVT, AF, and conduction blocks
• Evaluation of high-risk patients (CHD, cardiomyopathy, valvular disease, and pulmonary HTN)
• Guides therapy: drug effects, electrolyte imbalance, QT prolongation, and ischemia
• Perioperative and intrapartum safety: labour, cesarean, and anesthesia monitoring
• Protects maternal-fetal outcomes by early detection of cardiac instability

Table 11.
Clinical significance of ECG monitoring in pregnancy.

Pulse oximetry monitoring	
Indications	**Contraindications/limitations**
• Routine perioperative and anesthetic monitoring (labor and cesarean) • High-risk pregnancies (preeclampsia, eclampsia, and HELLP) • Maternal cardiac disease (valvular, cardiomyopathy, and pulmonary HTN) • Pulmonary disease (asthma, pneumonia, and embolism) • Critical illness/ICU (sepsis, hemorrhage, ARDS, and severe anemia) • Symptomatic patients (dyspnea, chest pain, cyanosis, and altered sensorium) • Fetal safety is indirectly ensured by ensuring maternal oxygenation	• No absolute contraindications (safe and noninvasive) • Interference: dyshemoglobins, IV dyes, nail polish, henna, ambient light, and motion • Poor accuracy: peripheral vasoconstriction, shock, severe PET, and hypothermia • Electrocautery interference during surgery

Table 12.
Pulse oximetry monitoring.

Pulse oximetry is a simple, non-invasive, and essential tool for monitoring hemodynamics during pregnancy. It allows rapid detection of hypoxemia, supports safe anesthetic care, guides management in high-risk situations, and protects both maternal and fetal outcomes. It measures tissue oxygen saturation; pulse oximetry provides continuous, noninvasive monitoring with modern devices that are autocalibrating and have fast response times. However, it is a poor indicator of ventilation, as oxygen desaturation is a late manifestation of apnea or respiratory insufficiency [26].

Assessment of arterial oxygenation is a vital component of anesthesia practice, as early recognition and timely management of hypoxemia help prevent serious complications. Clinical signs of hypoxemia—such as tachycardia, altered mental status, and cyanosis—are often subtle or masked during anesthesia, making pulse oximetry indispensable. Importantly, in addition to oxygen saturation, pulse oximetry also provides continuous heart rate monitoring, which further aids in assessing the clinical situation early and guiding timely management to prevent complications.

While pulse oximetry offers clear clinical benefits, its accuracy and reliability can be affected by several factors commonly encountered during anesthesia, including dyshemoglobins, intravenous dyes (such as methylene blue, indocyanine green, and indigo carmine), nail polish, ambient light, variability in light-emitting diodes, motion artifact, and background noise. Additionally, electrocautery may interfere with pulse oximeter function if radiofrequency emissions are detected by the photodetector.

6.3.1 Clinical significance

1. Early detection of hypoxemia: Pulse oximetry is essential in pregnancy as it detects early desaturation from respiratory or cardiovascular compromise, such as pulmonary embolism, pneumonia, asthma, pulmonary edema, sepsis, or cardiac failure, enabling timely interventions to prevent maternal decompensation and protect fetal well-being (**Figure 6**).

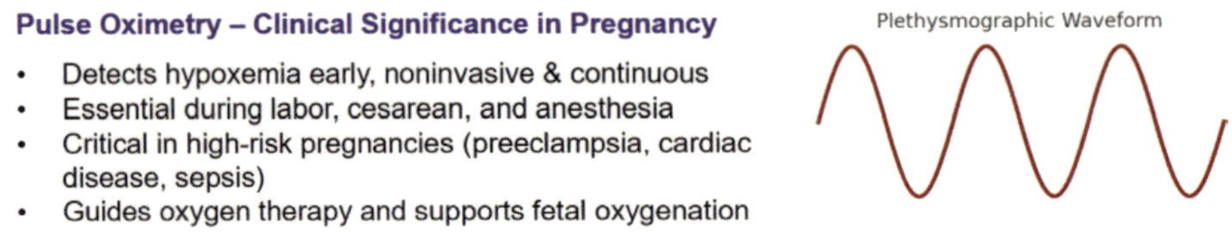

Figure 6.
Pulse oximetry clinical significance.

2. Intrapartum and anesthesia monitoring [27]: During labor, pulse oximetry is essential, particularly with neuraxial or general anesthesia, where hypoventilation or airway compromise may develop. It also helps detect hypoxemia resulting from hypotension-induced reductions in uteroplacental perfusion, ensuring timely corrective measures for maternal and fetal safety.

3. Maternal oxygenation monitoring: Pulse oximetry provides a continuous, noninvasive assessment of arterial oxygen saturation (SpO_2), offering real-time insight into maternal oxygenation status. Ensuring adequate maternal oxygen delivery plays a critical role in maintaining optimal uteroplacental blood flow and supporting fetal perfusion, thereby reducing the risk of hypoxic complications.

4. High-risk pregnancies: In high-risk pregnancies complicated by preeclampsia, cardiac disease, pulmonary hypertension, sepsis, or hemorrhage, pulse oximetry is particularly important as oxygen delivery is critical. Continuous monitoring in the ICU or operating room provides essential guidance for optimizing maternal hemodynamics and tailoring oxygen therapy to ensure maternal stability and fetal well-being [28].

5. Maternal-fetal safety: By maintaining adequate maternal SpO_2, pulse oximetry indirectly safeguards fetal oxygenation and helps reduce the risk of intrauterine hypoxia. It is especially valuable in emergencies, providing a rapid, non-invasive assessment of oxygenation status before invasive monitoring can be established.

6.4 Echocardiography

6.4.1 Role of echocardiography in pregnancy monitoring

Echocardiography provides a safe, accurate, and noninvasive method to assess cardiac structure and function throughout all stages of pregnancy. Both transthoracic and transesophageal echocardiography can be utilized to evaluate overall cardiac risk and guide management in pregnant women with heart disease. The echocardiographic parameter—left ventricular ejection fraction—remains unchanged during pregnancy. Diastolic function is most commonly assessed echocardiographically by evaluating mitral valve inflow, pulmonary venous flow, and myocardial tissue motion (tissue Doppler imaging).

In pregnancy, the hyperdynamic circulation can lead to misinterpretation of echocardiograms in women with cardiac disease, as cardiac impairment may be missed when ventricular function appears normal instead of appropriately hyperdynamic.

It is also valuable for assessing intravascular volume and may reduce the need for invasive right-sided heart catheterization to measure ventricular filling pressures.

6.4.2 Role of echocardiography in pregnancy

6.4.2.1 Diagnosis of cardiac disease

Echocardiography is a safe and reliable tool for evaluating both structural and functional heart abnormalities during pregnancy [29]. It plays a key role in identifying conditions such as congenital heart disease, valvular lesions, cardiomyopathy, and pulmonary hypertension (**Figure 7**). Beyond diagnosis, it is highly valuable for risk stratification and guiding individualized management planning, ensuring optimal maternal and fetal outcomes.

6.4.2.2 Assessment of cardiac function

Echocardiography effectively detects chamber enlargement, assesses ventricular function, and identifies abnormalities in wall motion. In normal pregnancy, the left ventricular ejection fraction (LVEF) typically remains unchanged, but the technique is crucial for evaluating the severity of stenotic or regurgitant lesions, which may be exacerbated by the altered hemodynamics of pregnancy [30].

6.4.2.3 Hemodynamic monitoring

Echocardiography provides a non-invasive method for assessing intravascular volume and cardiac filling pressures, often reducing the need for invasive right-sided heart catheterization. It is particularly valuable in critically ill pregnant women, where it helps guide fluid resuscitation and drug therapy safely and effectively.

6.4.2.4 Guidance in high-risk situations

Echocardiography is especially important for women with congenital heart disease, prosthetic valves, pulmonary hypertension, or severe valvular stenosis. In complex situations where detailed imaging is required, transesophageal echocardiography may be employed to provide more precise evaluation and management guidance.

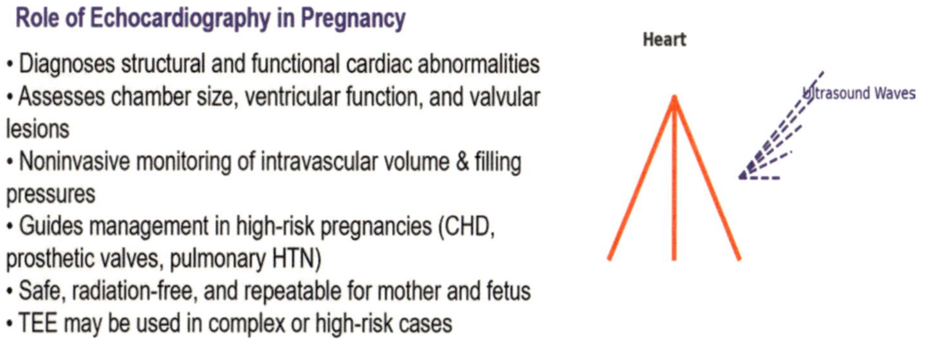

Figure 7.
Role of echocardiography in pregnancy.

6.4.2.5 Fetal and maternal safety

Echocardiography is noninvasive, radiation-free, and safe for both mother and fetus, making it an ideal tool in pregnancy [31]. Its wide availability and ability to be repeated as needed allow for effective ongoing monitoring throughout gestation.

7. Arterial line monitoring

Invasive ABP monitoring in pregnancy is reserved for critically ill or high-risk women where precise, continuous monitoring, and rapid therapeutic adjustments are essential to ensure maternal stability and fetal safety.

In summary, arterial BP monitoring in pregnancy is indicated in severe maternal disease, unstable hemodynamics, or when tight BP control and frequent ABG sampling are required. It should be avoided in patients with local infection, vascular compromise, or coagulation abnormalities.

Role of invasive arterial BP monitoring in pregnancy (**Table 13**)

- Continuous and accurate blood pressure monitoring [32]
    - o Provides beat-to-beat BP measurement, superior to non-invasive methods in unstable patients.
- High-risk pregnancies
    - o Indicated in women with severe preeclampsia, eclampsia, HELLP syndrome, or hemodynamic instability.
    - o Used in patients with significant cardiac disease, pulmonary hypertension, or severe hemorrhage.
- Intrapartum and perioperative safety

Invasive arterial blood pressure monitoring	
Indications	**Contraindications/ limitations**
• Severe preeclampsia, eclampsia, HELLP (tight BP control) • Maternal cardiac disease (valvular stenosis, cardiomyopathy, and pulmonary HTN) • Hemodynamic instability (hemorrhage, sepsis, and shock) • High-risk cesarean or obstetric anesthesia • Need for frequent ABG sampling • Major surgery in pregnancy (cardiac, neurosurgery, and non-obstetric) • Metabolic derangements and anticipated BP fluctuations	• Absolute: Infection at insertion site, distal limb ischemia, and severe peripheral vascular disease • Relative: Coagulopathy, thrombocytopenia, poor collateral circulation (failed Allen's test), and vascular trauma

Table 13.
Invasive blood pressure monitoring: indications and contraindications.

DOI: http://dx.doi.org/10.5772/intechopen.1013589

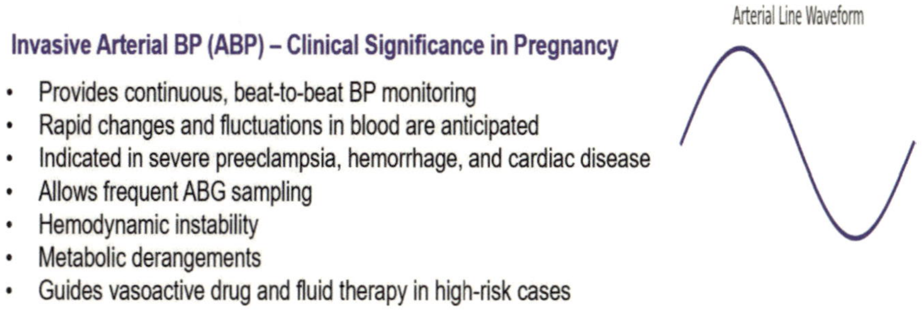

Figure 8.
Clinical significance of invasive blood pressure monitoring in pregnancy.

- o Recommended during high-risk cesarean deliveries, cardiac surgery, or procedures requiring tight BP control (e.g., neuraxial block in preeclampsia).

- Guiding therapy

    - o Allows precise titration of vasoactive drugs, fluids, and anesthetics [33].

    - o Facilitates monitoring during rapid hemodynamic shifts in labor, delivery, or postpartum autotransfusion (**Figure 8**).

- Additional benefits

    - o Enables arterial blood gas (ABG) sampling for oxygenation, ventilation, and acid-base balance.

    - o Provides early warning of maternal hypotension or hypertension, protecting uteroplacental perfusion and fetal oxygenation.

8. CVP and right heart pressure

CVP monitoring in pregnancy is indicated for high-risk monitoring of cardiac/obstetric patients, providing reliable vascular access and facilitating complex hemodynamic management, as well as guiding fluid therapy. However, contraindications such as infection, thrombosis, or severe coagulopathy must be carefully considered (**Figure 9**). Interpretation should always consider the physiological changes associated with pregnancy [34].

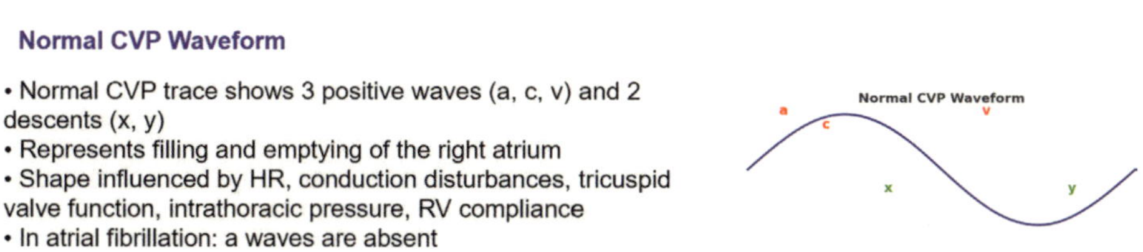

Figure 9.
Normal central venous pressure waveform.

Central venous cannulas provide essential intraoperative vascular access and facilitate assessment of intravascular volume status, rapid fluid administration, insertion of pulmonary artery or central venous oximetry catheters, placement of transvenous pacing electrodes, monitoring of central venous pressure (CVP), and serve as an access point for detection and management of venous air embolism.

8.1 Role of CVP in pregnancy

8.1.1 Assessment of intravascular volume

Central venous pressure (CVP) monitoring provides an estimate of right atrial pressure and venous return, reflecting right-sided hemodynamics. It is particularly useful in guiding fluid therapy for critically ill obstetric patients, such as those with sepsis, hemorrhage, or severe preeclampsia, and offers a less invasive and more cost-effective option compared to pulmonary artery monitoring.

8.1.2 Guidance in high-risk pregnancies

CVP monitoring is especially useful in women with cardiac disease, including valvular lesions, cardiomyopathy, or pulmonary hypertension. It helps guide fluid resuscitation while minimizing the risk of fluid overload and pulmonary edema, ensuring safer hemodynamic management (**Table 14**) [35].

8.1.3 Perioperative and critical care use

During major surgery, such as cesarean delivery in high-risk women or cardiac procedures during pregnancy, CVP monitoring allows close assessment of

CVP monitoring and clinical significance in pregnancy
• Guides fluid therapy in critically ill obstetric patients
• Useful in high-risk cardiac conditions (valvular disease, cardiomyopathy, and pulmonary HTN)
• Provides reliable access for fluids, drugs, and nutrition
• Supports perioperative management in high-risk surgery
• Interpretation requires caution due to pregnancy-related physiologic changes
• Trends are more valuable than single values
Functions of central venous cannulas
• Provide reliable intraoperative vascular access
• Facilitate assessment of intravascular volume status
• Enable rapid fluid and drug administration
• Insertion of PACs or central venous oximetry catheters
• Placement of transvenous pacing electrodes
• Monitoring of central venous pressure (CVP)
• Detection and management of venous air embolism

Table 14.
Monitoring and functions of the central venous cannula.

CVP monitoring in pregnancy – indications and contraindications	
Indications	**Contraindications/limitations**
• Severe preeclampsia/eclampsia with pulmonary edema or oliguria • HELLP syndrome with hemodynamic instability • Massive obstetric hemorrhage, transfusion • Sepsis/septic shock needing goal-directed fluids • Maternal cardiac disease (valvular lesions, cardiomyopathy, and pulmonary HTN) • High-risk cesarean or major surgery • Need for central venous access (vasoactive drugs, nutrition, and dialysis) • Detection/management of venous air embolism	• Absolute: local infection at the insertion site • Absolute: venous thrombosis or SVC obstruction • Relative: severe coagulopathy or thrombocytopenia • Relative: distorted anatomy (neck/mediastinal masses and prior surgery) • Pregnancy factors: aortocaval compression, ↑ intra-abdominal pressure • Does not reliably reflect left-sided filling pressures

Table 15.
Indications and contraindications of central venous pressure monitoring in pregnancy.

hemodynamic status. It also serves as a reliable access point for administering vasoactive drugs, rapid fluid resuscitation, and parenteral nutrition when required.

8.1.4 Limitations in pregnancy

CVP monitoring has important limitations, as it can be affected by factors such as aortocaval compression, increased intra-abdominal pressure, and mechanical ventilation. Single CVP readings are often unreliable, making trends over time and correlation with the clinical picture more meaningful [36]. As CVP is less predictive of left-sided filling pressures, echocardiography is often required for supplementation, and its accuracy is further reduced in the presence of cardiac or pulmonary parenchymal disease that alters pressure-volume relationships (**Table 15**).

9. Pulmonary artery catheterization

Pulmonary artery catheters (PACs) provide more comprehensive information than central venous monitoring, as they differentiate the function of the right heart, pulmonary circulation, and left heart. Pulmonary artery pulsatile pressures reflect right ventricular function, while pulmonary capillary wedge pressure (PCWP) closely approximates left ventricular end-diastolic pressure (LVEDP). With balloon inflation, the PAC wedges in the pulmonary vasculature. PACs are also utilized to measure cardiac output in structurally normal hearts. However, their routine utilization has declined significantly in recent years (**Figure 10**).

10. Left and right-sided heart catheterization

Cardiac interventions may occasionally be necessary during pregnancy for both diagnosis and treatment [37]. Cardiac catheterization for suspected coronary artery disease is considered safest in the second trimester, after completion of organogenesis and before activation of the fetal thyroid. Fetal radiation exposure can be minimized

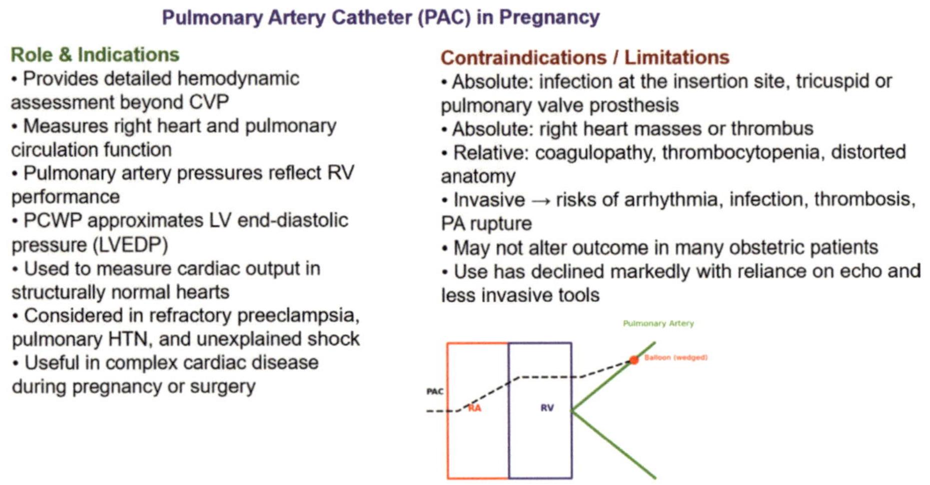

Figure 10.
Indications and contraindications of pulmonary artery catheter in pregnancy.

Principles of safe cardiac inverventions in pregnancy
• Cardiac interventions may be required for diagnosis or treatment during pregnancy
• Cardiac catheterization for coronary artery disease is safest in the second trimester
• By this stage, organogenesis is complete, and the fetal thyroid remains inactive
• Fetal radiation minimized with abdominal shielding
• Use of brachial or radial artery access is preferred over femoral
• Limit fluoroscopy time to reduce fetal exposure
Diagnostic cardiac catheterization in pregnancy
• Left-sided heart catheterization is the gold standard for diagnosing coronary artery disease
• Can be safely performed at any stage of pregnancy when clinically indicated
• Second trimester preferred for elective procedures (post-organogenesis and pre-fetal thyroid activation)
• Fetal radiation minimized with abdominal shielding and radial/brachial access
• Fluoroscopy time should be limited to reduce fetal exposure
• Reserved for women with suspected or confirmed ischemic heart disease during pregnancy

Table 16.
Principles of cardiac interventions in pregnancy.

by using abdominal shielding, brachial or radial artery access, and limiting the time spent on fluoroscopy (**Table 16** and **Figure 11**).

11. Advanced hemodynamic monitoring – PICCO

The PiCCO system provides advanced, minimally invasive hemodynamic monitoring during pregnancy and is particularly valuable in critically ill obstetric patients, especially when precise assessment of fluid and cardiac performance is crucial (**Table 17**).

Right vs Left Heart Catheterization

Feature	Right Heart Catheterization	Left Heart Catheterization
Access Route	Via venous system (jugular, subclavian, femoral)	Via arterial system (radial, femoral)
Main Measurements	RA, RV, PA pressures, PCWP (estimates LVEDP)	LV pressures, coronary anatomy, wall motion
Primary Uses	Pulmonary HTN, severe preeclampsia, unexplained shock, RV function	Gold standard for CAD, LV dysfunction, ischemia evaluation
Pregnancy Applications	Guides fluid/vasopressor therapy in high-risk obstetrics	Reserved for suspected ischemic heart disease
Risks	Arrhythmia, infection, thrombosis, PA rupture	Radiation exposure, vascular injury, stroke

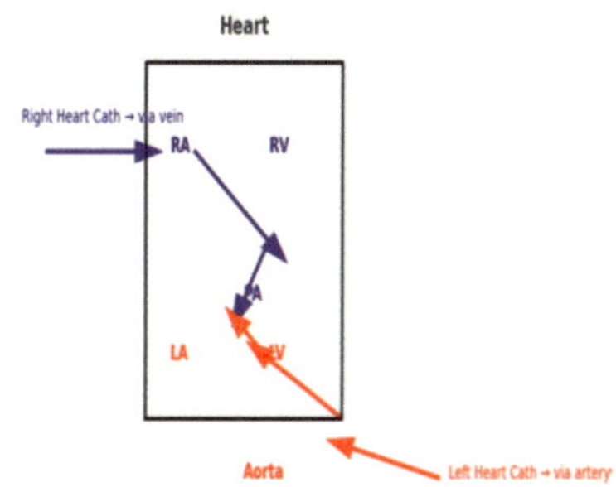

Figure 11.
Right vs. left heart catheterization.

PiCCO monitoring in pregnancy	
Role and indications	**Advantages and limitations**
• Advanced hemodynamic monitoring when standard tools are insufficient • Measures CO, SVV, SVR, GEDV, and EVLW • Useful in severe preeclampsia/eclampsia with pulmonary edema • Guides fluid resuscitation in sepsis, septic shock, massive hemorrhage • Monitors cardiac performance in cardiomyopathy or complex cardiac disease	• Less invasive than pulmonary artery catheter (PAC) • Provides continuous, dynamic, real-time data • Helps balance fluids vs. risk of overload • Requires arterial + central venous access (still invasive) • Interpretation affected by pregnancy physiology (↑CO, ↓SVR) • Limited evidence base in obstetric patients

Table 17.
PICCO monitoring in pregnancy.

11.1 FloTrac monitoring in pregnancy

FloTrac offers a less-invasive alternative for advanced hemodynamic monitoring in pregnancy, especially valuable in high-risk obstetric and cardiac patients, guiding fluid and vasoactive therapy while reducing the need for invasive catheters. It analyzes the arterial pressure waveform to calculate [38].

- Cardiac output (CO)
- Stroke volume (SV)
- Stroke volume variation (SVV)
- Systemic vascular resistance (SVR)

FloTrac monitoring in pregnancy	
Role and indications	**Advantages & limitations**
• Provides minimally invasive, continuous hemodynamic monitoring • Calculates CO, SV, SVV, and SVR from arterial waveform • Useful in severe preeclampsia/eclampsia with instability • Guides management in obstetric hemorrhage and massive transfusion • Helps in sepsis, septic shock, cardiomyopathy, or valvular disease • Supports perioperative monitoring in high-risk cesarean or cardiac surgery	• Less invasive – requires only an arterial line (no central line) • Quick setup, continuous real-time data • Integrates easily into anesthesia and ICU workflows • Accuracy reduced in arrhythmias, severe vasodilation, and extreme states • May be influenced by pregnancy physiology (↑CO and ↓SVR) • Limited validation and evidence in obstetric patients

Table 18.
FloTrac monitoring in pregnancy.

11.2 Role in pregnancy

FloTrac provides continuous maternal hemodynamic monitoring without the need for a pulmonary artery catheter, making it especially valuable in high-risk obstetric conditions such as severe preeclampsia, obstetric hemorrhage, sepsis, or peripartum cardiomyopathy [39]. It guides fluid and vasopressor therapy to balance perfusion while avoiding overload and can be effectively applied perioperatively during cesarean section, cardiac surgery in pregnancy, and in critical care settings (**Table 18**).

12. Cardioversion

Cardioversion (synchronized or unsynchronized) is safe and effective in pregnancy for managing unstable arrhythmias, with maternal safety prioritized and continuous FHR monitoring recommended (**Figure 12**) [40].

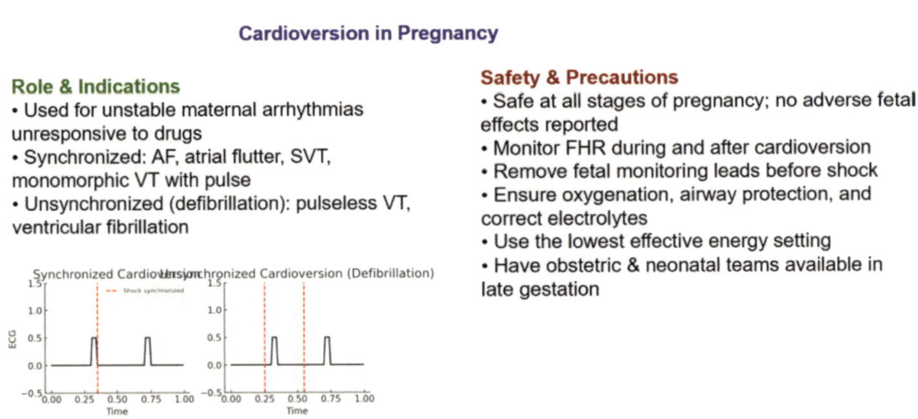

Figure 12.
Cardioversion in pregnancy.

12.1 Synchronized cardioversion

Synchronized cardioversion involves delivering an electric shock timed with the QRS complex. It is utilized to treat supraventricular arrhythmias (such as atrial fibrillation, atrial flutter, and atrial tachycardia) and monomorphic ventricular tachycardia with a pulse.

12.2 Unsynchronized cardioversion

Pulseless and polymorphic ventricular tachycardia are managed with unsynchronized cardioversion (defibrillation).

13. Defibrillation

Defibrillation is the delivery of electric energy to terminate ventricular fibrillation [41]. Biphasic automatic external defibrillators (AEDs) are more effective at terminating ventricular fibrillation using lower energy levels (**Table 19**).

14. Implantable cardiac devices

Pacemakers and ICDs are safe and effective in pregnancy, ensuring maternal rhythm stability and improving outcomes. Care requires multidisciplinary planning, intrapartum monitoring, and electrocautery precautions to prevent complications.

Hemodynamic instability due to symptomatic bradycardia, asystole lasting more than 3 seconds, or escape rhythms below the AV node with rates under 40 beats per minute [42] requires a temporary venous pacemaker in pregnant women (**Table 20**).

Congenital heart disease with advanced second- or third-degree AV block is uncommon in pregnancy but may necessitate temporary pacing. The choice to implant a temporary or permanent device should be made collaboratively by a multidisciplinary team.

Defibrillation in pregnancy	
Role and indications	**Safety and precautions**
• Indicated for pulseless ventricular tachycardia (VT) and ventricular fibrillation (VF) • Follows standard ACLS protocols – no pregnancy-specific modifications to energy levels • Immediate intervention is critical for maternal survival, which optimizes fetal survival	• Defibrillation is safe at all stages of pregnancy • Transthoracic impedance unchanged → standard energy levels apply • Remove external/internal fetal monitoring leads before shock delivery • FHR should be monitored after defibrillation • Maternal resuscitation remains the priority • Prepare for emergency delivery if maternal resuscitation is unsuccessful

Table 19.
Defibrillation in pregnancy.

Implantable cardiac devices in pregnancy	
Role and indications	**Safety and peripartum precautions**
• Pacemakers for bradyarrhythmias (e.g., high-grade AV block) • ICDs for prevention of life-threatening ventricular arrhythmias • Indications remain the same as the non-pregnant population • Ensure rhythm stability, reduce maternal/fetal risk • Maternal stabilization improves fetal outcomes	• Generally safe during pregnancy; fetal exposure minimal • Device reprogramming may be required for physiologic changes • During cesarean: ICD shock function may be deactivated • External defibrillator/pacing equipment should be available • Use bipolar electrocautery; keep grounding pad away from device • Breastfeeding is safe; normal postpartum device checks apply

Table 20.
Implantable cardiac devices in pregnancy.

1. Types of Devices

   - Pacemakers (PM): for management of bradyarrhythmia (e.g., advanced AV block) (**Figure 13**).

   - Implantable cardioverter-defibrillators (ICD): for prevention or termination of life-threatening ventricular arrhythmias.

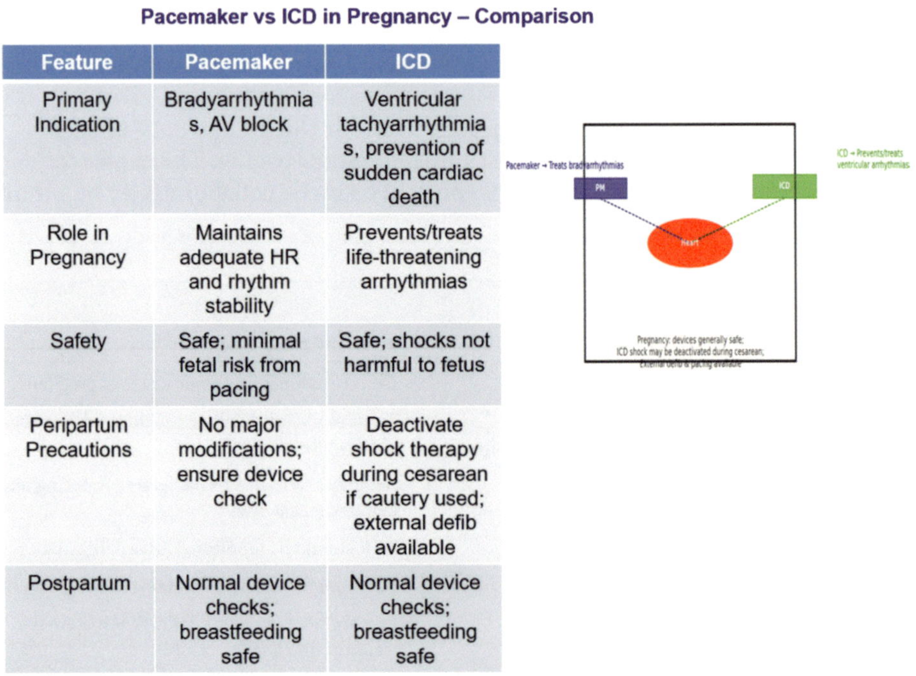

Feature	Pacemaker	ICD
Primary Indication	Bradyarrhythmias, AV block	Ventricular tachyarrhythmias, prevention of sudden cardiac death
Role in Pregnancy	Maintains adequate HR and rhythm stability	Prevents/treats life-threatening arrhythmias
Safety	Safe; minimal fetal risk from pacing	Safe; shocks not harmful to fetus
Peripartum Precautions	No major modifications; ensure device check	Deactivate shock therapy during cesarean if cautery used; external defib available
Postpartum	Normal device checks; breastfeeding safe	Normal device checks; breastfeeding safe

Figure 13.
Comparison of pacemakers vs. implantable cardioverter-defibrillators (ICD) in pregnancy.

15. Cardiopulmonary bypass

Cardiopulmonary bypass can be performed safely during pregnancy when essential, ideally in the second trimester, with strategies to maintain maternal hemodynamic stability and uteroplacental perfusion to protect the fetus.

The second trimester is considered the optimal time for cardiopulmonary bypass during pregnancy, whereas procedures done immediately postpartum or on an emergency basis carry a higher risk of maternal mortality (**Figure 14**).

Intraoperative FHR monitoring is essential. Fetal outcomes improve with normothermic CPB at >2.4 L/min/m^2, maintaining MAP >70–75 mmHg, left uterine displacement, and hematocrit >28%.

15.1 Cardiopulmonary resuscitation in pregnancy

Standard BLS and ACLS principles apply in pregnancy. CPR in pregnancy requires early recognition, left uterine displacement, a higher hand position for compressions, standard defibrillation, and rapid perimortem cesarean if no ROSC by 4 minutes.

15.1.1 Incidence

Maternal cardiac arrest occurs in approximately 1 in 20,000–30,000 pregnancies and may result from pregnancy-specific complications such as amniotic fluid embolism, severe hemorrhage or uterine atony, eclampsia, and placental abruption. Non-obstetric causes, including cardiomyopathy, arrhythmia, sepsis, and trauma, also contribute significantly to maternal collapse.

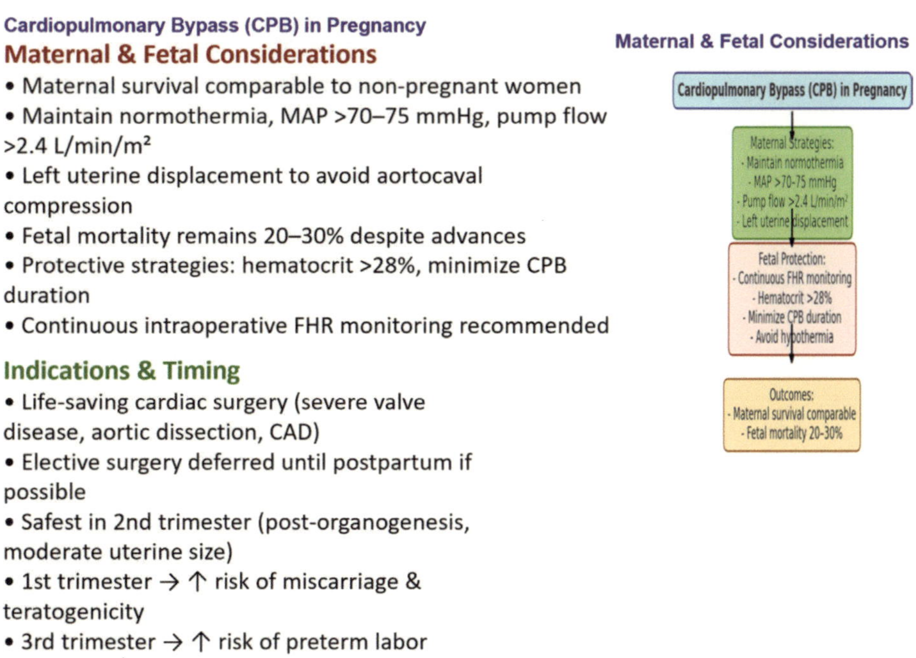

Figure 14.
Maternal and fetal considerations in cardiopulmonary bypass in pregnancy.

15.1.2 Modifications to standard CPR

During maternal cardiac arrest, modifications to standard CPR are required. Chest compressions should be performed with manual left uterine displacement or a 15–30° tilt to relieve aortocaval compression, placing the hands slightly higher on the sternum due to the cephalad displacement of the diaphragm. Early intubation is recommended due to the increased risk of aspiration, and IV or IO access should be established above the diaphragm to ensure effective drug delivery.

15.1.3 Defibrillation in pregnancy

Defibrillation in pregnancy is performed using the same energy levels as in non-pregnant adults and is considered safe at all gestational ages. Fetal monitoring leads should be removed before shock delivery, and continuous fetal heart rate monitoring is essential after return of spontaneous circulation (ROSC) to assess fetal well-being.

15.1.4 Emergency hysterotomy/perimortem cesarean delivery

Emergency hysterotomy/perimortem cesarean delivery: If return of spontaneous circulation (ROSC) is not achieved within 4 minutes of maternal cardiac arrest, an

CPR in pregnancy – overview	*Modifications of CPR in pregnancy*
• Incidence: ~1 in 20,000–30,000 pregnancies • Pregnancy-specific causes: AFE, hemorrhage/uterine atony, eclampsia, and abruption • Non-obstetric causes: cardiomyopathy, arrhythmia, sepsis, and trauma • Maternal survival is the strongest predictor of fetal survival	• Left uterine displacement (15–30 degrees) • Airway o Consider airway edema associated with pregnancy • Breathing o Be aware of the impact of decreased functional residual capacity in pregnancy • Circulation o Perform chest compressions higher on the sternum than in nonpregnant patients • Defibrillation o May use automated external defibrillator (AED) o Apply same energies as in nonpregnant patients o Remove all fetal monitoring probes and leads • Drugs o Drugs (and doses) are the same as those used in nonpregnant patients
Perimortem cesarean delivery	*Defibrillation in pregnancy*
• If no ROSC within 4 minutes → perform cesarean by 5 minutes • Improves maternal resuscitation (relieves aortocaval compression) • Increases chance of neonatal survival • Requires coordinated team response (OB, anesthesia, neonatology, and ICU)	• Same energy levels as non-pregnant adults • Safe in all trimesters; impedance unchanged • Remove fetal monitoring leads before shock • FHR monitoring recommended after ROSC

Table 21.
Cardiopulmonary resuscitation modifications in pregnancy.

emergency hysterotomy or cesarean delivery should be performed by 5 minutes. This intervention not only improves maternal resuscitation by relieving aortocaval compression but also significantly enhances the chances of neonatal survival, making it a critical component of maternal cardiac arrest management.

15.1.5 Key principles

Maternal survival remains the strongest predictor of fetal survival, emphasizing the need to prioritize maternal resuscitation efforts. Standard BLS and ACLS protocols apply (**Table 21**) during pregnancy but require specific modifications to account for physiological changes and the presence of the gravid uterus (**Table 21**). Effective management also relies on close multidisciplinary coordination among obstetric, anesthesia, neonatal, and critical care teams to optimize both maternal and fetal outcomes.

16. Summary

Pregnancy induces significant cardiovascular and physiological adaptations—such as an expanded blood volume, increased cardiac output, and decreased systemic vascular resistance—that can exacerbate or mask underlying heart disease. Accurate hemodynamic monitoring is therefore essential to distinguish normal gestational changes from pathology, maintain maternal stability, and safeguard fetal well-being.

Standard noninvasive monitoring (NIBP, ECG, pulse oximetry, and capnography) provides continuous surveillance, while advanced modalities—arterial lines, central venous pressure, pulmonary artery catheters, and contemporary arterial waveform/thermodilution systems (e.g., FloTrac, PiCCO)—support timely diagnosis, guide fluid and vasoactive therapy, and help prevent complications in higher-risk scenarios. In line with ASA standards, anesthesiologists are responsible for continuous monitoring of oxygenation, ventilation, circulation, and temperature during routine and high-risk obstetric care. A tailored, risk-stratified monitoring strategy, interpreted through the lens of pregnancy physiology, reduces morbidity and mortality, optimizes intrapartum management, and improves maternal-fetal outcomes. This chapter integrates current evidence, guideline recommendations, and practical considerations into a concise framework for perioperative and critical care in pregnancy.

16.1 Key messages

- Pregnancy produces significant cardiovascular changes that can mask or mimic disease.

- Correct interpretation of hemodynamic data requires explicit knowledge of normal gestational adaptations.

- Standard monitoring (NIBP, ECG, pulse oximetry, and capnography) is foundational for all obstetric patients.

- Advanced monitoring (arterial line, CVP, PAC, arterial pressure analysis, FloTrac, and PiCCO) is adjunctive for high-risk or unstable cases.

- Adherence to ASA standards ensures continuous monitoring of oxygenation, ventilation, circulation, and temperature.
- Individualized, risk-based monitoring improves detection of deterioration, guides timely intervention, and enhances maternal and fetal outcomes.
- Differentiating physiologic vs. pathologic change is critical to avoid misdiagnosis and mismanagement.

Acknowledgements

The authors acknowledge Dr. Nissar Sheikh for providing us with this opportunity, as well as the institutions that supported the preparation of this chapter.

The author acknowledges the use of QuillBot for language polishing of the manuscript.

Author details

Seema Nahid[1*], Fateen Shareef[2], Umm E. Amara[2], Salma Mehjabeen[3], Umme Nashrah[2], Roshan Afsha[4], M. Abdul Wasay[2] and Azha Fatima[5]

1 Hamad Medical Corporation, Doha, Qatar

2 Deccan College of Medical Sciences, Hyderabad, India

3 Yashoda Hospital, Somajiguda, Hyderabad, India

4 University of Michigan, Michigan, United States of America

5 Kamineni Institute of Medical Sciences, Hyderabad, India

*Address all correspondence to: snahid@hamad.qa

References

[1] Cunningham FG, Leveno KJ, Bloom SL, Dashe JS, Hoffman BL, Casey BM, et al. Williams Obstetrics. 26th ed. New York: McGraw Hill; 2022

[2] Datta S, Norris MC, Arkoosh VA, Ostheimer GW. Obstetric Anesthesia: Principles and Practice. 5th ed. Philadelphia: Elsevier; 2018

[3] Creasy RK, Resnik R, Iams JD, Lockwood CJ, Moore TR, Greene MF. Creasy and Resnik's Maternal-Fetal Medicine: Principles and Practice. 9th ed. Philadelphia: Elsevier; 2022

[4] Chestnut DH, Wong CA, Tsen LC, Kee WD, Beilin Y, Mhyre J, et al. Chestnut's Obstetric Anesthesia: Principles and Practice. 6th ed. Philadelphia: Elsevier; 2020

[5] Oakley C, Warnes CA. Heart Disease in Pregnancy. 2nd ed. Oxford: Blackwell Publishing; 2007

[6] Pinsky MR, Broch O, Mebazaa A. Hemodynamic Monitoring. Berlin: Springer; 2018

[7] Gaiser R, Datta S, Shnider SM. Shnider and Levinson's Anesthesia for Obstetrics. 5th ed. Philadelphia: Wolters Kluwer; 2012

[8] Arulkumaran S, Regan L, Farquharson D. Oxford Handbook of Obstetrics and Gynaecology. 3rd ed. Oxford: Oxford University Press; 2011

[9] Ngan Kee WD. Obstetric Anesthesia and Uncommon Disorders. Cambridge: Cambridge University Press; 2012

[10] Yentis SM, Hirsch NP, Smith GB. Anaesthesia and Intensive Care A–Z: An Encyclopaedia of Principles and Practice. 6th ed. Edinburgh: Elsevier; 2013

[11] Hegewald MJ, Crapo RO. Respiratory physiology in pregnancy. Clinics in Chest Medicine. 2011;**32**(1):1

[12] American Society of Anesthesiologists (ASA). Standards for Basic Anesthetic Monitoring. Schaumburg (IL): American Society of Anesthesiologists; 2015

[13] Goldkrand JW, Jackson MJ. Blood pressure measurement in pregnant women in the left lateral recumbent position. American Journal of Obstetrics and Gynecology. 1997;**176**(3):642-643. DOI: 10.1016/s0002-9378(97)70562-3

[14] American College of Obstetricians and Gynecologists (ACOG). Postpartum hemorrhage: Practice Bulletin No. 183. Obstetrics and Gynecology. 2017;**130**(4):e168-e186

[15] World Health Organization (WHO). WHO Recommendations: Intrapartum Care for a Positive Childbirth Experience. Geneva: WHO; 2018

[16] World Health Organization (WHO). WHO Recommendations for Prevention and Treatment of Maternal Peripartum Infections. Geneva: WHO; 2015

[17] World Health Organization (WHO). Maternal Mortality: Evidence Brief. Geneva: WHO; 2019

[18] American Heart Association (AHA). 2020 American Heart Association guidelines for cardiopulmonary resuscitation and emergency cardiovascular care. Circulation. 2020;**142**(16_suppl. 2):S337-S357

[19] American Heart Association (AHA). Cardiac arrest in pregnancy: A scientific statement. Circulation. 2015;**132**(18):1747-1773

[20] European Society of Cardiology (ESC), Regitz-Zagrosek V, et al. ESC guidelines on the management of cardiovascular diseases during pregnancy. European Heart Journal. 2018;**39**(34):3165-3241

[21] National Institute for Health and Care Excellence (NICE). Intrapartum Care for Healthy Women and Babies. NICE Clinical Guideline CG190. London: NICE; 2014

[22] Barash PG, Cullen BF, Stoelting RK, Cahalan MK, Stock MC, Ortega R. Clinical Anesthesia. 9th ed. Philadelphia: Wolters Kluwer; 2021

[23] Angeli F, Angeli E, Verdecchia P. Electrocardiographic changes in hypertensive disorders of pregnancy. Hypertension Research. 2014;**37**(11):973-975

[24] Miller RD, Cohen NH, Eriksson LI, Fleisher LA, Wiener-Kronish JP, Young WL. Miller's Anesthesia. 9th ed. Philadelphia: Elsevier; 2020

[25] Habib AS, Gambling DR, et al. Essentials of Obstetric Anesthesia. Cambridge: Cambridge University Press; 2018

[26] Hines RL, Marschall KE. Stoelting's Anesthesia and Co-Existing Disease. 7th ed. Philadelphia: Elsevier; 2018

[27] Farquharson D, Arulkumaran S. Handbook of Obstetric Medicine. 5th ed. Boca Raton (FL): CRC Press; 2019

[28] Hughes P, Arulkumaran S. Best Practice in Labour and Delivery. Cambridge: Cambridge University Press; 2007

[29] Clark SL, Cotton DB, Hankins GD, Phelan JP. Critical Care Obstetrics. 6th ed. Hoboken (NJ): Wiley-Blackwell; 2018

[30] Goudie RJ, Houghton FD, Redfern RE. Handbook of Obstetric Medicine. 6th ed. Boca Raton: CRC Press; 2021

[31] Myles PS, Smith JA. Monitoring in Anesthesia and Perioperative Care. Cambridge: Cambridge University Press; 2018

[32] Webb AR, Angus DC, Finfer S, Gattinoni L, Singer M. Oxford Textbook of Critical Care. 2nd ed. Oxford: Oxford University Press; 2016

[33] National Institute for Health and Care Excellence (NICE). Hypertension in Pregnancy: Diagnosis and Management. (NICE Guideline NG133). London (UK): National Institute for Health and Care Excellence; 2019

[34] American College of Cardiology Foundation/AHA. 2013 ACCF/AHA guideline for the management of heart failure. Circulation. 2013;**128**:e240-e327

[35] National Institute for Health and Care Excellence (NICE). Caesarean Section. (NICE Clinical Guideline CG132). London (UK): National Institute for Health and Care Excellence; 2011

[36] Society for Obstetric Anesthesia and Perinatology (SOAP). Consensus Statement on Neuraxial Anesthesia in Obstetric Patients. Schaumburg (IL): Society for Obstetric Anesthesia and Perinatology; 2017

[37] ACOG. Gestational diabetes mellitus: Practice Bulletin No. 190. Obstetrics and Gynecology. 2018;**131**(2):e49-e64

[38] WHO. Managing Complications in Pregnancy and Childbirth: A Guide for Midwives and Doctors. Geneva: WHO; 2017

[39] AHA. Guidelines for the management of hypertension. Hypertension. 2017;**71**:e13-e115

[40] Cauldwell M et al. Direct current cardioversion in pregnancy: A multicentre study. BJOG: An International Journal of Obstetrics & Gynaecology. 2023;**130**(10):1269-1274. DOI: 10.1111/1471-0528.17457

[41] European Society of Cardiology (ESC). Guidelines on the management of valvular heart disease. European Heart Journal. 2021;**42**:407-465

[42] ASA Task Force. Practice guidelines for obstetric anesthesia. Anesthesiology. 2016;**124**:270-300